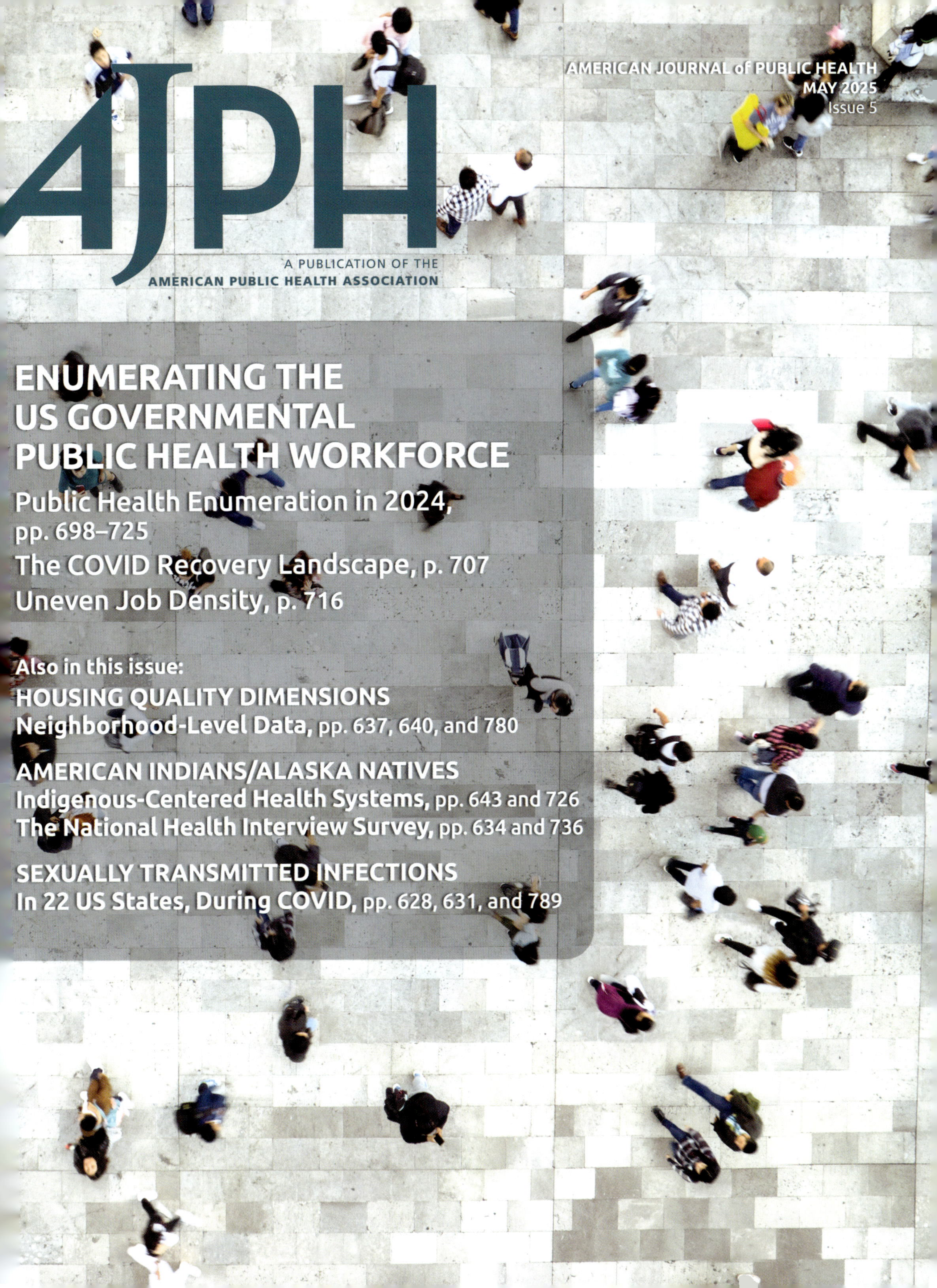

AMERICAN JOURNAL of PUBLIC HEALTH
MAY 2025
Issue 5

AJPH

A PUBLICATION OF THE
AMERICAN PUBLIC HEALTH ASSOCIATION

ENUMERATING THE US GOVERNMENTAL PUBLIC HEALTH WORKFORCE

Public Health Enumeration in 2024, pp. 698–725
The COVID Recovery Landscape, p. 707
Uneven Job Density, p. 716

Also in this issue:

HOUSING QUALITY DIMENSIONS
Neighborhood-Level Data, pp. 637, 640, and 780

AMERICAN INDIANS/ALASKA NATIVES
Indigenous-Centered Health Systems, pp. 643 and 726
The National Health Interview Survey, pp. 634 and 736

SEXUALLY TRANSMITTED INFECTIONS
In 22 US States, During COVID, pp. 628, 631, and 789

APHA
AMERICAN PUBLIC HEALTH ASSOCIATION
For science. For action. For health.

AJPH®, published monthly, is the official Journal of the American Public Health Association®, 800 I St NW, Washington, DC 20001-3710; (202) 777- APHA; TDD (202) 777-2500. APHA is a nongovernmental professional society founded in 1872, representing all disciplines and specialties in public health.

The *American Journal of Public Health*® (*AJPH*) (print ISSN: 0090-0036; electronic ISSN: 1541- 0048), first published in 1911, is the official journal of the American Public Health Association® (APHA). The oldest and largest organization of public health professionals in the world, APHA represents approximately 30 000 members from more than 50 occupations of public health.

Submissions: Visit www.editorialmanager.com/ajph or ajph.edmgr.com for online manuscript preparation and submission guidelines. Contributions of original unpublished research, social science analyses, scholarly essays, critical commentaries, departments, and letters to the editor are welcome. Questions? Write ajph.submissions@apha.org or call APHA at (202) 777-2469.

Print plus online subscriptions: Institutional price (print copy with online access for a single institution and all authorized users, regardless of geographic location) varies by size of organization and ranges from $993–$1445 for US organizations, and $1073–$1526 for international organizations (air delivery); multiple campuses not permitted without special arrangement. Details of the tiered pricing system at https://subscriptionoffice.com/pages/apha-landing-page. To order, write apha.subscriptions@apha.org.

Online-only subscriptions: Institutional price for one institution and its authorized users (regardless of geographic location) is $878–$1307. To order, write apha.subscriptions@apha.org. For academic consortia or multisite corporate subscriptions, contact apha.subscriptions@apha.org.

Print-only subscriptions: Institutional price is US $701, $782 international.

Back print issues: A limited number of print issues are for sale. Single copies are US $65, $75 international (air delivery). Shipping included; prepay only. To order, write apha.subscriptions@apha.org.

Reprints: For prices and ordering information on 50 or more reprints, check the Reprints section at www.ajph.org. To order smaller quantities of reprints (rush delivery), use the "Purchase Article" link on the article site itself.

Electronic access: Online articles more than 10 years old are available free for personal use at www.ajph.org. Recent articles are available through pay-per-view: single PDF article for $24, single issue access for 24 hours for $33, or entire site access for 24 hours for $38.

Postal information: Periodicals postage paid at Washington, DC, and additional mailing offices. Postmaster: Send address changes to American Journal of Public Health, 800 I St NW, Washington, DC 20001-3710.

Address changes: Send to AJPH, Membership Department (members) or AJPH Subscriptions (subscribers), APHA, 800 I St NW, Washington, DC 20001-3710. Or write to membership.mail@apha.org (members) or apha.subscriptions@apha.org (subscribers).

Indexes: Publications that index or abstract articles from *AJPH* include the following: Ageline, Assia (Applied Social Science Index and Abstracts), Biological Abstracts, Chemical Abstracts, CINAHL, Criminal Justice Abstracts, EMBASE, EMCare, Environmental Abstracts, e-psyche, ERIC, ETOH (Alcohol and Alcohol Problems Science Database), Excerpta Medica, Food Science and Technology, General Science Index, Grateful Med, Hospital Literature Index, Human Resources Abstracts, International Pharmaceutical Abstracts (IPA), Medline, Physical Education Index, Pollution Abstracts, Psychological Abstracts, PsychINFO, Safety Science Abstracts, Sage Family Studies Abstracts, Sage Human Resources Abstracts, Science Citation Index, SCOPUS, SIIC Data Bases, Social Work Research and Abstracts, and Statistical Reference Index (SRI)/LexisNexis.

AJPH
A PUBLICATION OF THE
AMERICAN PUBLIC HEALTH ASSOCIATION

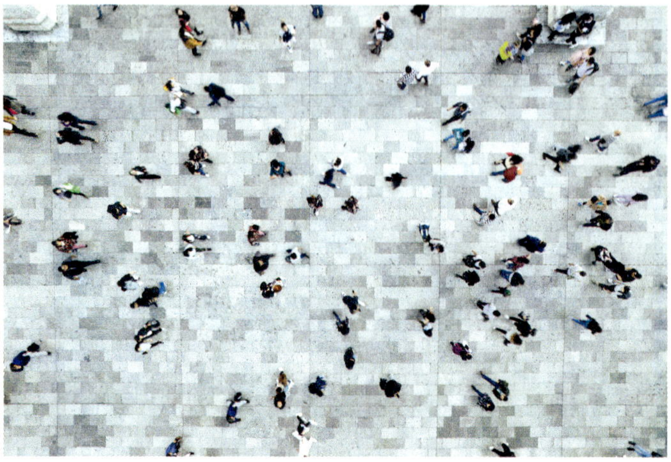

COVER: How many public health workers were in the United States before the current decimation of the federal public health workforce? Where were they, and what occupations did they fill? Answering and understanding these questions is crucial for creating a benchmark for evaluating the impact of the current administration, but also planning for its replacement and development. In this issue of *AJPH*, we consider the monumental task of enumerating public health workers—the heart of the US pubic health system.

Cover concept and selection by Aleisha Kropf. Image by Orbon Alina / Getty, printed with permission.

APHA
AMERICAN PUBLIC HEALTH ASSOCIATION
For science. For action. For health.

Promoting public health research, policy, practice, and education is the *AJPH* mission. As we widen our scope to embrace global issues, we also sharpen our focus to support the needs of public health practitioners. We invite contributions of original unpublished research, opinion and commentary, and letters to the editor.

The *Journal* is printed on acid-free recycled paper.

OPEN ACCESS | ONLINE ONLY | PODCAST | DATA SUPPLEMENT AVAILABLE

EDITOR'S CHOICE

622 With New Editors, *AJPH* History Section Forges Forward
M. M. Jones and C. Roth

BOOKS & MEDIA

624 A Magnificent Example of Why We Need Multilateral Organizations Such as WHO
C. Victora

OPINIONS, IDEAS, & PRACTICE

EDITORIALS

626 *AJPH* and the Threat of Political Interference in Scientific Publishing
A. Morabia

628 Sexually Transmitted Infection Cases During COVID-19: Implications for Public Health
T. S. Fitzpatrick and J. D. Tucker

631 COVID-19 Policies and the Impact on STIs: Context, Equity, and Innovation
C. N. Pinto, S. B. Griner, and R. D. Hubach

634 Exploring Indigenous Health and Employment: Methods to Capture Diversity and Intersecting Factors
V. Gunn, P. O'Campo, and C. Muntaner

637 Housing as a Determinant of Health: A Population-Level Approach
A. Fenelon

640 Advancing a Research and Policy Agenda on Housing and Health
G. Routhier

643 Why Achieving Health Equity for Indigenous Peoples Requires Indigenizing the Social Determinants of Health
V. Blue Bird Jernigan and T. L. Maudrie

646 Polysubstance Use Is Not Synonymous With Poly Substance Use Disorder
K. Y. Xu, L. (Allison) Lin, and R. A. Grucza

649 Addressing the Mechanisms of the Long-Term Effects of Racial Housing Inequalities
L. C. Winling

651 Leveraging Lessons Learned From the COVID-19 Pandemic to Support Vaccine Adherence
S. R. MacEwan

PERSPECTIVES

654 To Arms, Public Health Citizens!
A. Braggion and A. Flahault

656 Monitoring Is Not Enough
A. Chiolero

658 Changing Ecosystems and the Role of One Health: Engaging Public Health Professionals
H. J. Chapman, M. Akpinar-Elci, L. H. Kahn, and T. J. Doker

663 The Murder of Black Women in the United States: A Public Health Crisis
T. L. Gillum, A. Sheffield, A. D. Norton, and C. J. Hampton

668 Mitigating Medical Debt as a Public Health Equity Issue: Challenges and Opportunities in New York City
D. Maru, R. E. Schwartz, J. Fordjuoh, E. W. Wiewel, R. K. Sood, E. Clippinger, J. Jackson, A. Ayedun, D. Flynn, A. Vasan, and M. Morse

673 Age Restricted Location Policies: A Potential Strategy for Advancing the Tobacco Endgame
M. E. Roberts, J. G. Lee, M. E. Morean, G. Kong, A. K. Ferketich, P. F. Craigmile, R. C. Ceasar, V. B. Spinola, and M. L. Berman

RADICAL HOPE

678 Forging Radical Hope: Waiting for the World to Change, or Changing the World?
R. J. Kim-Farley

681 A Love Letter to Hope
M. Zaragoza

682 We Don't Give Hope, We Build It Together
I. I. Bradeanu

EDITOR'S CORNER

685 "We Who Believe in Freedom Cannot Rest": Affirming the Call to Critically Engage Public Health
L. Bowleg

687 Protecting Public Health in the Courts
W. E. Parmet

NOTES FROM THE FIELD

689 Addressing Unsheltered Homelessness and Substance Use Disorder From Tent Encampment to Safe Spaces, Boston 2021–2022
M. Bharel, M. N. Clark, D. Dooley, and B. O. Ojikutu

693 Going Places: An Active Transportation Intervention to Increase Youth Physical Activity, Durham, North Carolina, 2023–2024
E. M. D'Agostino, C. D. Neshteruk, T. Li, J. Davis, I. Granados, A. Kumar, J. Forde, and C. P. Hornik

PUBLIC HEALTH ENUMERATION IN 2024

698 Public Health Enumeration in 2024: Who Is Keeping the Public Healthy?
A. C. Young, C. L. Chung, and L. A. Dauphin

701 Enumerating the US Governmental Public Health Workforce
C. P. Balio, N. A. Dockery, and R. Hogg-Graham

RESEARCH & ANALYSIS

PUBLIC HEALTH ENUMERATION IN 2024

707 Enumeration 2024: What We Know and What We Wish We Knew About the Governmental Public Health Workforce in a COVID-19 Recovery Landscape
J. P. Leider, C. P. Balio, R. Hogg-Graham, N. M. Weiss, A. Vogel, S. O. Onal, X. Zang, P. Kett, J. Edmonds, H. Karnik, N. Dockery, B. Joseph, M. Pak, A. B. Thomas, and B. Bekemeier

716 Enumerating the State and Local Public Health Workforce During the COVID-19 Response
A. Vogel, S. O. Onal, N. M. Weiss, X. Zang, M. Pak, B. Joseph, and J. P. Leider

PERSPECTIVES FROM THE SOCIAL SCIENCES

726 Developing Indigenous-Centered Healing, Health, and Wellness Frameworks to Strengthen Indigenous Health Systems, Decolonize Public Health, and Achieve Health Equity
C. E. Oré, E. Loerzel, E. Marziale, and M. Parker

POLICY

732 Immigrant Inequities in Uninsurance and Postpartum Medicaid Extension: A Quasi-Experimental Study in New York City, 2016–2021
T. Janevic, L. Birnie, K. Belfon, L. Glenn, S. Maru, S. Reynolds, F. Eniola, H. Kim, F. M. Howell, A. Fox, and E. Weber

METHODS

736 Occupational Determinants of Health and Well-Being for Indigenous Populations in the United States: Findings From the National Health Interview Survey, 2020–2022
B. Shannon, C. Ryder, C. Abasilim, K. S. Almberg, T. Bonney, L. Forst, and L. S. Friedman

747 Polysubstance Use Profiles Among the General Adult Population, United States, 2022
K. M. Rockhill, J. C. Black, J. Iwanicki, and A. Abraham

OPEN-THEMED RESEARCH

758 Behavioral Interventions for Increasing Seat Belt Use and Decreasing Distracted Driving Using Telematics: A National Randomized Trial
J. P. Ebert, R. Yan, S. Friday, D. Small, C. C. McDonald, K. Bartolozzi, and M. K. Delgado

769 How and Why Does Redlining Matter for Present-Day Health? Critical Perspectives on Causality, Cartography, and Capitalism
C. Swope, S. Markley, S. Whittaker, and A. Hillier

780 Housing Quality Metric (HQM): Neighborhood-Level Data, Housing Quality, and Population Health
V. Garrison, P. J. Ashley, A. J. Moran, T. K. M. Cudjoe, E. M. Perrin, and C. E. Pollack

789 COVID-19 Policies and Sexually Transmitted Infections in 22 US States, January 2020–December 2021
C. C. Pollack, G. H. Redd, C. M. Timm, and Y. C. Manabe

799 Sexually Transmitted Infection Disparities and Social Determinants of Health in California, 2013–2021
E. E. Gotlieb, N. O. Burghardt, J. Hu, K. Jacobson, and R. E. Snyder

BACKMATTER

OTHER DEPARTMENTS

808 Subscription Form

With New Editors, *AJPH* History Section Forges Forward

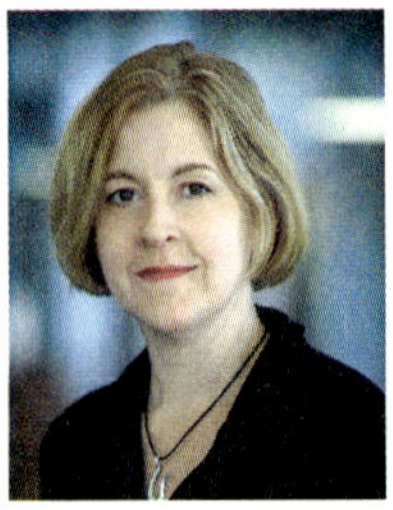
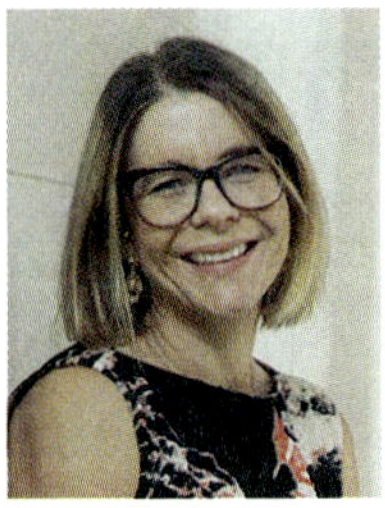

Marian Moser Jones, PhD, MPH
AJPH History Editor
Cassia Roth, PhD, MPH
AJPH History Editor

As the new history editors for *AJPH*, we seek to illuminate histories of public health beyond the well-developed, institutionally focused historiography of the urban United States. We welcome scholarship that highlights the perspectives of historical actors who were often silenced because of their social, cultural, economic, or geographic locations; studies that challenge accepted narratives about the nature and operation of public health; work that critically examines the role of colonialism and anticolonial resistance in shaping public health within the United States and abroad; and other new authors, voices, and histories that have been absent from the pages of *AJPH*. In at least one future call for papers, we will offer more details on the scholarship we are seeking.

We acknowledge that we have big shoes to fill. Since its launch in 1971, the "Public Health: Then and Now" (PHTN) section has successfully engaged the history of public health in conversation with the latest developments in the field. When Elizabeth Fee became *AJPH*'s history editor in 1990, she transformed the section into one of the most dynamic aspects of the journal. Fee, and soon coeditor Theodore (Ted) M. Brown, made this section the go-to venue for cutting-edge history of public health scholarship. These essays covered a range of issues: pandemics, social histories of chronic and infectious diseases, occupational health, social movements, substance use and misuse, and data collection. They highlighted ways that public health institutions have sometimes reinforced racial and social stereotypes and stigmas, and explored grassroots health movements that have challenged such inequities. Fee and Brown also created the "Voices From the Past" section, which reprinted original sources authored by past public health thinkers, researchers, leaders, and activists. Fee's death in 2018 and Brown's transition to Editor Emeritus in 2023 led to a leadership transition of the History section of the *AJPH*.

We will continue the mission of our predecessors by publishing excellent and accessible historical scholarship that speaks to current public health concerns and links history to public health practice. We seek work that tells stories; highlights the enduring importance of power relationships, personalities, and political dynamics in shaping our field and the public's health; and challenges dominant

Continued on page 623...

HISTORY CORNER

3 YEARS AGO

Enumeration of Public Health Nurses in the United States: Limits of Current Standards

[E]numeration surveys have been plagued by highly variable criteria for determining whether to "count" a nurse as a member of the PHN workforce. This lack of precision has severely impeded our ability to determine the actual number or supply of public health nurses in the workforce. Moreover, it has left us unable to assess if communities meet the recommended national minimum standard of a public health nurse-to population ratio of 1 to 5000 in the United States, and, as COVID-19 has so painfully taught us, it rendered us unable to determine if this standard is adequate to meet the needs of the population during regular times and in times of crisis.

From *AJPH*, Supplement 3, 2022, p. S293

16 YEARS AGO

Public Health Workforce Enumeration

The most recent national public health enumeration counted approximately 450 000 workers in 2000. This effort and the critiques of the reported findings illustrate the need for a system that produces national data on a regular basis, thereby allowing the monitoring trends and the measuring longitudinally of the impact of activities on the workforce, rather than the current intermittent efforts using diverse approaches. . . . Advancing the field of public health requires aligning fragmented efforts to collect workforce data and updating much needed narratives, perspectives, and assumptions.

We bring varied expertise to this project. Marian Moser Jones (The Ohio State University) is a historian of US public health, with a PhD and an MPH in sociomedical sciences. Her historical research has investigated public health institutional development and racial inequities in the context of public health crises. Her scholarship on disasters, wars, nursing, pandemics, homelessness, unintentional injuries, and infant mortality also extends into the health policy sphere. Cassia Roth (University of California, Riverside) has a PhD in Latin American history, with a focus on Brazil, and an MPH in epidemiology. Her historical research has focused on people's lived experience of reproductive health and health care from the 18th century to today. Her non-US focus expands "American" beyond the borders of the United States to encompass the entire hemisphere. Her training as both a historian and an epidemiologist further melds the "Then and Now" of the section.

Overall, our expertise lends itself to cultivating diverse voices in public health history and seeking out new historical scholarship that builds upon *AJPH*'s existing tradition of excellence. We are reminded how George Rosen, the section's founder, emphasized the need to publish historical public health pieces with direct relevance to the present and future. We continue that mission, remembering that the country we are today is not the same it was in 1971, and that needs to be reflected in the stories we tell. AJPH

DOI: https://doi.org/10.2105/AJPH.2024.307993

HISTORY CORNER

statistics on the size and composition of the workforce. The results of this alignment and updating will inform national and nationwide activities to recruit and retain a strong public health workforce.

From *AJPH*, May 2009, p. 787

99 YEARS AGO

Census of Public Health Nurses

In keeping with its earliest tradition—to ascertain the number of public health nurses in the United States and where they are employed—the National Organization for Public Health Nursing has taken a census. . . . There is still a wide field untouched by public health nursing. The census shows that 59 per cent of the total number of counties in the United States were without any public health nursing service. Of the remaining 41 per cent of the counties a relatively small number of them had nursing services available to the entire county. Public health nursing was largely confined to the towns and cities, for 74 per cent of the public health nurses in the United States were working in cities of 10,000 or more population.

From *AJPH*, August 1926, pp. 822–823

A Magnificent Example of Why We Need Multilateral Organizations Such as WHO

Cesar Victora, MD, PhD

ABOUT THE AUTHOR

Cesar G. Victora is with the International Center for Equity in Health, Federal University of Pelotas, Pelotas, Brazil.

AJPH May 2025, Vol. 115, No. 5

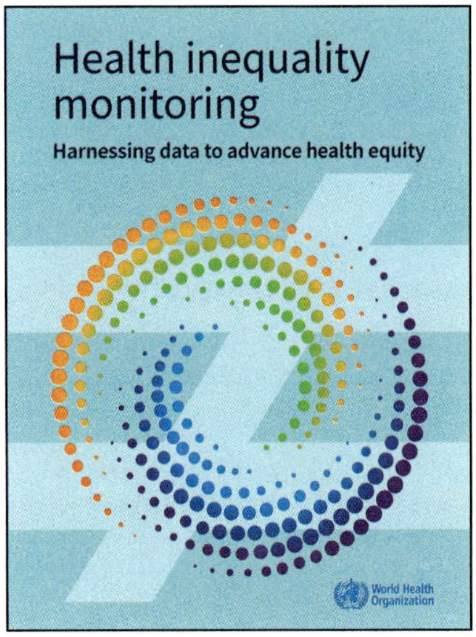

World Health Organization
Health Inequality Monitoring: Harnessing Data to Advance Health Equity
Geneva: World Health Organization; 2024
425 pages, open access
ISBN 978-9-24010-260-6

The World Health Organization (WHO) has recently released a much-needed, timely resource: *Health Inequality Monitoring: Harnessing Data to Advance Health Equity*. Having worked in equity-focused epidemiological research since the 1970s, I only regret that a similar publication was not made available earlier, as it would have saved much of the time it took me to learn—by consulting multiple separate sources—how to carry out and disseminate health equity analyses.

Studies of inequalities in health started to appear in Western Europe and North America in the 1840s,[1] mostly relying on occupation and geography to describe wide disparities. Chadwick, Engels, Virchow, and Villermé were among the pioneers in this new discipline. Over time, the science of health inequalities progressed rather slowly. By the second half of the 20th century, economists and epidemiologists analyzed health inequalities independently, with limited interactions or dialogue. In the health field, we mainly focused on geographic, educational, ethnic, gender, and occupational inequalities, whereas economists tended to favor household expenditure and income levels as stratifiers. Yet, data on expenditure require lengthy fieldwork, and income information is often unreliable and of limited relevance for the informal sector and rural inhabitants.

A breakthrough occurred around the end of the 20th century when World Bank economists employed survey data on household assets and on building characteristics to calculate continuous wealth indices through principal component analyses. These indices allowed the classification of households into equal-sized groups (typically wealth quintiles), a feature much appreciated by data analysts.[2] The wealth indices were rapidly adopted to provide massive documentation of socioeconomic inequalities—for example, in the health and nutrition of women and children—using data from national population-based surveys from low- and middle-income countries (LMICs).[3] This was a significant development because, whereas health inequalities among rich and poor countries were widely acknowledged, within-country disparities in LMICs were ignored because of an unspoken assumption that families in these countries were uniformly poor.[3,4] Wealth indices are currently used in equity analyses of data from hundreds of surveys from most LMICs, with results being readily available on web sites such as the WHO Health Inequality Data Repository (https://www.who.int/data/inequality-monitor/data), to which my group in Brazil contributes with analyses of within-country disparities in the health and nutrition of women and children (www.equidade.org).

This historical recap will help us understand the importance of the book being reviewed here. It is driven by the WHO-led team of researchers and analysts behind the Repository, who felt the need to disseminate the methodology used in their work. In doing so, they were both ambitious and meticulous. With over 400 pages, the report's multifaceted approach covers theoretical foundations, practical methods, and ethical considerations. Particular attention is given to reliance on multiple sources of health information, critical appraisal of data quality, selection and calculation of equity stratifiers and outcome indicators, principles of simple and complex analyses of disparities, and translation of results to the population and decision-makers.

To achieve its objectives, the book covers different dimensions of health inequality, including stratifiers that may be usefully compared across countries, such as age, economic position, education level, place of residence, sex, and subnational region. It also covers context-specific indicators, including ethnicity, language, marital status, migratory status, occupation, religion, sexual orientation, and gender identity. Although many examples are provided of these multiple dimensions, the most substantial emphasis is given to socioeconomic position—for example, the expression "wealth quintiles" appears 244 times in the book, considerably more than any other stratification variable. Such emphasis is well in line with WHO's recent work on the importance of social determinants of health and how such knowledge can be employed to build more equitable societies.[5] The methodological contents of the book are essential for helping countries monitor progress in health not only in aggregate terms but also to identify whether such progress is contributing to closing the health and well-being gaps among different subgroups of their societies. They will allow, for example, reporting progress by the poorest or most vulnerable population subgroups rather than by the country as a whole.[6]

I particularly appreciate the book's focus on translating the robust results of equity analyses to a broad audience, ensuring that dissemination is user-friendly and accessible to health managers and policymakers who seldom received substantial training in epidemiology or statistics. This book will become an indispensable resource for policymakers, researchers, and public health professionals willing to implement evidence-informed, equity-oriented strategies.

This book and the Health Inequality Data Repository would certainly have been welcomed by the 1840s cohort of health equity pioneers such as Chadwick, Engels, Virchow, Villermé, and several others. The book and the Repository are also magnificent examples of why we need multilateral organizations such as WHO, as no other types of institutions could make such resources widely available to high-, middle-, and low-income countries and, more importantly, could promote and support its widespread use by countries. At a time when an epidemic of right-wing populist governments is threatening the very existence of multilateralism, let this effort remain an example of how the world should function. AJPH

CORRESPONDENCE

Correspondence should be sent to Cesar G. Victora, Centro Internacional de Equidade em Saúde, Rua Marechal Deodoro 1160, Pelotas, RS 96220, Brazil (e-mail: cvictora@equidade.org). Reprints can be ordered at https://www.ajph.org by clicking the "Reprints" link.

PUBLICATION INFORMATION

Full Citation: Victora C. A magnificent example of why we need multilateral organizations such as WHO. *Am J Public Health*. 2025;115(5):624–625.

Acceptance Date: January 3, 2025.

DOI: https://doi.org/10.2105/AJPH.2025.308013

CONFLICTS OF INTEREST

C. G. Victora is a member of the WHO Science Committee and received research grants from WHO in the past.

REFERENCES

1. Krieger N, Birn AE. A vision of social justice as the foundation of public health: commemorating 150 years of the spirit of 1848. *Am J Public Health*. 1998;88(11):1603–1606. https://doi.org/10.2105/AJPH.88.11.1603
2. Filmer D, Pritchett LH. Estimating wealth effects without expenditure data—or tears: an application to educational enrollments in states of India. *Demography*. 2001;38(1):115–132.
3. Gwatkin D, Rutstein S, Johnson K, Pande R, Wagstaff A. *Socioeconomnic Differences in Health, Nutrition and Population*. Washington, DC: World Bank; 2000.
4. Victora CG, Wagstaff A, Schellenberg JA, Gwatkin D, Claeson M, Habicht JP. Applying an equity lens to child health and mortality: more of the same is not enough. *Lancet*. 2003;362(9379):233–241. https://doi.org/10.1016/S0140-6736(03)13917-7
5. *Closing the Gap in a Generation: Health Equity Through Action on the Social Determinants of Health: Final Report of the Commission on Social Determinants of Health*. Geneva, Switzerland: World Health Organization; 2008.
6. Gwatkin DR, Bhuiya A, Victora CG. Making health systems more equitable. *Lancet*. 2004;364(9441):1273–1280. https://doi.org/10.1016/S0140-6736(04)17145-6

AJPH and the Threat of Political Interference in Scientific Publishing

Alfredo Morabia, MD, PhD

ABOUT THE AUTHOR

Alfredo Morabia is AJPH *editor-in-chief and is with the Barry Commoner Center for Health and the Environment, Queens College, City University of New York, and the Department of Epidemiology, Mailman School of Public Health, Columbia University, New York, NY.*

Since taking office, the new US administration has issued numerous executive orders (e.g., order 14151 and 14168 of January 20, 2025) that significantly impact public health research. They restrict the scope of federally funded research in areas already understudied and limit public health data collection and availability, among other imposed limitations. Officially, many of these measures aim to eliminate research perceived as promoting diversity, equity, and inclusion. In practice, however, if allowed to stand, they may weaken the foundation of governmental and academic research.

These executive orders have direct implications for the *American Journal of Public Health* (*AJPH*) and the scientific press. In recent weeks, several requests have been made to *AJPH* mentioning these orders. Officials from federal institutions have requested the withdrawal of articles supported by federal funds, citing concerns that they address politically sensitive topics such as transgender health. Authors have sought to modify accepted or in-press articles by removing their names from the author list. Other requests include modifying specific wording or eliminating sentences after the article has been accepted.

These requests do not stem from scientific concerns about methodological rigor or scientific merit but rather reflect external pressures related to 2025 presidential executive orders. In this editorial, I outline why *AJPH* has consistently declined requests motivated by political and ideological pressure and explain why doing so is necessary to preserve the integrity of the scientific record.

WHAT CONSTITUTES A PUBLISHED SCIENTIFIC ARTICLE?

An accepted article is a scholarly work that has undergone rigorous peer review to ensure its validity and originality. Once accepted, it undergoes additional revisions, copyediting, and production. At this stage, the *Journal* has added substantial value to the article, ensuring its clarity and scientific integrity.

Thus, a final article is not solely the work of the authors but a vetted scientific contribution in which the *Journal* plays a crucial role. While *AJPH* does not necessarily hold the copyright to every article, it has an obligation to maintain the integrity of the published record. This responsibility includes declining requests for any modifications after an article has been accepted except when such modifications are justified by rigorous, state-of-the-art scientific reasoning.

It is also important to distinguish between articles under review and those that have been accepted. While authors may revise their work during the peer review process, once an article has been accepted, it represents a finalized contribution to scientific knowledge and should only be corrected or withdrawn under extraordinary circumstances.

Allowing, after an article has been accepted, name removals or content modifications for ideological or political reasons fundamentally undermines the long-term integrity of the scientific record. The listed authors met authorship criteria at the time of submission, and their names reflect accountability for the work. Accommodating these requests based on shifting political priorities risks setting a dangerous precedent—one in which research findings can be altered retroactively because of ideological pressures rather than scientific integrity.

THE PRECEDENT FOR POLITICALLY MOTIVATED CENSORSHIP

The suppression of scientific research for political reasons is not unprecedented in American history. Examples include McCarthy-era blacklisting of scientists suspected of communist affiliations, which led to academic dismissals and funding cuts; neglect and underfunding of AIDS research in the 1980s, which hindered studies on LGBTQ+ health; government-imposed restrictions on discussing contraception and reproductive health in federally funded public health programs; and censorship of climate change science, notably between 2017 and 2021, when references to climate change were systematically removed from multiple federal agency websites and political interference affected climate research.

These historical instances of suppression of scientific research for political reasons resulted in censored or manipulated research to align with political agendas, stagnation in public health advancements, and inadequate responses to health crises, such as the AIDS epidemic. These historical instances show how small concessions to political pressures can snowball into broader suppression of research, censorship of public health information, and obstructions to scientific progress.

The current situation follows the same fundamental pattern: scientific findings are being challenged not based on evidence but based on ideological considerations. We must therefore consider what actions—however small—are necessary to counter tactics that create a chilling effect on scientific discourse and, ultimately, risk corrupting the integrity of science.

Granting name removals or content modification on a case-by-case basis may turn into a routine concession, ultimately weakening the *Journal's* role as an independent arbiter of science.

WHY *AJPH* MUST REJECT CENSORSHIP

Scientific journals must remain committed to editorial independence and the integrity of the published record. If *AJPH* were to accommodate politically motivated modifications, it would set a dangerous precedent—one that could be exploited to reshape the scientific record based on ideology rather than evidence, ultimately resulting in harm to populations. The *Journal* has a duty to ensure that scientific publications remain independent, based on methodological rigor and scientific merit, and are not a product of political expediency. AJPH

CORRESPONDENCE

Correspondence should be sent to Alfredo Morabia, Professor of Epidemiology, Queens College, Barry Commoner Center, 65-30 Kissena Blvd, Remsen #311, Flushing, NY 11367 (e-mail: editorajph@apha.org). Reprints can be ordered at https://www.ajph.org by clicking the "Reprints" link.

PUBLICATION INFORMATION

Full Citation: Morabia A. *AJPH* and the threat of political interference in scientific publishing. *Am J Public Health*. 2025;115(5):626–627.

Acceptance Date: February 25, 2025.

DOI: https://doi.org/10.2105/AJPH.2025.308100

CONFLICTS OF INTEREST

The author has no conflicts of interest to report.

Sexually Transmitted Infection Cases During COVID-19: Implications for Public Health

Thomas S. Fitzpatrick, MD, MPH, and Joseph D. Tucker, MD, AM, PhD

ABOUT THE AUTHORS

Thomas S. Fitzpatrick is with the Division of Infectious Diseases, University of Washington School of Medicine, Seattle. Joseph D. Tucker is with the Institute for Global Health and Infectious Diseases, University of North Carolina at Chapel Hill, and the Clinical Research Department, Faculty of Infectious and Tropical Diseases, London School of Hygiene and Tropical Diseases, London, England.

See also Pinto et al., p. 631, and Pollack et al., p. 789.

Early in the COVID-19 pandemic, sexual health care providers recognized that the global public health emergency would likely have an impact on sexually transmitted infections (STIs) in complex and conflicting ways. As hundreds of millions stayed at home and social activities were suspended, sexual behaviors fundamentally changed. People across the globe reported having less casual sex,[1] presumptively lowering their risk for acquiring and transmitting STIs.

However, the widespread social disruption caused by COVID-19 also prevented many people from seeking STI testing, STI treatment, and condoms.[2] Those who sought care during COVID-19 encountered limited sexual health care services hindered by reduced STI clinic hours, reallocated staff, and shortages in STI testing supplies. Dramatic temporary reductions in STI cases, sometimes exceeding 70%, were reported during the initial months of the pandemic.[3] What explains these trends and the implications for future public health programming remain important questions.

In this issue of *AJPH*, Pollack et al. (p. 789) examine bacterial STI case reports in the United States, comparing the periods before and during the COVID-19 pandemic. In its application of an interrupted time series approach to jurisdiction-level chlamydia, gonorrhea, and syphilis case counts, their analysis provides the clearest picture yet of how COVID-19 mitigation policies affected reported STI cases. Mandatory stay-at-home orders were associated with 25% fewer reported chlamydia cases and 15% fewer reported gonorrhea cases but did not have an impact on syphilis cases. These reductions were seen across regions, genders, and most racial groups. In addition, the most stringent restrictions on social gatherings, which limited gatherings to 10 people or fewer, were associated with fewer reported chlamydia cases but were not associated with changes in gonorrhea or syphilis cases. These findings are broadly consistent with earlier descriptive reports showing larger and more sustained reductions in chlamydia cases during the pandemic, with smaller and less sustained reductions in gonorrhea and syphilis cases.[3]

Although Pollack et al. provide convincing evidence that the most stringent lockdown measures at the beginning of the pandemic reduced reported chlamydia and gonorrhea cases, the extent to which this represents a true decrease in STI incidence or underreporting on the part of the disrupted sexual health care system remains uncertain. The authors reasonably contend that their results suggest the reductions were due to limited access to sexual health services because the effect of COVID-19 mitigation policies disappeared after exclusion of the period March through May 2020, when clinic closures were most pronounced. However, this same period may also have been when people most adhered to stay-at-home orders, decreasing the frequency of sex. The ineffectiveness of subsequent stay-at-home orders after this initial period may have been influenced by COVID-19 fatigue, with large numbers of people defying lockdowns to engage socially, including to have sex.[4]

Other researchers have attempted to disentangle these complexities by using symptomatic STI cases (e.g., male urethral gonorrhea) as proxies for sexual behavior and asymptomatic STI cases (e.g., early latent syphilis) as proxies for STI screening resulting from either health care service availability or health care seeking.[5] These studies identified reductions in both types of cases, with larger reductions in asymptomatic than symptomatic infections,[5–7] suggesting that issues impeding health care access may have been more important than changes in sexual behavior. Although changes in sexual behavior varied by region and demographics, the reduced STI testing access observed during COVID-19 may have driven decreased reported STI cases.

After decreasing during the initial months of the COVID-19 pandemic,

STI cases rebounded above prepandemic levels in most settings, a phenomenon also described by Pollack et al. Whether or not mandatory stay-at-home orders and gathering restrictions initially decreased STI transmission, they clearly proved transient.

Efforts to combat STIs through imposing top-down policies that aim to restrict sexual behaviors seem unlikely to succeed long term and may potentially backfire. Qualitative work with gay, bisexual, and other men who have sex with men during the pandemic revealed that lockdown measures were a substantial barrier to casual sex, but anxiety and hopelessness from social isolation ultimately drove some men to engage in riskier sexual behaviors. For example, one study showed that these men increased their number of sex partners after lockdowns ended.[8] Alternatively, grounds-up strategies that actively partner with those at higher risk of acquiring STIs (e.g., increased access to self-testing[9] and social network distribution of STI prevention measures) may ultimately be more sustainable during periods of social disruption.

Even if COVID-19 mitigation measures decreased STI transmission to some extent through preventing casual sex, we should still also be cautious about seeing decreases in STI case counts as a victory for sexual health. Multicountry behavioral survey research suggests that both men and women became less satisfied with their sex lives during the COVID-19 pandemic.[2] Gay, bisexual, and other men who have sex with men reported that lack of physical and sexual intimacy during COVID-19 lockdowns negatively affected their feelings of connectedness and worsened their mental health.[10]

There are several historical examples of other periods of social upheaval that transformed sexual behaviors and thereby resulted in dramatic reductions in STIs. Both the communist revolution in China[11] and the Islamic revolution in Iran[12] led to large-scale changes in social behaviors. In China, structural interventions that shuttered brothels, organized large-scale presumptive STI treatment, and fostered harsh social pressure were associated with substantial decreases in syphilis diagnoses within STI clinics.[11] By the 1950s and 1960s, syphilis was rarely encountered in STI clinics. The Iranian revolution of 1979 also wrought large-scale shifts in social norms and sexual behaviors, increasing stigma related to sex, promoting conservative sexual attitudes, and creating barriers to STI testing.[12] These historical examples remind us that decreases in STI case counts may herald worsening rather than improving sexual health.

Examining STI cases during COVID-19 underscores the limitations of existing surveillance systems and the need for more holistic metrics to assess sexual health. People-centered measures that include sexual satisfaction and related sex-positive items would be useful in this context. AJPH

CORRESPONDENCE

Correspondence should be sent to Joseph D. Tucker, MD, MPH, Bioinformatics Building, Mason Farm Rd, UNC Chapel Hill, Chapel Hill, NC 27599 (e-mail jdtucker@med.unc.edu). Reprints can be ordered at https://www.ajph.org by clicking the "Reprints" link.

PUBLICATION INFORMATION

Full Citation: Fitzpatrick TS, Tucker JD. Sexually transmitted infection cases during COVID-19: implications for public health. *Am J Public Health*. 2025;115(5):628–630.

Acceptance Date: January 6, 2025.

DOI: https://doi.org/10.2105/AJPH.2025.308024

ORCID iDs:
Thomas S. Fitzpatrick https://orcid.org/0000-0002-0852-7291

Joseph D. Tucker https://orcid.org/0000-0003-2804-1181

CONTRIBUTORS

T. S. Fitzpatrick wrote the first draft. Both authors edited the article.

ACKNOWLEDGMENTS

Joseph D. Tucker is supported by the National Institute of Allergy and Infectious Diseases (grant K24AI143471).

CONFLICTS OF INTEREST

The authors report no potential conflicts of interest.

REFERENCES

1. Schumacher CM, Thornton N, Wagner J, et al. Sexually transmitted infection transmission dynamics during the coronavirus disease 2019 (COVID-19) pandemic among urban gay, bisexual, and other men who have sex with men. *Clin Infect Dis*. 2022;75(1):e1137–e1144. https://doi.org/10.1093/cid/ciab1053
2. Toller Erausquin J, Tan RKJ, Uhlich M, et al. The International Sexual Health And REproductive Health during COVID-19 (I-SHARE) Study: a multicountry analysis of adults from 30 countries prior to and during the initial coronavirus disease 2019 wave. *Clin Infect Dis*. 2022;75(1):e991–e999. https://doi.org/10.1093/cid/ciac102
3. Pagaoa M, Grey J, Torrone E, Kreisel K, Stenger M, Weinstock H. Trends in nationally notifiable sexually transmitted disease case reports during the US COVID-19 pandemic, January to December 2020. *Sex Transm Dis*. 2021;48(10):798–804. https://doi.org/10.1097/OLQ.0000000000001506
4. Spiegel M. COVID NPIs and lockdown fatigue. Available at: https://europepmc.org/article/ppr/ppr659805. Accessed December 20, 2024.
5. Berzkalns A, Thibault CS, Barbee LA, Golden MR, Khosropour C, Kerani RP. Decreases in reported sexually transmitted infections during the time of COVID-19 in King County, WA: decreased transmission or screening? *Sex Transm Dis*. 2021;48(8s):S44–S49. https://doi.org/10.1097/OLQ.0000000000001463
6. Chow EPF, Hocking JS, Ong JJ, Phillips TR, Fairley CK. Sexually transmitted infection diagnoses and access to a sexual health service before and after the national lockdown for COVID-19 in Melbourne, Australia. *Open Forum Infect Dis*. 2021;8(1):ofaa536. https://doi.org/10.1093/ofid/ofaa536
7. Bonett S, Teixeira da Silva D, Lazar N, Makeneni S, Wood SM. Trends in sexually transmitted infection screening during COVID-19 and missed cases among adolescents. *Public Health*. 2022;213:171–176. https://doi.org/10.1016/j.puhe.2022.10.007
8. Loosier PS, Ogale YP, Smith RC, Kachur R, Nicolae L, Heumann C. Sexual behavior and sexual decision-making among gay, bisexual, and other men who have sex with men during the COVID-19

pandemic: observations from a rapid ethnographic assessment in Marion County, Indiana, October–November 2021. *Arch Sex Behav.* 2024;53(3):871–877. https://doi.org/10.1007/s10508-023-02795-0

9. Jiang H, Xie Y, Xiong Y, et al. HIV self-testing partially filled the HIV testing gap among men who have sex with men in China during the COVID-19 pandemic: results from an online survey. *J Int AIDS Soc.* 2021;24(5):e25737. https://doi.org/10.1002/jia2.25737
10. Seah XY, Tan RKJ, Yong XM, Asano M. Sexual and mental health of Singaporean gay, bisexual and other men who have sex with men in times of COVID-19: a qualitative study. *Int J Qual Stud Health Well-being.* 2024;19(1):2408816. https://doi.org/10.1080/17482631.2024.2408816
11. Chen XS, Yin YP, Wang QQ, Wang BX. Historical perspective of syphilis in the past 60 years in China: eliminated, forgotten, on the return. *Chin Med J (Engl).* 2013;126(14):2774–2779.
12. Simforoosh N. A decrease in the incidence of syphilis in Iran and the effect of Islamic rules in controlling sexually transmitted diseases. *Med J Islam Repub Iran.* 1989;2(4):283–285.

COVID-19 Policies and the Impact on STIs: Context, Equity, and Innovation

Casey N. Pinto, PhD, MPH, CRNP, Stacey B. Griner, PhD, MPH, CPH, RDH, and Randolph D. Hubach, PhD, MPH

ABOUT THE AUTHORS

Casey N. Pinto is with the Department of Public Health Sciences, Penn State University, Hershey, PA. Stacey B. Griner is with the College of Public Health, University of North Texas Health Science Center, Fort Worth, TX. Randolph D. Hubach is with the Department of Public Health, Purdue University, West Lafayette, IN.

See also Fitzpatrick and Tucker, p. 628, and Pollack et al., p. 789.

As public health professionals who research sexually transmitted infections (STIs), we value the recently published article by Pollack et al., experts in the field (p. 789). We agree that the relationship between COVID-19 policies and the potential impact on STI rates is complex, warranting further examination. The overarching policies described—specifically, lockdown measures—had an associated decrease with STI rates with some qualifications and nuances related to the stringency of the policies. The associations with STIs only held true when the COVID-19 policies were strict and people were required to stay home or were in lockdown, potentially limiting the ability of people to engage in sexual intercourse with partners outside their home. However, when policies were modified and people were provided with recommendations (not requirements) to stay home or limit gatherings to certain numbers, STI rates were no different or, in the case of gonorrhea, increased.

Moving forward, there are three major considerations for how these COVID-19 policies may have affected STI rates: context, equity, and innovation. Although many of the points discussed here were highlighted in the article, COVID-19 has changed not only the way Americans view public health, but also how they receive sexual health care.

CONTEXTUAL CONSIDERATIONS

Declining chlamydia rates during lockdown periods may be due in part to COVID-19 policies; however, the expected change in sexual behaviors may not be behind these declines. Other factors, including a lack of screening for STIs, will equate to a decline in rates, and there were significant decreases in STI screening during the COVID-19 lockdown.[1,2] This decline in screening was related to a combination of treating empirically,[3] lack of supplies for STI screening (many testing mediums were being used for COVID-19 testing),[4] and a lack of routine STI screening within primary care and other settings.[2,5] In addition, many public health STI clinics were closed or not providing STI care, and disease intervention specialists, our elite team of contact tracers who primarily focus on STIs, were transitioned to focus on COVID-19 contact tracing.[5] Thus, a key point plaguing the STI field is determining if the decreases in STI rates seen during COVID-19 are a true decrease in rates, or are representative of the use of empiric treatment or of significant changes in STI contact tracing, screening, and surveillance.

Despite national policies being enacted, implementation may not have been consistent across all jurisdictions. Although jurisdictions from multiple states were included in this analysis, there may be significant variations in implementation, enforcement, and perceptions of COVID-19 severity. For instance, New York City was the epicenter for COVID-19 in the United States, news coverage was high, and residents were invested in responding, likely improving the willingness to adhere to lockdown policies.[6] Other areas experienced COVID-19 to varying degrees.

Further complicating individual adherence included the extent to which COVID-19 infection affected one's social circle and one's personal belief about the benefit of social distancing. At the jurisdiction level, the policy implementation process may have varied in interpretation and application. For instance, the definition of who and what jobs were considered frontline or "essential" and exempt from lockdowns may have disproportionally affected people of color and women.[7] Consideration of contextual factors such as access to screening and inequities in policy implementation can contribute to a better understanding of the specific role these policies had on STI rates.

EQUITY CONSIDERATIONS

Some of the proposed contextual considerations related to the federal lockdown mandates and policies overlap with equity considerations, particularly those related to social

AJPH May 2025, Vol. 115, No. 5

determinants of health. Although many studies have found decreased sexual activity during lockdown periods, these findings were not universal for all marginalized populations. For example, some populations were prone to increased substance use during lockdown, which was also associated with increased sexual risk taking.[8] In addition, people with jobs that were amenable to shelter-in-place policies were able to transition to working from home, whereas others were laid off, or could not run their businesses because they could not be done from home and were reliant on federal aid. This inequity in economic stability related to the policies may have also affected STI rates. For instance, those who were able to safely transition to work from home without any major impact to their finances suddenly found themselves with no commute time, no socialization at work, and no extracurricular activities (especially for those living alone). These people may have been more likely to connect, socialize, or build relationships in other ways; one example of this is engaging in smaller, home-based dates. This is exemplified in research, and one study clearly quotes, "When you got nothing to do, you do somebody."[9] The pandemic highlighted many significant inequities and flaws within the health care system, but these issues become even more complex through the lens of COVID-19 policies and the contributions of the social determinants of health on STI rates.

In addition to the inequity in jobs transitioning to home, there were also inequities in access to STI care. Because health care was focused on COVID-19, primary care offices were limiting in-patient visits. Providers in urgent care centers were consolidating and using their staff for COVID-19 testing centers. Public health clinics were severely limiting STI services.[5] In many cases, there was a transition to online direct-to-consumer STI testing, which did improve access to care and filled a void in screening, but only for patients who could afford to pay the associated costs. Direct-to-consumer STI services and other services that were utilized during the lockdowns, such as virtual visits, may have benefits but may not reach some vulnerable populations. The dual impact of COVID-19 on the opioid epidemic is one example.[10] Although this population likely faced increased barriers to accessing care,[10] they were also probably unable to access direct-to-consumer testing because of high cost.

INNOVATION CONSIDERATIONS

Despite the inequities of direct-to-consumer testing, these tests are innovative in bringing access to patients who otherwise might not have accessed testing. Although direct-to-consumer testing was available for years before COVID-19, the lockdowns increased demand for alternative screening modalities, and industry responded. Post-COVID-19 direct-to-consumer tests are providing patients who face stigma or other access barriers a means to access care, especially in rural or underserved areas.[11]

The COVID-19 pandemic, coupled with policy mandates, have forced innovation for consumers, industry, health care, and research. Future STI-related diagnostic and preventive innovations are in the pipeline, indicating a strong focus to move the STI field forward. Health care providers, public health reporting and surveillance, and policymakers will be required to match the speed of this development and focus on rapid implementation in the future.

CONCLUSION

As the Greek philosopher Heraclitus opined, "The only constant in life is change." Although the pandemic-related policies did not have a clear relationship with or impact on STI rates, it is clear that COVID-19 has changed how Americans access health care, necessitating adaptation by the STI field as well. COVID-19 provided significant information about rapid policy implementation and the ability to "monitor and adjust" dissemination and implementation strategies. Overall, we saw innovation in rapid communication strategies to the general public, which can be used moving forward to address emerging STI epidemics such as mpox and congenital syphilis. However, because STI funding has been stagnant for decades,[12] this cannot be accomplished without an increase in funding to support a public health response. AJPH

CORRESPONDENCE

Correspondence should be sent to Casey N. Pinto, 90 Hope Dr, Hershey, PA 17033 (e-mail: Cnp113@psu.edu). Reprints can be ordered at https://www.ajph.org by clicking the "Reprints" link.

PUBLICATION INFORMATION

Full Citation: Pinto CN, Griner SB, Hubach RD. COVID-19 policies and the impact on STIs: context, equity, and innovation. *Am J Public Health*. 2025;115(5):631–633.

Acceptance Date: January 14, 2025.

DOI: https://doi.org/10.2105/AJPH.2025.308032

ORCID iDs:

Casey N. Pinto https://orcid.org/0000-0003-4355-7813

Stacey B. Griner https://orcid.org/0000-0002-2774-5841

CONTRIBUTORS

C. N. Pinto and S. B. Griner contributed to the conceptualization, drafting, revision, and final edits of the manuscript. R. D. Hubach assisted in conceptualization and editing of the manuscript.

CONFLICTS OF INTEREST

C. N. Pinto has received honoraria from Roche and funding from Hologic. S. B. Griner and R. D. Hubach do not have any conflicts to disclose.

REFERENCES

1. Pinto CN, Niles JK, Kaufman HW, et al. Impact of the COVID-19 pandemic on chlamydia and gonorrhea screening in the US. *Am J Prev Med.* 2021;61(3):386–393. https://doi.org/10.1016/j.amepre.2021.03.009
2. Tao G, Dietz S, Hartnett KP, Jayanthi P, Gift TL. Impact of the COVID-19 pandemic on chlamydia and gonorrhea tests performed by a large national laboratory—United States, 2019 to 2020. *Sex Transm Dis.* 2022;49(7):490–496. https://doi.org/10.1097/OLQ.0000000000001638
3. Centers for Diseases Control and Prevention. Dear colleague letter: STD treatment options. April 2020. Available at: https://stacks.cdc.gov/view/cdc/149809/cdc_149809_DS1.pdf. Accessed December 31, 2024.
4. Centers for Diseases Control and Prevention. Dear colleague letter: DSTDP lab and drug shortages [press release]. 2020. Available at: https://stacks.cdc.gov/view/cdc/149808/cdc_149808_DS1.pdf. Accessed December 31, 2024.
5. National Coalition of STD Directors. COVID-19 and the state of the STD field I. 2020. Available at: https://ncsddc.org/resource/covid-19-and-the-state-of-the-std-field. Accessed December 31, 2024.
6. City Lens NY. Things fall apart. Available at: https://covid19.nycitylens.com. Accessed December 31, 2024.
7. Centers for Disease Control and Prevention. Interim list of categories of essential workers mapped to standardized industry codes and titles. 2020. Available at: https://archive.cdc.gov/www_cdc_gov/vaccines/covid-19/categories-essential-workers.html. Accessed January 2, 2025.
8. Lehmiller JJ, Garcia JR, Gesselman AN, Mark KP. Less sex, but more sexual diversity: changes in sexual behavior during the COVID-19 coronavirus pandemic. *Leis Sci.* 2021;43(1-2):295–304. https://doi.org/10.1080/01490400.2020.1774016
9. Akers AY, Muhammad MR, Corbie-Smith G. "When you got nothing to do, you do somebody": a community's perceptions of neighborhood effects on adolescent sexual behaviors. *Soc Sci Med.* 2011;72(1):91–99. https://doi.org/10.1016/j.socscimed.2010.09.035
10. Ghose R, Forati AM, Mantsch JR. Impact of the COVID-19 pandemic on opioid overdose deaths: a spatiotemporal analysis. *J Urban Health.* 2022;99(2):316–327. https://doi.org/10.1007/s11524-022-00610-0
11. Exten C, Pinto CN, Gaynor AM, Meyerson B, Griner SB, Van Der Pol B. Direct-to-consumer sexually transmitted infection testing services: a position statement from the American Sexually Transmitted Diseases Association. *Sex Transm Dis.* 2021;48(11):e155–e159. https://doi.org/10.1097/OLQ.0000000000001475
12. Karnabi I. As STD funding stagnates, rates rise to all-time highs. National Coalition of STD Directors. 2019. Available at: https://ncsddc.org/as-std-funding-stagnates-rates-rise-to-all-time-highs. Accessed January 2, 2025.

Exploring Indigenous Health and Employment: Methods to Capture Diversity and Intersecting Factors

Virginia Gunn, PhD, Patricia O'Campo, PhD, and Carles Muntaner, PhD

ABOUT THE AUTHORS

Virginia Gunn is with the School of Nursing, Cape Breton University, Sydney, Nova Scotia, Canada and the Unit of Occupational Medicine, Institute of Environmental Medicine, Karolinska Institute, Stockholm, Sweden. Patricia O'Campo is with the MAP Centre for Urban Health Solutions, St. Michael's Hospital and Dalla Lana School of Public Health, University of Toronto, Toronto, Ontario, Canada. Carles Muntaner is with the Lawrence S. Bloomberg School of Nursing and the Dalla Lana School of Public Health, University of Toronto, Toronto, Ontario, Canada.

See also Shannon et al., p. 736.

The political, economic, and cultural problems faced by Indigenous populations in the United States, including American Indian and Alaska Native (AIAN) communities, are the consequence of a history of settler colonialism, contemporary injustices, systemic discrimination, oppression, genocide, and inequitable policies.[1,2] These political and social determinants, compounded by ongoing harmful federal policies and interventions, manifest themselves in extreme poverty rates and limited access to employment, or overrepresentation in precarious employment.[1,3,4] The consequences of historic and ongoing colonization for Indigenous populations—contributing to their limited rights and access to services, systematic exclusion from property ownership, and reduced participation in the labor market—are linked to numerous negative physical and mental health outcomes and health inequities.[5,6] Because of concerns over the range of health inequities affecting Indigenous populations in the United States and elsewhere around the world, their causes and mechanisms are examined in a growing body of research.[5–7]

Improving the social and health status of Indigenous populations requires corrective action to address structural inequities. This can be accomplished through policies focused on honoring self-determination, restoring tribal sovereignty, providing reparation for land dispossession, and ensuring that tribes have control over their lands and resources, along with steady investments in infrastructure, health care, and education.[1,2,4,6] In this issue, Shannon et al. (p. 736) focus on employment as an avenue for intervention, discussing occupational determinants of Indigenous health and well-being, identified through an analysis of 2020–2022 US National Health Interview Survey data. The focus is on three Indigenous groups: (1) non-Hispanic AIAN, (2) Hispanic AIAN, and (3) AIAN and other race. The findings revealed distinct employment characteristics and obstacles to employment among the three Indigenous groups examined. In addition to responding to a data gap regarding occupational-related factors affecting AIAN populations, Shannon et al. highlight several important methodological considerations regarding Indigenous health and employment research.

First, the authors use their findings to highlight the heterogeneous character of Indigenous populations and warn against using definitions, data collection, and analysis approaches that do not differentiate among subgroups and, as a result, do not facilitate accurate assessments of unique health outcomes and needs of distinct populations. Because their findings revealed that both demographic profiles and employment characteristics varied among the three Indigenous subgroups studied, they argue that a lack of disaggregated data and analysis approaches hinders the potential of public health research to address the range of health inequities affecting Indigenous groups. They advocate for a redefining of Indigenous groups in national US surveys to capture currently missed subpopulations (e.g., major tribes).

Using methodologies with the potential to capture the diversity of Indigenous populations aligns with calls from other researchers who highlight their potential to identify different factors and mechanisms causing Indigenous subgroups' ill health.[6,8] The need to collect granular data that enable disaggregated analyses and the examination of compounding effects of power and social identity are not specific to Indigenous populations. Such approaches

AJPH May 2025, Vol. 115, No. 5

have the potential to advance public health research and benefit all population subgroups, especially those suffering from poor health outcomes, often masked and undistinguishable when detailed subgroup data are lacking and only aggregated analyses are conducted.[9] There is growing recognition among public health researchers that a limited access to racial/ethnic data,[9] and a lack of intersectional approaches to data collection and analysis[7] or to the study of power and social justice,[10] could preclude progress on decreasing structural health inequities and improving population health.

Second, by examining the occupational determinants of health and well-being for Indigenous populations, Shannon et al. show concern for the role of employment and the opportunity it presents for interventions to improve health and reduce health inequities. Reflecting on the finding that employment-related outcomes differed among the three Indigenous groups examined, the authors reinforce the need for occupational health research to study population subgroups separately to accurately distinguish the effect of cultural and social factors on the health and well-being of each subgroup.

Public health researchers' concern for examining the role of employment on health is not new or limited to Indigenous populations. In recent decades, employment, a key social determinant of health and well-being, garnered increased attention, in the context of well-documented decreases in employment quality and the intensification of nonstandard and precarious forms of employment.[11,12] In this context, the range of theoretical and methodological approaches used by researchers to examine the impact of employment on workers has expanded significantly, reflecting intensified efforts to capture the diversity of effects caused by low-quality employment and their interactions.[3,11,12] Additionally, there is increased acknowledgment among public health researchers that low-quality employment does not affect all population subgroups equally, but places a heavier toll on the health and well-being of individuals and groups from underrepresented and underserved communities.[3,11,12] For example, historically deprived or oppressed groups, including Indigenous populations, are exposed to numerous sources of oppression, including the individual and combined effects of social determinants such as colonial violence and displacement, treaty violations and resource exploitation, cultural suppression (e.g., boarding schools), and systemic racism.[1,4,7] Accordingly, research approaches should demonstrate attention to interwoven issues of power and structural inequalities and avoid using compartmentalized approaches[10] to study the causes of economic and social inequities, environmental health risks, trauma and mental disorders, and overall ill health.

The study by Shannon et al. is a relevant and timely contribution to this journal issue, a convincing reminder of the complex links between employment and population health. We make several additional recommendations, building on arguments made by the authors. First, we believe the redefining of Indigenous groups must consider ongoing debates about the use of pan-ethnic terms (e.g., American Indian). For example, although the strategy to use pan-ethnic identities is meant to unite groups against discrimination, this approach could hide important historical, cultural, and economic differences among groups. Related to this, the use of the term Hispanic is rejected by many Latino/Latinx communities who argue that it hides the variety of "Hispanic" subgroups with distinct cultures and history. Additionally, the mere use of labels, without political, economic, and cultural explanations, to facilitate an understanding of the contextual nature of current differences in health profiles among Indigenous groups in the United States could lead to further stigmatization of certain tribes. Further, a focus on the demographic traits of individuals or groups without situating them in the political, economic, and cultural context in which the root causes of inequities lie, is misplaced and will impede real change. In addition to collecting information on individuals or groups, obtaining data on context and upstream root causes of ill health and inequities is a priority for action and structural changes if we are to improve inequities between groups.

Second, we argue that a thorough understanding of the impact of employment on health requires the study of employment and working conditions, in addition to a focus on occupational factors. Additionally, taking stock of specific employment-related factors and processes influencing the health of diverse population subgroups is not sufficient. Implementation research is equally important to facilitate targeted action to improve employment and occupational outcomes among Indigenous populations through addressing the risk factors identified for each subgroup or strengthening aspects recognized for their health-enhancing potential.

Because employment is increasingly recognized as a significant determinant of health, contributing to health and social inequities, a thorough understanding of employment-related determinants of health is a key prerequisite for improving population health.[11,12]

Accordingly, public health researchers interested in improving health and well-being among diverse populations, including Indigenous nations, should expand their focus from occupational determinants to the impact of employment and working conditions. Additionally, public health researchers could strengthen their contribution to the elimination of health inequities through adopting intersectional approaches that reveal the heterogeneity of factors and processes influencing people's health and well-being[7,10] and participatory community-led research that captures the diversity of the populations studied and channels their voices.[8] AJPH

CORRESPONDENCE

Correspondence should be sent to Virginia Gunn, 1250 Grand Lake Rd, Sydney, Nova Scotia B1P 6L2, Canada (e-mail: virginia.gunn@cbu.ca). Reprints can be ordered at https://www.ajph.org by clicking the "Reprints" link.

PUBLICATION INFORMATION

Full Citation: Gunn V, O'Campo P, Muntaner C. Exploring Indigenous health and employment: methods to capture diversity and intersecting factors. *Am J Public Health*. 2025;115(5):634–636.

Acceptance Date: January 11, 2025.

DOI: https://doi.org/10.2105/AJPH.2025.308030

ORCID iD:
Virginia Gunn https://orcid.org/0000-0003-3104-9539

CONTRIBUTORS

V. Gunn conceptualized and drafted the initial version of the manuscript. P. O'Campo and C. Muntaner contributed written entries and provided critical feedback, supported the identification of relevant references, and helped revise drafts of the manuscript. All authors read and approved the final manuscript, and are responsible for the overall content.

CONFLICTS OF INTEREST

The authors have no conflicts of interest in regard to this study.

REFERENCES

1. Dunbar-Ortiz R. *An Indigenous Peoples' History of the United States.* Boston,MA: Beacon Press; 2023.
2. United Nations General Assembly. United Nations Declaration on the Rights of Indigenous Peoples. Available at: https://www.un.org/development/desa/indigenouspeoples/wp-content/uploads/sites/19/2018/11/UNDRIP_E_web.pdf?v=010703. Accessed January 3, 2025.
3. Cubrich M, Tengesdal JA, Ugueto-Rey G, Stahl R, Crow Brauer M. Pandemics and precarious work: translating research to practice for marginalized workers. *Transl Issues Psychol Sci.* 2022;8(3):416–430. https://doi.org/10.1037/tps0000327
4. Warne D, Frizzell LB. American Indian health policy: historical trends and contemporary issues. *Am J Public Health.* 2014;104(suppl 3):S263–S267. https://doi.org/10.2105/AJPH.2013.301682
5. King MP, Smith AMD, Gracey MP. Indigenous health part 2: the underlying causes of the health gap. *Lancet.* 2009;374(9683):76–85. https://doi.org/10.1016/S0140-6736(09)60827-8
6. Valeggia CR, Snodgrass JJ. Health of Indigenous peoples. *Annu Rev Anthropol.* 2015;44(1):117–135. https://doi.org/10.1146/annurev-anthro-102214-013831
7. World Health Organization. COVID-19 and the social determinants of health and health equity: evidence brief. 2021. Available at: https://iris.who.int/handle/10665/348333. Accessed January 3, 2025.
8. Wilkinson CF. *Blood Struggle: The Rise of Modern Indian Nations.* New York, NY: WW Norton & Company; 2005.
9. Kauh TJ. Read JG, Scheitler AJ. The critical role of racial/ethnic data disaggregation for health equity. *Popul Res Policy Rev.* 2021;40(1):1–7. https://doi.org/10.1007/s11113-020-09631-6
10. Bowleg L. Evolving intersectionality within public health: from analysis to action. *Am J Public Health.* 2021;111(1):88–90. https://doi.org/10.2105/AJPH.2020.306031
11. International Labour Organization. Non-standard employment around the world: understanding challenges, shaping prospects. Available at: https://www.ilo.org/sites/default/files/wcmsp5/groups/public/%40dgreports/%40dcomm/%40publ/documents/publication/wcms_534326.pdf. Accessed August 10, 2021.
12. Benach J, Muntaner C. Precarious employment and health: developing a research agenda. *J Epidemiol Community Health.* 2007;61(4):276–277. https://doi.org/10.1136/jech.2005.045237

Housing as a Determinant of Health: A Population-Level Approach

Andrew Fenelon, PhD

ABOUT THE AUTHOR

The author is with the Division of Epidemiology and Community Health, the Minnesota Population Center, and the Life Course Center for the Demography and Economics of Aging, University of Minnesota-Twin Cities, Minneapolis.

See also Routhier, p. 640, and Garrison et al., p. 780.

Housing is a well-known social determinant of population health, and the effects of housing on health are multidimensional and occur at multiple levels.[1] The nationwide housing affordability crisis has brought renewed scholarly and legislative attention to the importance of housing. Half of renters nationwide struggle to afford their housing, paying more than 30% of income toward rent.[2] As the cost of housing has risen, it has eclipsed other household expenses including food and transportation and represents the largest expenditure for all but the wealthiest households.

Historically, housing quality in the United States has been comparatively poor; one fifth of housing units in 1934 were so poor that they were considered "unfit for habitation," and another one fifth lacked modern plumbing or heat.[3] During much of the 19th and 20th centuries, studies linking housing and health focused heavily on improving the quality of the physical structure.[4] As average housing quality improved, the research focus shifted to less direct pathways such as affordability and neighborhood context. But the distinction between physical quality and other aspects of housing is not as clear as it may seem.

In this issue of *AJPH*, Garrison et al. adeptly synthesize the importance of the physical characteristics of housing with the economic and contextual considerations. In doing so, they produce arguably the most comprehensive spatial assessment to date of housing circumstances at the neighborhood level, an index term "housing quality dimensions" (HQD). Focusing on physical inadequacy, housing cost burdens, and poor neighborhood perceptions, they produce a nationwide census tract–level data source of the state of housing quality. They skillfully highlight that housing affordability, physical quality, and neighborhood context, far from being independent aspects of housing, are deeply interrelated issues. Indeed, families struggling financially often sacrifice on housing or neighborhood quality to stay within their budget.

The authors draw on detailed American Housing Survey housing quality metrics and use observable household characteristics to model the presence of housing quality concerns. Once modeled, they apply those results to national data from the American Community Survey in a detailed spatial analysis, identifying census tracts with high predicted levels on the three dimensions. The results are striking: individuals in 63% of housing units experience at least one housing quality concern, more than 40% of US census tracts are in the top quartile on at least one dimension, and 10% of tracts are in the top quartile on all three dimensions.

They also identify associations between HQD and geospatially referenced measures of adult health conditions that might be expected to respond to poor housing quality. Residents of the most housing-distressed neighborhoods report rates of fair or poor health that are two to three times those of residents of the least distressed neighborhoods, net of demographic and socioeconomic composition. Connecting these housing quality dimensions to population health is a significant contribution, particularly given increasing recognition of the importance of secure, high-quality housing as a platform for investments in health and well-being.

Innovative research on housing and health that is sufficiently high quality to inform successful interventions requires creative data integration. Because the United States lacks a comprehensive registry of housing quality issues, researchers must join multiple data sources to develop one. The American Housing Survey and American Community Survey are inadequate in isolation but provide significant value when combined.

The HQD index has several strengths—including coverage, comprehensiveness, and interoperability—with immediate benefits for various constituencies. For example, nationwide coverage permits local public health agencies to identify neighborhoods in their jurisdictions at the greatest need of resource investment related to housing and infrastructure. In addition, comprehensive assessments of many dimensions of housing quality can be valuable to public housing agencies in identifying hotspots of housing quality concerns. Finally, the interoperability of the index allows researchers to merge their own data, including data on residential segregation, environmental exposures, medical records, and housing program participation. Thus, developing the metric itself is a significant contribution, with myriad applications for both research and practice.

However, an equally significant and more nuanced contribution is conceptual: recognizing that forces beyond the individual are responsible for structuring exposure to housing-related concerns. Census tracts with more housing quality issues also have residents who experience other dimensions of economic disadvantage, and these residents report more health problems. Even if not directly causally related, the co-occurrence of these measures of disadvantage is troubling from the perspective of health equity. Garrison and colleagues' article joins recent work that seeks to reconceptualize housing concerns, not as a result of individual-level choices but as a reflection of unjust sociopolitical forces that constrain household decision making and heighten adverse exposures.[5,6] The population-level focus of the HQD reminds us that these forces operate at levels beyond the individual or family.

What is missing from the HQD? If anything, it is the importance of housing stability, which is difficult to measure with the American Housing Survey. Unstable housing can be deadly; work by Graetz et al.[7] draws attention to the severe health effects of experiencing an eviction, which is both a consequence and a cause of economic precarity. Families at risk of eviction may be hesitant to push landlords to improve housing conditions for fear that it will precipitate displacement. Similarly, families struggling to afford their housing are at higher risk of an eviction.[8] Housing instability may have unique linkages to health, particularly if frequent moves make it difficult to develop health-related routines, invest in connections to care providers, or maintain employment or schooling.

Where do we go from here? As housing has gained renewed appreciation for its enduring impact on health, federal rental assistance policies have largely prioritized neighborhood context through an emphasis on the housing choice voucher program. Housing vouchers offer the possibility to move to higher opportunity neighborhoods, but the program relies on private landlords who may have little incentive to improve the physical quality of units beyond meeting basic standards.

In contrast, public housing offers the opportunity to directly invest in the quality of housing. Despite large improvements in physical housing quality over the past century, exposure to substandard housing remains a significant disparity mechanism. Although just 2% of renter households experience severely inadequate housing, 54% of these households have incomes below 50% of their area median.[9] Tenant organizers recognize the importance of working with a public entity to improve housing conditions, as private landlords are often unresponsive to tenant concerns. A push for broader public ownership and management of affordable housing would be a welcome development, one bolstered by evidence that public housing may be more effective than other housing programs in reducing resident lead exposure.[10] Public housing's primary source of criticism—that it tends to be located in disadvantaged neighborhoods[11]—highlights the importance of building public housing developments in areas of economic opportunity and linking them with high-quality public services.

Secure access to housing at an affordable price in a safe neighborhood represents a bundle of goods that has multifaceted effects on health but proves difficult to achieve given the housing affordability crisis nationwide. As scholars and policymakers work to address challenges such as the rising cost of housing, unaccountable private landlords, and distressed neighborhoods isolated from the economic dynamism of large cities, the index developed by Garrison et al. promises to be extremely valuable in directing the conversation. AJPH

CORRESPONDENCE

Correspondence should be sent to Andrew Fenelon, PhD, Division of Epidemiology and Community Health, West Bank Office Building, 1300 S 2nd St Suite 300, Minneapolis, MN 55454 (e-mail: afenelon@umn.edu). Reprints can be ordered at https://www.ajph.org by clicking the "Reprints" link.

PUBLICATION INFORMATION

Full Citation: Fenelon A. Housing as a determinant of health: a population-level approach. *Am J Public Health*. 2025;115(5):637–639.

Acceptance Date: January 31, 2025.

DOI: https://doi.org/10.2105/AJPH.2025.308053

ORCID iD:
Andrew Fenelon https://orcid.org/0000-0001-7097-1679

ACKNOWLEDGMENTS

I gratefully acknowledge support from the University of Minnesota Life Course Center on the Demography and Economics of Aging (grant P30AG066613), funded through the National Institute on Aging, and from the Minnesota Population Center (grant P2C HD041023), funded through the Eunice Kennedy Shriver National Institute for Child Health and Human Development.

CONFLICTS OF INTEREST

The author reports no conflicts of interest.

REFERENCES

1. Swope CB, Hernández D. Housing as a determinant of health equity: a conceptual model. *Soc*

Sci Med. 2019;243:112571. https://doi.org/10.1016/j.socscimed.2019.112571

2. Joint Center for Housing Studies. The state of the nation's housing 2023. Available at: https://www.jchs.harvard.edu/sites/default/files/reports/files/Harvard_JCHS_The_State_of_the_Nations_Housing_2023.pdf. Accessed February 7, 2024.
3. Bauer C. Housing in the United States—problems and policy. *Int Labour Rev*. 1945;52:1–28.
4. Riis J. *How the Other Half Lives: Studies among the Tenements of New York*. Charles Scribner's Sons; 1890. https://doi.org/10.1037/12986-000
5. Schwartz GL, Leifheit KM, Arcaya MC, Keene D. Eviction as a community health exposure. *Soc Sci Med*. 2024;340:116496. https://doi.org/10.1016/j.socscimed.2023.116496
6. Keene DE, Blankenship KM. The affordable rental housing crisis and population health equity: a multidimensional and multilevel framework. *J Urban Health*. 2023;100(6):1212–1223. https://doi.org/10.1007/s11524-023-00799-8
7. Graetz N, Gershenson C, Porter SR, Sandler DH, Lemmerman E, Desmond M. The impacts of rent burden and eviction on mortality in the United States, 2000–2019. *Soc Sci Med*. 2024;340:116398. https://doi.org/10.1016/j.socscimed.2023.116398
8. Hepburn P, Louis R, Fish J, et al. US eviction filing patterns in 2020. *Socius*. 2021;7(22):237802312110099. https://doi.org/10.1177/23780231211009983
9. Alvarez TA, Steffen BL. Worst case housing needs: 2023 report to Congress. Available at: https://www.huduser.gov/portal/publications/Worst-Case-Housing-Needs-2023.html. Accessed January 6, 2025.
10. Chu MT, Fenelon A, Rodriguez J, Zota AR, Adamkiewicz G. Development of a multidimensional housing and environmental quality index (HEQI): application to the American Housing Survey. *Environ Health*. 2022;21(1):56. https://doi.org/10.1186/s12940-022-00866-8
11. Newman SJ, Holupka CS. Race and assisted housing. *Hous Policy Debate*. 2017;27(5):751–771. https://doi.org/10.1080/10511482.2017.1311275

Advancing a Research and Policy Agenda on Housing and Health

Giselle Routhier, PhD, MSW

ABOUT THE AUTHOR

Giselle Routhier is with the Department of Population Health, NYU Grossman School of Medicine, New York, NY.

See also Fenelon, p. 637, and Garrison et al., p. 780.

There is ample evidence that housing and health are intertwined in many ways. Experiencing an eviction is linked to poor child health outcomes.[1] Homelessness is associated with increased mortality and premature aging.[2,3] Living in unaffordable or crowded housing is associated with worse physical and mental health, as well as more chronic health conditions.[4,5] Poor-quality housing, which may include mold, allergens, inadequate ventilation, and pests, is linked with chronic health conditions such as asthma and cardiovascular disease.[6] However, research on housing and health has been hindered by data availability, which limits studies to look at only one aspect of housing at a time, a limited geographic area, or certain populations.

In their article "Housing Quality Dimensions (HQD): Neighborhood-Level Data, Housing Quality, and Population Health," Veronica Garrison et al. (p. 780) leverage three large data sets to present a new nationwide measure of multiple housing challenges at the census tract level, combining indicators of poor physical conditions, unaffordability, and poor neighborhood perceptions into a multidimensional measure. The resulting Housing Quality Dimensions (HQD) shows a link between higher HQD scores (indicating worse quality housing) and poor self-rated health, poor physical health, and poor mental health.

Several important points emerge from the authors' approach to quantifying housing challenges across the United States. First, this research confirms that the prevalence of housing challenges is high, bolstering findings from previous work[7,8] and underscoring the urgent need for research and policy interventions to improve housing conditions, stability, and affordability. Second, how we define housing insecurity matters. Garrison et al. found variation across the country in HQD, with poor physical conditions most prevalent on the West Coast and in the Southwest and a high prevalence of housing cost burden concentrated in the Northeast. Additionally, there was variation in the multidimensional nature of the HQD, with some tracts showing high rates of just one dimension and other tracts showing all three. Third, we lack precise, nationwide data on multidimensional housing insecurity and health at the individual and small geographic levels. Garrison et al. provide a novel approach to filling this gap by combining multiple data sets with advanced statistical methods. At the same time, their work highlights the lack of nationwide data collected on both housing and health.

To move toward a better collective understanding of the relationship between housing and health, as well as where to intervene to improve housing and health outcomes, a robust research and policy agenda is warranted and should consider the following points.

1. Public health and housing researchers should work toward a standardized way of measuring housing challenges. Recent scholarship has begun to define housing challenges (also variably labeled as housing insecurity, instability, quality, or hardship) in a multidimensional way, including using measures of physical quality, unaffordability, crowding, forced or frequent moves, and neighborhood conditions.[4,7,9] Some housing dimensions, such as affordability and crowding, for the most part have been measured consistently across research, using housing cost burden and persons per room. Others, such as unit conditions, instability, and neighborhood perceptions, vary considerably in their operationalization. Consensus on what measures to use and when can help lay a foundation for a better understanding of the relationships between housing and health. Recently, the US Department of Housing and Urban Development (HUD) developed and validated an index measure of housing insecurity using data from the American Housing Survey and a one-time supplemental survey module, the Housing Insecurity Research Module, administered in 2019.[10] It included measures

AJPH May 2025, Vol. 115, No. 5

of cost, frequent and forced moves, safety, quality, and crowding. However, they noted a need for further testing to ensure applicability and consistency across data sets and populations. Regardless of operationalization, multiple dimensions of housing challenges must be examined collectively, as they may affect health in different ways and in different directions, and households may experience some or all of these challenges simultaneously.

2. Researchers and policymakers should root their work in an understanding of the role that systemic racism and historical and contemporary policies have played in furthering housing challenges and their unequal distribution. Redlining, restrictive racial covenants, neighborhood displacement, disinvestment in public housing, and subprime loans, among other policies, have deeply shaped the prevalence and distribution of housing challenges in the United States. Swope and Hernández[11] and Leifheit et al.[12] put forth useful conceptual models toward understanding the pathways through which housing and health are intertwined within the context of these systemic factors.
3. Large-scale individual-level longitudinal data are needed to understand causality and the direction of relationships between housing and health metrics. Some researchers have leveraged longitudinal data sets with different primary goals to understand health and housing relationships for specific populations, including young people[9] and older adults,[7] but Garrison et al.'s work highlights the dearth of data that focus on simultaneously understanding housing challenges and health at the population level. In addition to understanding causality, examining the compounding effects of housing challenges over time and the life course is important, given emerging trends showing increasing homelessness among both children and older adults.
4. The perspectives of people with lived experience of housing insecurity should be promoted alongside academic research. Hearing directly from affected people is crucial to illustrating and deepening our understanding of the mechanisms by which housing influences specific health outcomes, and vice versa. The Health x Housing ("health by housing") Lab at NYU Grossman School of Medicine, which I codirect, recently launched a Speakers Bureau and Peer Network comprising 10 individuals with lived experience of housing insecurity, with the aim of connecting researchers, policymakers, and health care providers with people with direct experience of housing insecurity. Such partnerships are crucial to furthering understanding and inclusiveness in research on housing and health and to developing solutions that are feasible, acceptable, and effective.

With severe housing shortages affecting nearly every region of the country and record-setting levels of homelessness, interventions are urgently needed to address the high prevalence of housing challenges across the nation toward the goal of safe, secure, and affordable housing for all. The proposed research and policy agenda could be advanced in several ways. Researchers at HUD have taken important steps toward operationalizing housing insecurity and could act as a convener of researchers in the public health and housing realms to advance a consistent measurement of the concept. Simultaneously, academic institutions should work toward building large-scale cohort data with the specific intent of studying the relationship between housing and health metrics. Ideally, federal funding would support such work focused on US population health, but in the absence of federal support, philanthropic organizations interested in housing, racial and economic justice, and social determinants of health should step in. On an individual level, researchers and policymakers should partner with community organizations and individuals with lived experience to create inclusive and collaborative environments to advance research and policymaking at the intersection of housing and health. AJPH

CORRESPONDENCE

Correspondence should be sent to Giselle Routhier, 180 Madison Ave, 9th Fl, New York, NY 10016 (e-mail: giselle.routhier@nyulangone.org). Reprints can be ordered at https://www.ajph.org by clicking the "Reprints" link.

PUBLICATION INFORMATION

Full Citation: Routhier G. Advancing a research and policy agenda on housing and health. *Am J Public Health*. 2025;115(5):640–642.

Acceptance Date: January 31, 2025.

DOI: https://doi.org/10.2105/AJPH.2025.308054

ORCID iD:
Giselle Routhier https://orcid.org/0000-0003-2435-2396

ACKNOWLEDGMENTS

This work was supported in part by the Community Service Plan at NYU Langone Health.

CONFLICTS OF INTEREST

The author has no conflicts of interest to report.

REFERENCES

1. Ramphal B, Keen R, Okuzuno SS, Ojogho D, Slopen N. Evictions and infant and child health outcomes: a systematic review. *JAMA Netw Open.* 2023;6(4):e237612. https://doi.org/10.1001/jamanetworkopen.2023.7612
2. Fowle MZ, Routhier G. Mortal systemic exclusion yielded steep mortality-rate increases in people experiencing homelessness, 2011–20. *Health Aff (Millwood).* 2024;43(2):226–233. https://doi.org/10.1377/hlthaff.2023.01039
3. Brown RT, Hemati K, Riley ED, et al. Geriatric conditions in a population-based sample of older homeless adults. *Gerontologist.* 2017;57(4):757–766. https://doi.org/10.1093/geront/gnw011
4. Bhat AC, Almeida DM, Fenelon A, Santos-Lozada AR. A longitudinal analysis of the relationship between housing insecurity and physical health among midlife and aging adults in the United States. *SSM Popul Health.* 2022;18:101128. https://doi.org/10.1016/j.ssmph.2022.101128
5. Nakphong MK, Bright DJ, Koreitem A, et al. Housing instability patterns among low-income, urban black young adults in California and associations with mental health outcomes: baseline data from a randomized waitlist-controlled trial. *BMC Public Health.* 2024;24(1):2492. https://doi.org/10.1186/s12889-024-19948-y
6. Krieger J, Higgins DL. Housing and health: time again for public health action. *Am J Public Health.* 2002;92(5):758–768. https://doi.org/10.2105/AJPH.92.5.758
7. Paredes LG, Wang Y, Keene DE, Gill TM, Becher RD. Population-based estimates of major forms of housing insecurity among community-living older Americans. *J Am Geriatr Soc.* 2024;72(12):3773–3783. https://doi.org/10.1111/jgs.19167
8. Routhier G. Beyond worst case needs: measuring the breadth and severity of housing insecurity among urban renters. *Hous Policy Debate.* 2019;29(2):235–249. https://doi.org/10.1080/10511482.2018.1509228
9. Pierce KA, Mendelsohn A, Smith B, Johnson SB, Duh-Leong C. Trajectories of housing insecurity from infancy to adolescence and adolescent health outcomes. *Pediatrics.* 2024;154(2):e2023064551. https://doi.org/10.1542/peds.2023-064551
10. Murdoch J, Brahmachari M, Okyere D, Moumen F, Streiff S. Measuring housing insecurity: index development using American Housing Survey data. US Dept of Housing and Urban Development. Available at: https://www.huduser.gov/portal/publications/Measuring-Housing-Insecurity-Index-Development-Using-AHS-Data.html. Accessed January 23, 2025.
11. Swope CB, Hernández D. Housing as a determinant of health equity: a conceptual model. *Soc Sci Med.* 2019;243:112571. https://doi.org/10.1016/j.socscimed.2019.112571
12. Leifheit KM, Schwartz GL, Pollack CE, Linton SL. Building health equity through housing policies: critical reflections and future directions for research. *J Epidemiol Community Health.* 2022;76(8):759–763. https://doi.org/10.1136/jech-2021-216439

Why Achieving Health Equity for Indigenous Peoples Requires Indigenizing the Social Determinants of Health

Valarie Blue Bird Jernigan, DrPH, MPH, and Tara L. Maudrie, PhD, MSPH

ABOUT THE AUTHORS

Valarie Blue Bird Jernigan is with the Center for Indigenous Health Research and Policy, Oklahoma State University Center for Health Sciences, Tulsa. At the time of this research, Tara L. Maudrie was with the Johns Hopkins School of Public Health, Baltimore, MD.

See also Oré et al., p. 726.

Indigenous peoples in the United States experience significant health disparities. American Indians and Alaska Natives (AI/ANs) have the highest prevalence of type 2 diabetes of any population group in the country[1]; higher incidence rates of liver, stomach, kidney, lung, colorectal, and breast cancers than other populations[2]; and the highest age-adjusted suicide rates of any population group.[3] The life expectancy of AI/ANs is seven years less than that of the US general population,[4] declining from 72 years in 2019 to 65 years in 2021.[4] Although the COVID-19 pandemic led to a dramatic drop in life expectancy among AI/ANs, COVID-19 alone does not account for this disparity.[5] During the two decades before COVID-19, the life expectancy of AI/ANs remained stagnant while continuing to rise in all other population groups.[5] Similar trends have been observed in Canada, New Zealand, and Australia, where gaps in health outcomes between Indigenous and non-Indigenous people are stagnating and, in some cases, even worsening.[6]

The social determinants of health (SDOH)—the social conditions in which people are born, grow, live, and age—are widely recognized as the primary influences of health. The World Health Organization and others expand on these determinants to include structural determinants such as governance, macroeconomic policies, social policies, culture, and societal values.

In this issue of *AJPH*, Oré et al. (p. 726) assert that the pervasive nature of AI/AN health disparities highlights limitations of the current framing of the SDOH for Indigenous peoples. The authors describe interconnected social contexts and conditions beyond the mainstream SDOH that shape the health and well-being of Indigenous peoples. They propose four important constructs to guide an Indigenous SDOH framework: sovereignty and governance, language and identity, land and kinship, and Indigenous knowledge, worldviews, and practices. They argue that incorporating these constructs into an SDOH framework is necessary to eliminate Indigenous health disparities and provides a lens to recognize the unique histories, strengths, and challenges faced by Indigenous communities. The authors emphasize the importance of co-creating SDOH frameworks alongside Indigenous communities using a collaborative approach to ensure that Indigenous knowledge systems and lived experiences are centered, positioning this work as a critical contribution to decolonizing public health and eliminating disparities.

We agree with this important reframing and extend the authors' perspective to include two additional points. First, structural racism and settler colonialism are interrelated, ongoing, and enduring forces that undermine the health of Indigenous peoples and other racial groups and must be included in SDOH frameworks to more effectively address health disparities.[7] Second, an Indigenous SDOH model such as that proposed by Oré et al. offers lessons not just for Indigenous health but also for reimagining health systems for all peoples.

The current SDOH framework fails to include many of the integral factors causing health disparities, perhaps most important structural racism. Yearby[8] argues that structural racism, the way systems are structured to advantage the majority and disadvantage racial and ethnic minorities, is the root cause of racial health disparities. Yearby outlines several ways in which US law structures the employment system in a racially discriminatory way, resulting in racial health disparities.[8] For Indigenous populations, who globally experience the greatest disparities in health, settler colonialism is identified as the most important determinant of health and further elucidates racism's impact on health.[7] Even modern racialization is seen as an extension of

AJPH May 2025, Vol. 115, No. 5

settler colonialism and serves to solidify colonial powers.[7]

All of the determinants of health for Indigenous peoples—social and structural—interact with and are affected by settler colonialism as it manifests in both historical and contemporary ways. For example, Indigenous erasure, the process whereby settler societies disregard and eliminate the presence of AI/AN peoples, cultures, knowledges, and sovereignty, is evidenced in the ongoing exclusion of AI/ANs from national health data sets and the narrative that all AI/ANs have long vanished.[9] Efforts to eliminate tribal sovereignty,[10] assimilate AI/AN culture,[11] and pollute and exploit AI/AN lands[12–14] are continuous and persistent. Because structural racism and settler colonialism are intertwined—one cannot exist without the other—these powerful forces continue to threaten and undermine the health of Indigenous people as well as the health of the planet. Explicitly naming these forces in SDOH frameworks alone is not sufficient, but it will allow the opportunity to further understand health disparities from Indigenous perspectives and develop interventions that can more effectively eliminate Indigenous health disparities.

Oré et al. propose constructs of sovereignty, identity, kinship, and intergenerational knowledge that are rooted in Indigenous experiences, worldviews, and intergenerational wisdom. However, these constructs hold resonance for more than just Indigenous peoples. Indigenous frameworks and conceptualizations of health often emphasize the interconnectedness of physical, spiritual, emotional, and relational health as inseparable components of well-being. This holistic approach to health recognizes the complexity of human health and offers an approach rooted in health as a collective value and responsibility, addressing gaps in Western health systems that often compartmentalize care and neglect relational and environmental dimensions of health.

As noted by Ore at al., for Indigenous peoples the physical world is inseparable from human experience. Extending this perspective beyond Indigenous peoples, it becomes clear that all people are inextricably linked to their environments through the food they eat, the water they drink, and the air they breathe. Indigenous peoples, as the original stewards of Turtle Island (now North America), hold invaluable knowledge about how to live in reciprocity with land and waterways to promote holistic health, not only for humans but for all of our relations. Indigenous teachings and worldviews remind us that health, rather than being an individual endeavor, is a collective responsibility that requires reciprocity with ourselves, one another, and the natural world. By applying values from these Indigenous-centered frameworks, public health systems can move toward more comprehensive and relational strategies to improve the health of all people.

The constructs proposed by Oré et al. and other Indigenous-centered frameworks are crucial not only for their potential to eliminate health disparities in Indigenous communities but also because they offer perspectives to guide the field of public health to be a more inclusive, effective, and socially just discipline that serves the holistic health needs of all people. Indigenous health frameworks are not just for Indigenous peoples; they are powerful blueprints for building holistic and sustainable health systems that benefit all people.

To translate Indigenous-centered frameworks into meaningful change, the public health community must take deliberate, collaborative, and sustained actions. Policymakers, researchers, and public health practitioners have an opportunity—and a responsibility—to create environments where Indigenous health frameworks can thrive. Long-term investments in Indigenous-led health initiatives, including research, education, and program development, are essential for creating systems that align with Indigenous values and knowledge. Public health systems should seek to learn from and integrate Indigenous knowledge and practices while ensuring that these collaborations are equitable and rooted in mutual respect. Educational initiatives that elevate Indigenous perspectives in public health curricula, such as the Indigenous SDOH training developed by Oré et al., can help train the next generation of practitioners to approach public health work with cultural humility and relational accountability.

Finally, public health must embrace its role in addressing the structural inequities, including settler colonialism, that perpetuate health disparities. By centering Indigenous health frameworks, we can reimagine public health systems that honor the interconnectedness of people, communities, and the natural world and the transformative power in these connections. The time for action is now, and the path forward is clear: build with, listen to, and amplify Indigenous voices so that good health becomes a shared reality for all. AJPH

CORRESPONDENCE

Correspondence should be sent to Valarie Blue Bird Jernigan, DrPH, MPH, Center for Indigenous Health Research and Policy, 5310 E 31st St, Suite 1011, Tulsa, OK 74135 (e-mail: bluebird.jernigan@okstate.edu). Reprints can be ordered at https://www.ajph.org by clicking the "Reprints" link.

PUBLICATION INFORMATION

Full Citation: Blue Bird Jernigan V, Maudrie TL. Why achieving health equity for Indigenous peoples requires indigenizing the social determinants of health. *Am J Public Health*. 2025;115(5):643–645.

Acceptance Date: February 4, 2025.

DOI: https://doi.org/10.2105/AJPH.2025.308059

ORCID iD:
Valarie Blue Bird Jernigan https://orcid.org/0000-0002-3965-8518

CONTRIBUTORS

The authors contributed equally to this work.

ACKNOWLEDGMENTS

This work would not have been possible without the collective effort and collaboration of those who recognize the vital importance of centering Indigenous knowledge and self-determination in public health, miigwetch, yakoke—thank you. To the knowledge keepers, community leaders, researchers, and advocates who tirelessly work to uplift the voices of our peoples—your wisdom and resilience are the foundation upon which we build pathways to equity and healing. To the elders who share teachings rooted in intergenerational wisdoms, and to the young people who carry these teachings forward with courage, we honor your role in connecting us across time to shape a brighter future for Indigenous health. To the communities whose lived realities inspire and guide Indigenous health frameworks, thank you for your strength and for entrusting the world with your stories and solutions. May we all continue this journey together, grounded in relational accountability, to ensure that the frameworks we build reflect the richness and diversity of Indigenous ways of knowing and being.

CONFLICTS OF INTEREST

The authors have no conflicts of interest to report.

REFERENCES

1. Villarroel MA, Clark TC, Norris T. Health of American Indian and Alaska Native adults, by urbanization level: United States, 2014–2018. *NCHS Data Brief*. 2020;372:1–8.
2. Melkonian SC, Weir HK, Jim MA, Preikschat B, Haverkamp D, White MC. Incidence of and trends in the leading cancers with elevated incidence among American Indian and Alaska Native populations, 2012–2016. *Am J Epidemiol*. 2020;190(4):528–538. https://doi.org/10.1093/aje/kwaa222
3. Stone D, Mack K, Qualters J. Recent changes in suicide rates, by race and ethnicity and age group—United States, 2021. *MMWR Morb Mortal Wkly Rep*. 2023;72(6):160–162. https://doi.org/10.15585/mmwr.mm7206a4
4. Arias E, Tejada-Vera B, Ahmad F, Kochanek KD. Provisional life expectancy estimates for January through June, 2020. Available at: https://stacks.cdc.gov/view/cdc/100392. Accessed December 20, 2024.
5. Dwyer-Lindgren L, Kendrick P, Kelly YO, et al. Life expectancy by county, race, and ethnicity in the USA, 2000–19: a systematic analysis of health disparities. *Lancet*. 2022;400(10345):25–38. https://doi.org/10.1016/S0140-6736(22)00876-5
6. Mitrou F, Cooke M, Lawrence D, et al. Gaps in Indigenous disadvantage not closing: a census cohort study of social determinants of health in Australia, Canada, and New Zealand from 1981–2006. *BMC Public Health*. 2014;14(1):201. https://doi.org/10.1186/1471-2458-14-201
7. Wispelwey B, Tanous O, Asi Y, Hammoudeh W, Mills D. Because its power remains naturalized: introducing the settler colonial determinants of health. *Front Public Health*. 2023;11:1137428. https://doi.org/10.3389/fpubh.2023.1137428
8. Yearby R. Structural racism and health disparities: reconfiguring the social determinants of health framework to include the root cause. *J Law Med Ethics*. 2020;48(3):518–526. https://doi.org/10.1177/1073110520958876
9. Orr R, Sharratt K, Iqbal M. American Indian erasure and the logic of elimination: an experimental study of depiction and support for resources and rights for tribes. *JEMS*. 2019;45(11):2078–2099. https://doi.org/10.1080/1369183X.2017.1421061
10. VanSickle A. Supreme Court upholds Native American adoption law. Available at: https://www.nytimes.com/2023/06/15/us/supreme-court-native-american-children-tribes.html. Accessed December 20, 2024.
11. Levitt Z, Parshina-Kottas Y, Romero S, Wallace T. War against the children. Available at: https://www.nytimes.com/interactive/2023/08/30/us/native-american-boarding-schools.html. Accessed December 20, 2024.
12. Macmillan L. Uranium mines dot Navajo land, neglected and still perilous. Available at: https://www.nytimes.com/2012/04/01/us/uranium-mines-dot-navajo-land-neglected-and-still-perilous.html. Accessed December 20, 2024.
13. Friedman L. Standing Rock Sioux tribe wins a victory in Dakota access pipeline case. Available at: https://www.nytimes.com/2020/03/25/climate/dakota-access-pipeline-sioux.html. Accessed December 20, 2024.
14. Blue Bird Jernigan V, Peercy M, Branam D, et al. Beyond health equity: achieving wellness within American Indian and Alaska Native communities. *Am J Public Health*. 2015;105(suppl 3):S376–S379. https://doi.org/10.2105/AJPH.2014.302447

Polysubstance Use Is Not Synonymous With Poly Substance Use Disorder

Kevin Y. Xu, MD, MPH, Lewei (Allison) Lin, MD, MS, and Richard A. Grucza, PhD

ABOUT THE AUTHORS

Kevin Y. Xu is with the Department of Psychiatry, Washington University School of Medicine, and the Institute for Public Health, Washington University, Saint Louis, MO. Lewei (Allison) Lin is with the Department of Psychiatry, University of Michigan Medical School, and the Center for Clinical Management Research, VA Ann Arbor Healthcare System, Ann Arbor, MI. Richard A. Grucza is with the Department of Family and Community Medicine, Saint Louis University School of Medicine, Saint Louis, MO.

See also Rockhill et al., p. 747.

The term polysubstance use can be defined in a multitude of ways, including any combination of two or more psychoactive drug exposures.[1,2] Unsurprisingly, such a wide-ranging definition of polysubstance use—typically agnostic to the continuum of substance use patterns that exists among people who use drugs—has been difficult to conceptualize in both research studies and clinical encounters. On the one hand, polysubstance use may conjure images of polydrug exposures implicated in overdoses (i.e., co-use of novel synthetic opioids and xylazine[3] in people with multiple substance use disorders). On the other hand, polysubstance use can potentially encompass the usage of psychoactive drugs without the functional impairment conventionally attributable to "addiction" (i.e., recreational cannabis and nicotine vaping). In some cases, polysubstance use may even represent an effort by people seeking to overcome functional impairment from addiction (i.e., using nonprescribed buprenorphine and antidepressants through a lack of access to substance use disorder treatment).[4]

In recent years, our long-standing definitions of polysubstance use have come under rightful critique for their ambiguity and coarseness of exposure measurement.[1,2] However, efforts to develop a rigorous conceptual model for polysubstance use, particularly one that accounts for the nuanced clinical context underlying each polydrug combination,[1,2] are hindered by a lack of nationally representative empirical data. Against this backdrop, the latent class analysis performed by Rockhill et al. (p. 747) identifies four latent classes of polysubstance use in a large nationally representative survey in the United States, the Survey of Non-Medical Use of Prescription Drugs data set. The two largest classes, identified as people with "medically-guided" (class 1) and "self-guided" (class 2) polysubstance exposures, were characterized predominantly by exposure to psychoactive medications either prescribed or taken not as prescribed, especially opioid medicines; class 3 was principally characterized by cannabis exposure; class 4 was marked by heterogeneous patterns of drug exposures (i.e., illicit opioids, recreational drugs, cannabis, controlled and noncontrolled psychoactive prescription medications). Although class 4's drug exposure patterns, described as "indiscriminate," may be consistent with the volatile drug supply landscape in the United States, they also reflect the tremendous diversity of reasons and motives for using different types of psychoactive substances (prescribed or not), including as evidence-based treatments to alleviate undertreated disorders (e.g., the prescribing of routine antidepressants that are not known to be addictive).[3,4]

Whereas polysubstance use is often regarded as synonymous with poly substance use disorders, Rockhill et al. provide data illustrating why these two terms should not be used interchangeably. The authors use a particularly broad definition for polysubstance use that expands beyond drugs typically regarded as "addictive" (i.e., alcohol, opioids) to also encompass noncontrolled medications such as prescription antidepressants. They appropriately differentiate between prescribed and nonprescribed drug exposures, as well as outline the crucial distinction between drug use (drug exposures without functional impairment) and use disorder (drug use patterns that meet clinical criteria for addiction). Importantly, they observed that most people classified as having polysubstance use did not meet the threshold for canonical substance use disorder, with the exception of class 4 (58.9%). By contrast, the authors suggest that people using opioids and other psychoactive medications as prescribed (class 1) have a relatively low risk of any substance use disorder (6.7%) via the Drug Abuse Screening Test (DAST-10), which is known to detect substance use disorders at comparable rates as measured by the National Survey on Drug Use and Health.[5] Notably, people in class 2 (consisting heavily of individuals who use prescription opioids nonmedically) were still at relatively low risk of any substance use disorder (14.5%). Although a considerable proportion of people in class 2 appear to co-use opioids with other substances that raise their risk for drug-related adverse events (i.e., alcohol), illicit drug use was uncommon among people receiving psychoactive medications via prescriptions and nonprescribed routes (classes 1 and 2). Admittedly, Rockhill et al.'s findings do not permit us to assess whether receipt of prescribed or nonprescribed opioids is causing the specific substance use disorders detected via the DAST-10 scale. However, these findings overall do not lend support to the recent concern that individuals receiving prescription opioids are at a substantial risk for transition to "iatrogenic" opioid use disorder, illicit opioids, and other aspects of severe substance use disorder.[6]

Rockhill et al.'s analyses also shed light on a high prevalence of polydrug exposure marked predominantly by cannabis use. Cannabis, which is not typically implicated as the cause for polysubstance-related overdose deaths,[3] is seldom the focus of existing studies on polysubstance use (a largely opioid-centric literature base[3,7–10]). Yet with nearly one fifth (latent class 3) of the sample consisting of individuals with predominant cannabis exposure, it is evident that harm reduction frameworks for cannabis[11] will need to account for complex patterns of polydrug exposures beyond cannabis itself. Although the reasons for observed cannabis use patterns are beyond the scope of Rockhill et al.'s analysis, cannabis has seen rising popularity as an opioid "alternative" (including among people experiencing opioid tapering).[12] Additional studies are needed to clarify how underlying pain-related disorders (50% of the cannabis-predominant latent class; 60% of the overall sample) may influence polydrug exposures and outcomes in people using cannabis.

Looking forward, data-intensive research is urgently needed to study emerging trends, reasons and impacts of co-use, health outcomes, new treatment options, and barriers to care for people with multiple co-occurring substance use disorders. Addiction researchers have traditionally conceptualized substances in isolation, and efforts are needed to develop more rigorous definitions of polysubstance use,[1,2] including clarification of what class 4's "indiscriminate" exposures mean. Further work is particularly needed to understand different patterns of polysubstance use and the often bidirectional factors involved that are difficult to disentangle (e.g., mental health disorders may be a risk factor for polysubstance use, a cause for receiving psychoactive medications, a cause for nonmedical use especially if undertreated,[4] and a potential outcome associated with polysubstance use). Co-occurring substance use disorders as a whole remain understudied and undertreated, with much of the focus on treating individual substances.[7–10]

In conclusion, we think it is crucial for researchers and clinicians to not assume that everyone who uses multiple substances meets criteria for a substance use disorder, as Rockhill et al.'s data clearly show that many people with polysubstance use do not meet criteria for poly substance use disorders. Given the lack of consensus on what polysubstance use means,[1,2] researchers and clinicians should consider being as specific as possible in describing what they mean when they employ the term polysubstance use (i.e., prescribed vs nonprescribed, use vs use disorder). AJPH

CORRESPONDENCE

Correspondence should be sent to Kevin Young Xu, MD, MPH, Assistant Professor of Psychiatry, Renard 3007A, 4940 Children's Place, St. Louis, MO 63110 (e-mail: xukeviny@wustl.edu). Reprints can be ordered at https://www.ajph.org by clicking the "Reprints" link.

PUBLICATION INFORMATION

Full Citation: Xu KY, Lin LA, Grucza RA. Polysubstance use is not synonymous with poly substance use disorder. *Am J Public Health*. 2025;115(5):646–648.

Acceptance Date: February 10, 2025.

DOI: https://doi.org/10.2105/AJPH.2025.308070

ORCID iDs:

Kevin Y. Xu https://orcid.org/0000-0001-6595-695X

Richard A. Grucza https://orcid.org/0000-0002-8191-6875

CONTRIBUTORS

K. Y. Xu, L. Lin, R. A. Grucza conceptualized the article, revised it for important intellectual content, and approved the final version. K.Y. Xu wrote the initial draft. All authors agree to be accountable for all aspects of the work in ensuring that questions related to the accuracy or integrity of any part of the work are appropriately investigated and resolved.

ACKNOWLEDGMENTS

K. Y. Xu is supported by grant NIH K08DA061258. L. Lin is supported by grant R01DA05759.

We thank Matthew Ellis, PhD (assistant professor of psychiatry, Washington University) for his feedback on our initial draft.

CONFLICTS OF INTEREST

R. A. Grucza reported receiving grants from the National Institutes of Health (NIH) and Arnold Ventures LLC during the conduct of the study, consulting for Janssen Pharmaceuticals, and receiving personal fees for grant reviews from the NIH outside the submitted work. We declare no financial interests/personal relationships that may be considered as potential competing interests.

REFERENCES

1. Bunting AM, Shearer R, Linden-Carmichael AN, et al. Are you thinking what I'm thinking? Defining what we mean by "polysubstance use." *Am J Drug Alcohol Abuse*. 2024;50(1):1–7. https://doi.org/10.1080/00952990.2023.2248360
2. Shearer RD, Bart G, Reznikoff C. Rethinking the use of "polysubstance" to describe complex substance use patterns. *J Gen Intern Med*. 2022;37(12):3174–3175. https://doi.org/10.1007/s11606-022-07424-5

3. Shover CL, Friedman JR, Romero R, et al. Leveraging pooled medical examiner records to surveil complex and emerging patterns of polysubstance use in the United States. *Int J Drug Policy.* 2024;104397. https://doi.org/10.1016/j.drugpo.2024.104397
4. May T, Holloway K, Buhociu M, Hills R. Not what the doctor ordered: motivations for nonmedical prescription drug use among people who use illegal drugs. *Int J Drug Policy.* 2020;82:102823. https://doi.org/10.1016/j.drugpo.2020.102823
5. Black JC, Rockhill K, Forber A, Amioka E, May KP, Haynes CM, Dart RC. Redesign of survey of non-medical use of prescription drugs program improves benchmark estimates. RADARS System Technical Report, 2019-Q1. 2019. Available at: https://www.radars.org/system/publications/2019%201Q%20QTR.pdf. Accessed December 28, 2024.
6. Kolodny A, Bohler RM. Screened out—how a survey change sheds light on iatrogenic opioid use disorder. *N Engl J Med.* 2024;391(23):2183–2184. https://doi.org/10.1056/NEJMp2410911
7. Compton WM, Valentino RJ, DuPont RL. Polysubstance use in the US opioid crisis. *Mol Psychiatry.* 2021;26(1):41–50. https://doi.org/10.1038/s41380-020-00949-3
8. Lin LA, Bohnert ASB, Blow FC, et al. Polysubstance use and association with opioid use disorder treatment in the US Veterans Health Administration. *Addiction.* 2021;116(1):96–104. https://doi.org/10.1111/add.15116
9. Cicero TJ, Ellis MS, Kasper ZA. Polysubstance use: a broader understanding of substance use during the opioid crisis. *Am J Public Health.* 2020;110(2):244–250. https://doi.org/10.2105/AJPH.2019.305412
10. Xu KY, Mintz CM, Presnall N, Bierut LJ, Grucza RA. Comparative effectiveness associated with buprenorphine and naltrexone in opioid use disorder and cooccurring polysubstance use. *JAMA Netw Open.* 2022;5(5):e2211363. https://doi.org/10.1001/jamanetworkopen.2022.11363
11. Lin LA, Bonar EE, Coughlin LN. Toward a harm reduction approach to cannabis use disorder. *Am J Psychiatry.* 2024;181(2):98–99. https://doi.org/10.1176/appi.ajp.20230381
12. Nguyen T, Li Y, Greene D, Stancliff S, Quackenbush N. Changes in prescribed opioid dosages among patients receiving medical cannabis for chronic pain, New York State, 2017–2019. *JAMA Netw Open.* 2023;6(1):e2254573. https://doi.org/10.1001/jamanetworkopen.2022.54573

Addressing the Mechanisms of the Long-Term Effects of Racial Housing Inequalities

LaDale C. Winling, PhD

ABOUT THE AUTHOR

The author is with the Department of History and the Public History Program, Virginia Polytechnic Institute and State University, Blacksburg.

See also Swope et al., p. 769.

Perhaps no discipline has been bolder or more expansive than public health in interrogating the effects of redlining and the legacy of the Home Owners' Loan Corporation in modern life. A wide array of researchers in numerous disciplines have used the publicly available geographic information system layer files created from the corporation's maps to correlate historical data with present-day inequality and ascertained an explanation of the endurance of inequality that points to the federal government's actions from the 1930s.

Their efforts have been so successful that discussions of structural inequality abound in the popular press and in numerous academic and professional circles. The reparations movement may be at its most robust and operational point in decades if not ever. In part, the reason is that many disciplines to this point have been confounded by a lack of historical discussions of inequality or have not had a mechanism for connecting past wrongs to present-day conditions. Given an opportunity to make these connections in their research, many scholars jumped at the chance to consider the historical roots of the phenomena they see in the present.

As has been explained, however, in many instances these inquiries and publications lack a few key pieces of explanatory connective tissue that help illustrate how we moved from the conditions of the 1930s to those of the present. Among the most important pieces of connective machinery are a theoretical discussion of racial capitalism and a historical explanation of change over time.

Swope et al. (p. 769) posit that racial capitalism is an important element in understanding the maintenance of inequality in racialized spaces. Far more salient than the actual biological races of a neighborhood's residents is the way the neighborhood is marked or labeled and how the area marked by race is either starved of resources or given easy access to them. This racecraft is then repeated again and again to draw out a system of consistent profits for White investors and produce consistent losses and depreciation for Black investors.[1]

A historical account and explanation may be as important as a theoretical discussion of racial capitalism. The theoretical account can explain how the monetization of race has played out in the home finance sector as a whole, whereas a historical account can explain how the discriminatory decisions of the 1930s led to specific legislative choices, to the implementation of public programs, and to a new array of private practices in the subsequent decades. These explanations draw on historical contingencies, the specific conditions of each community, and the agency of individuals to act and make decisions that reinforce or transform discriminatory assessments of private appraisers and federal officials.

Either way, the essential elements are the explanatory tools to connect past to present rather than simply pointing to the correlation between redlining in the past and negative health conditions in the present. Environmental scientists and economists Hoffman and colleagues, for example, explained the connection between the environmental conditions of the 1930s, especially the tree cover and assessments of open space, parkland, and canopy tree cover, and the urban heat islands of the 21st century.[2] In this instance, wealthier and more highly rated neighborhoods had more green space historically and then saw greater investments in creating and maintaining green spaces in the subsequent decades, which led to more shade and less absorption of summer heat. By contrast, the low rating of a C-rated or D-rated "redlined" neighborhood meant the withholding of both public investment and private investment from public parks and the planting of street trees in favor of concrete, blacktop, and other absorptive, unshaded substances and surfaces.

Park planning and planting and maintenance of trees are the necessary connections between historical conditions and present-day circumstances. This illustrates the point made by Swope et al. that redlining maps and redlining in general are not determinative; discrimination and the maintenance of inequality require years and decades of decisions, actions, and investments that reinforce inequalities in both new and continuing ways. By the same token, any meaningful reparative intervention must grapple with the application of racialized labels to residential spaces and must roll back and untangle, in many iterations over decades, programs and unequal investments in racialized neighborhoods. Recognizing that there are actions to be undone or that there is an ideology to be unraveled may be far more difficult than deciding what is to be done to counter these public health inequalities. AJPH

CORRESPONDENCE

Correspondence should be sent to LaDale C. Winling, PhD, 431 Major Williams Hall, 220 Stranger St, Blacksburg, VA 24061 (e-mail: lwinling@vt.edu). Reprints can be ordered at https://www.ajph.org by clicking the "Reprints" link.

PUBLICATION INFORMATION

Full Citation: Winling LC. Addressing the mechanisms of the long-term effects of racial housing inequalities. *Am J Public Health*. 2025;115(5): 649–650.

Acceptance Date: February 12, 2025.

DOI: https://doi.org/10.2105/AJPH.2025.308074

ORCID iD:

LaDale C. Winling https://orcid.org/0009-0008-9495-6244

CONFLICTS OF INTEREST

The author declares that there are no known conflicts of interest because of grant support or funding relationships.

REFERENCES

1. Fields K, Fields B. *Racecraft: The Soul of Inequality in American Life*. Verso; 2012.
2. Hoffman JS, Pendleton N, Shandas V. The effects of historical housing policies on resident exposure to intra-urban heat: a study of 108 US urban areas. *Climate*. 2020;8(1):12. https://doi.org/10.3390/cli8010012

Leveraging Lessons Learned From the COVID-19 Pandemic to Support Vaccine Adherence

Sarah R. MacEwan, PhD

ABOUT THE AUTHOR

Sarah R. MacEwan is with the Division of General Internal Medicine, College of Medicine, The Ohio State University Wexner Medical Center, Columbus.

Over 1.2 million deaths have been attributed to COVID-19 in the United States as of November 2024.[1] More than three million additional deaths have been avoided through the implementation of COVID-19 vaccines,[2] which effectively reduce the risk of severe COVID-19 illness. Although COVID-19 vaccines have played a major role in mitigating the COVID-19 pandemic, their development, distribution, and promotion have also sparked concerns and questions, leading to an increase in vaccine hesitancy in some populations.

Sources of hesitancy toward COVID-19 vaccines have been the subject of extensive research, with reasons for refusing or delaying vaccination including uncertainty about the safety, efficacy, and necessity of the vaccine. Underlying sources of hesitancy reflect mistrust in government and medical organizations, mishandled communication, and misjudged vaccine mandates. As the COVID-19 pandemic evolved, these perceptions of COVID-19 vaccines were also affected by individuals' experiences with COVID-19 infection and continuing opportunities to receive updated vaccines and booster doses.

Bai et al. explored the predictors of persistent COVID-19 vaccine refusal following COVID-19 infection.[3] They found that individuals that cited lack of institutional confidence, philosophical objections, or religious exemptions were more likely to not be vaccinated at six months following a COVID-19 infection, compared with individuals that cited lack of vaccine accessibility or general vaccine uncertainty as the reason for not receiving an initial vaccine. These findings distinguish individuals open to receiving a COVID-19 vaccine despite initial reservations from individuals that persistently refuse a COVID-19 vaccine based on ideologies reflective of mistrust and prioritization of personal freedoms.

For individuals that have remained unvaccinated at this time, it appears that efforts to encourage uptake of the COVID-19 vaccine would likely have limited impact. A more impactful focus may be found in efforts to encourage adherence to updated COVID-19 vaccines and booster doses for those who received initial COVID-19 immunization. Multiple booster doses have now been recommended in the United States by the Centers for Disease Control and Prevention, including updated vaccines tailored to evolving variants. Uptake of these additional booster doses, important for providing protection when immunity has waned since a previous immunization or infection, has been low and decreasing over time.[4] For example, although 81% of the US population had received at least one dose of a COVID-19 vaccine as of May 2023,[5] only 48% of adults received or intended to receive the 2023–2024 updated vaccine as of October–November 2023[6] and 39% received or intend to receive the 2024–2025 updated vaccine as of October 2024.[7] These most recent rates are comparable to current flu vaccine coverage, with approximately 43% of US adults receiving a flu vaccine in the 2024–2025 flu season.[8] The decline in acceptance of COVID-19 vaccines over time likely involves multiple factors that reflect a "return to normal" as the pandemic transitioned to an endemic phase, including individuals' ongoing experiences of COVID-19 infection, perceptions of reduced COVID-19 risk, and unclear need for revaccination.

This attrition in COVID-19 vaccine booster adherence presents a challenge distinct from encouraging initial vaccination and likely requires unique approaches of messaging to reach individuals whose motivation to receive booster doses may be increasingly exhausted. Similar to the research question posed by Bai et al. in their work surrounding initial vaccination,[3] researchers also need to consider the factors contributing to the decisions to receive or not receive subsequent

AJPH May 2025, Vol. 115, No. 5

booster doses, where these factors likely include experiences with COVID-19 infection (e.g., severity of symptoms), experiences of COVID-19 vaccination (e.g., convenience, side effects), and perspectives about vaccine efficacy within the context of personal COVID-19 risk (e.g., potential exposure, risk of severe illness). It should also be recognized that as severe illness and death caused by COVID-19 infection has thankfully become less common over time, the benefits of COVID-19 vaccines and boosters may unfortunately be less persuasive. Poor communication distinguishing the efficacy of COVID-19 vaccines to reduce severe illness versus the efficacy to prevent contracting or transmitting COVID-19 has also contributed to perceptions that vaccines are ineffective when immunized individuals continue to experience COVID-19 infections. What is clear is that continued messaging is needed to communicate compelling benefits of updated COVID-19 vaccines and booster doses, such as decreased risk of experiencing Long COVID symptoms.

Although messages that relay the ongoing need and current benefits of COVID-19 vaccines are valuable in encouraging uptake of updated COVID-19 vaccines and booster doses, it is important to not overlook the underlying ideologies that may be driving vaccine refusal, as Bai et al.'s work alluded to.[3] One additional factor not considered by Bai et al. that appears to be contributing to the divergence of attitudes toward COVID-19 vaccines is the heightened degree of political polarization that has been incited throughout the pandemic.[9] Vaccination rates varied between political affiliations, as 90% of individuals identifying as Democrats received at least one dose of a COVID-19 vaccine as of September 2021 compared with 58% of individuals identifying as Republicans.[10] Perceptions of updated COVID-19 vaccines continue to be politically polarized, with 62% of individuals identifying as Democrats reporting having received or intending to receive the 2024–2025 updated COVID-19 vaccine compared with 18% of individuals identifying as Republicans.[7] Polarization of the media may play a role in communicating information that contributes to vaccine refusal or attrition. For example, communication of COVID-19 risk varied across politically leaning news sources and personal endorsement of vaccine misinformation,[9,11] and social media were used to promote targeted messaging, including misinformation and conspiracy theories.[9,12]

Although efforts are still certainly needed to bridge the gap in differing COVID-19 vaccine perceptions, it would be remiss to not also recognize the need to address perceptions of other vaccines that appear to have been affected since the onset of the COVID-19 pandemic. For example, adherence to childhood vaccines such as the measles, mumps, and rubella (MMR) vaccine has declined since 2019, as 39 US states failed to meet the 95% vaccination rate target among kindergarteners in the 2023–2024 school year, compared with 28 states in the 2019–2020 school year.[13] Similar to COVID-19 perceptions, opinions regarding childhood vaccination also appear to have gained a growing political polarization. For example, beliefs that childhood vaccines are extremely important have diverged over time; in a 2024 Gallup poll, 63% of individuals identifying as Democrats believed this to be true compared with 26% of individuals identifying as Republicans.[14] Outbreaks of illnesses such as measles demonstrate the potential repercussions of declining vaccination rates and the threat posed to the health of our communities if we cannot maintain the high vaccination rates required to support herd immunity.[15]

Ultimately, this polarization of vaccine attitudes has led to a call to action by some to implement strategies tailored to address sources of vaccine politicization.[16] Among recommended strategies is a clear need to change the foundational ways in which we understand and communicate scientific processes and public health measures. This requires enrichment of public knowledge about the biological science of infectious disease and pharmaceutical development as well as awareness of social marketing, behavioral science, and political science, which affect the sources, environments, and mechanisms through which we often consume information used to make personal health decisions. For example, increasing general knowledge about pharmaceutical discovery and development, as well as providing accessible and transparent communication about evolving research findings, are nonpartisan steps that can begin to include the general public in this scientific process, rather than expecting them to blindly accept the outcomes of these endeavors communicated through public officials that may or may not align with their political identity. Delivery of information through trusted messengers, who also dispel misinformation, can add further power to this effort.

Time will tell how our collective pandemic experiences will shape adherence to currently established immunizations, including the COVID-19 vaccine. The lessons we continue to learn from the successes and missteps of the COVID-19 vaccine campaign can help inform strategies to support acceptance of novel vaccines developed in response to future infectious disease–related public health emergencies. Bridging ideological differences in vaccine beliefs through increasing public engagement in science is one step we can take to help strengthen a united front for public health. AJPH

CORRESPONDENCE

Correspondence should be sent to Sarah R. MacEwan, 700 Ackerman Rd, Suite 4100, Columbus, OH 43202 (e-mail: Sarah.MacEwan@osumc.edu). Reprints can be ordered at https://www.ajph.org by clicking the "Reprints" link.

PUBLICATION INFORMATION

Full Citation: MacEwan SR. Leveraging lessons learned from the COVID-19 pandemic to support vaccine adherence. *Am J Public Health*. 2025; 115(5):651–653.

Acceptance Date: February 17, 2025.

DOI: https://doi.org/10.2105/AJPH.2025.308078

ORCID iD:
Sarah R. MacEwan https://orcid.org/0000-0002-4365-6232

ACKNOWLEDGMENTS

S. R. MacEwan receives support from the Center for Serological Testing to Improve Outcomes from Pandemic COVID-19 (STOP-COVID), funded by the National Cancer Institute (U54CA260582).

CONFLICTS OF INTEREST

The author has no conflicts of interest.

REFERENCES

1. Centers for Disease Control and Prevention. Trends in United States COVID-19 deaths, emergency department (ED) visits, and test positivity by geographic area. 2024. Available at: https://covid.cdc.gov/covid-data-tracker/#trends_totaldeaths_select_00. Accessed December 5, 2024.
2. Fitzpatrick MC, Moghadas SM, Pandey A, Galvani AP. Two years of US COVID-19 vaccines have prevented millions of hospitalizations and deaths. Commonwealth Fund. 2022. Available at: https://doi.org/10.26099/whsf-fp90. Accessed December 5, 2024.
3. Bai H, Brett-Major D, Du Y, et al. Predictors of persistent COVID-19 vaccine refusal among previously infected patients in Nebraska. *Am J Public Health*. 2025;115(3):414–424. https://doi.org/10.2105/AJPH.2024.307921
4. Tyson A, Pasquini G. How Americans view the Coronavirus, COVID-19 vaccines amid declining levels of concern. Pew Research Center. 2024. Available at: https://www.pewresearch.org/science/2024/03/07/how-americans-view-the-coronavirus-covid-19-vaccines-amid-declining-levels-of-concern. Accessed December 6, 2024.
5. USAFacts. US Coronavirus vaccine tracker. 2024. Available at: https://usafacts.org/visualizations/covid-vaccine-tracker-states. Accessed December 19, 2024.
6. Sparks G, Kirzinger A, Kearney A, Valdes I, Hamel L. KFF COVID-19 Vaccine Monitor November 2023: with COVID concerns lagging, most people have not gotten latest vaccine and half say they are not taking precautions this holiday season. KFF. 2023. Available at: https://www.kff.org/coronavirus-covid-19/poll-finding/vaccine-monitor-november-2023-with-covid-concerns-lagging-most-people-have-not-gotten-latest-vaccine. Accessed December 5, 2024.
7. Tyson A, Pasquini G. 60% of Americans say they probably won't get an updated COVID-19 vaccine. Pew Research Center. 2024. Available at: https://www.pewresearch.org/short-reads/2024/11/19/60-of-americans-say-they-probably-wont-get-an-updated-covid-19-vaccine. Accessed December 5, 2024.
8. Centers for Disease Control and Prevention. Weekly Flu Vaccination Dashboard. 2025. Available at: https://www.cdc.gov/fluvaxview/dashboard/index.html. Accessed January 22, 2025.
9. Bolsen T, Palm R. Politicization and COVID-19 vaccine resistance in the US. *Prog Mol Biol Transl Sci*. 2022;188(1):81–100. https://doi.org/10.1016/bs.pmbts.2021.10.002
10. Hamel L, Lopes L, Sparks G, et al. KFF COVID-19 Vaccine Monitor: September 2021. KFF. 2021. Available at: https://www.kff.org/coronavirus-covid-19/poll-finding/kff-covid-19-vaccine-monitor-september-2021. Accessed January 22, 2025.
11. Hamel L, Lopes L, Kirzinger A, Sparks G, Stokes M, Brodie M. KFF COVID-19 Vaccine Monitor: media and misinformation. KFF. 2021. Available at: https://www.kff.org/health-misinformation-and-trust/poll-finding/kff-covid-19-vaccine-monitor-media-and-misinformation. Accessed December 19, 2024.
12. Unlu A, Truong S, Tammi T, Lohiniva A-L. Exploring political mistrust in pandemic risk communication: mixed-method study using social media data analysis. *J Med Internet Res*. 2023;25:e50199. https://doi.org/10.2196/50199
13. Williams E, Kates J. Childhood vaccination rates continue to decline as Trump heads for a second term. KFF. 2024. Available at: https://www.kff.org/policy-watch/childhood-vaccination-rates-continue-to-decline-as-trump-heads-for-a-second-term. Accessed January 22, 2025.
14. Jones JM. Far fewer in US regard childhood vaccinations as important. Gallup. 2024. Available at: https://news.gallup.com/poll/648308/far-fewer-regard-childhood-vaccinations-important.aspx. Accessed January 22, 2025.
15. Phadke VK, Bednarczyk RA, Salmon DA, Omer SB. Association between vaccine refusal and vaccine-preventable diseases in the United States: a review of measles and pertussis. *JAMA*. 2016;315(11):1149–1158. https://doi.org/10.1001/jama.2016.1353
16. Sharfstein JM, Callaghan T, Carpiano RM, et al. Uncoupling vaccination from politics: a call to action. *Lancet*. 2021;398(10307):1211–1212. https://doi.org/10.1016/S0140-6736(21)02099-7

To Arms, Public Health Citizens!

Axelle Braggion, MD, and Antoine Flahault, MD, PhD

ABOUT THE AUTHORS

Axelle Braggion is with the Population Health Laboratory, University of Fribourg, Fribourg, Switzerland, and the Swiss School of Public Health, Zurich, Switzerland. Antoine Flahault is with the Institute of Global Health, University of Geneva, Geneva, Switzerland, and the Swiss School of Public Health, Zurich.

In an era of distrust in population health sciences and after a pandemic having revealed weaknesses in our surveillance systems,[1] we argue that abandoning the term "surveillance" for "monitoring"[2] could, symbolically, disarm public health. Such a proposal might not be timely.

Diving into the etymology and semantics of public health terms makes us realize that many of these terms are borrowed from military language, and public health surveillance is no exception.[3,4] Public health conducts activities related to surveillance, which comes from French "to watch over" and is defined as "the persistent monitoring of a target" by the North Atlantic Treaty Organization.[5] The terms "alert" and "alarm" come from the primitive Italian terms *all'erta* and *all'arme*, meaning, respectively, "to the watchtower" and "to arms" in the presence of an enemy or danger.

Public health practitioners plan vaccination and cancer screening campaigns on the model of armies. Epidemiologists often monitor epidemic "fronts" and label field epidemiologists as those investigating outbreaks on the "front line." "Sentinel" physicians are fighting and combating outbreaks of emerging infectious diseases or, for example, the obesity pandemic, whereas statisticians are computing attack rates, aiming to provide "early warning, alert, and response." Of course, public health surveillance is not a military activity, but in their own jargon epidemiology and public health take many of their roots from military language.

More than just being an analogy, public health is deeply anchored in the military culture. In the United States, many employees of the Centers for Disease Control and Prevention belong to the uniformed service branch of the US Public Health Service Commissioned Corps.[6,7] These officers wear navy-style uniforms when in duty. In France, the corps of public health doctors has grades of "inspector" and "general," also mimicking the army.[8]

Public health often taps into polysemic terminology because it aims to protect populations against different foreign enemies such as infectious agents, alcohol, tobacco, and sugar, and there are many similarities with military battles involving soldiers, arms, and munitions. Armed forces have historically faced many epidemics among their troops, leading to innovations in the combating of infectious diseases.[3,9] Malaria transmission pathways and communicable disease control measures are examples of important discoveries made by military doctors. In times of public health emergencies such as the COVID-19 pandemic, or when addressing posttraumatic stress syndrome, the military provides great support to public health,[3] the battles faced by both disciplines being in some aspects intertwined.

Because public health and the military share many terms and practices, their common objective is clearly defined: defending the well-being of the population, regardless of whether it is achieved through surveillance or monitoring. Public health surveillance is a meaningful term that should be kept for maintaining an effective and powerful arsenal of weapons against public health threats.[2] By exclusively using the term monitoring, we would abandon parts of our public health culture rooted in its own history and could ultimately lose firepower. AJPH

CORRESPONDENCE

Correspondence should be sent to Axelle Braggion, MD, Population Health Laboratory, University of Fribourg, Route des Arseneaux 41, 1700 Fribourg, Switzerland (e-mail: axelle.braggion@unifr.ch). Reprints can be ordered at https://www.ajph.org by clicking the "Reprints" link.

PUBLICATION INFORMATION

Full Citation: Braggion A, Flahault A. To arms, public health citizens! *Am J Public Health.* 2025; 115(5):654–655.

Acceptance Date: January 28, 2025.

DOI: https://doi.org/10.2105/AJPH.2025.308049

ORCID iDs:

Axelle Braggion https://orcid.org/0009-0007-0852-2312

Antoine Flahault https://orcid.org/0000-0002-6957-2977

CONTRIBUTORS

A. Braggion and A. Flahault wrote the article together on the basis of an original idea of A. Flahault.

CONFLICTS OF INTEREST

The authors report no conflicts of interest.

REFERENCES

1. Brownson RC, Burke TA, Colditz GA, Samet JM. Reimagining public health in the aftermath of a pandemic. *Am J Public Health.* 2020;110(11):1605–1610. https://doi.org/10.2105/AJPH.2020.305861
2. Morabia A, Dasgupta N, Thorpe L. Public health surveillance, monitoring, or data? Time to decide. *Am J Public Health.* 2024;114(7):661–662. https://doi.org/10.2105/AJPH.2024.307709

3. Falconer Hall T, Bricknell M, Ross D. Public health and military health. *J Public Health (Oxf)*. 2022;44(suppl 1):i88–i93. https://doi.org/10.1093/pubmed/fdac101
4. Tulchinsky TH, Varavikova EA. A history of public health. Available at: https://pmc.ncbi.nlm.nih.gov/articles/PMC7170188/pdf/main.pdf. Accessed December 20, 2024.
5. North Atlantic Treaty Organization. Joint intelligence, surveillance, and reconnaissance. Available at: https://www.nato.int/cps/en/natohq/topics_111830.htm. Accessed December 20, 2024.
6. Centers for Disease Control and Prevention. Commissioned Corps. Available at: https://jobs.cdc.gov/working-at-cdc/commissioned-corps.html. Accessed December 20, 2024.
7. US Public Health Service. Commissioned Corps of the US Public Health Service. Available at: https://www.usphs.gov. Accessed December 20, 2024.
8. Légifrance. Décret N° 2020-500 du 29 Avril 2020 modifiant le Décret N° 91-1025 du 7 Octobre 1991 relatif au statut particulier des médecins inspecteurs de santé publique. Available at: https://www.legifrance.gouv.fr/jorf/id/JORFTEXT000041841343. Accessed December 20, 2024.
9. Herron JBT, Dunbar JAT. The British Army's contribution to tropical medicine. *Clin Med (Lond)*. 2018;18(5):380–383. https://doi.org/10.7861/clinmedicine.18-5-380

Monitoring Is Not Enough

Arnaud Chiolero, MD, PhD

ABOUT THE AUTHOR

Arnaud Chiolero is with the Population Health Laboratory of the University of Fribourg, Switzerland; the School of Population and Global Health of McGill University, Montreal, Canada; and the Swiss School of Public Health, Zurich, Switzerland.

Should we replace the term "surveillance" with "monitoring"?[1] While "public health monitoring" seems appealing, it may not be sufficient to describe the full range of public health surveillance activities. I argue here that the term "surveillance" should be kept because, first, it encompasses not only monitoring but also reporting and, second, because accountability is a defining feature of surveillance activities not implied by monitoring.

Public health surveillance is traditionally defined as the ongoing systematic collection, analysis, and interpretation of data, closely integrated with the timely dissemination of the resulting information to those responsible for preventing and controlling disease and injury.[2,3] Within an evidence-based public health approach, surveillance is a cardinal element of public health policymaking and population health decisions.[4] A key strength of this definition is its comprehensiveness, encompassing both data collection and analysis (monitoring) and information dissemination (reporting). Data do not speak for themselves; transforming them into information, knowledge, and wisdom—following the DIKW information pyramid—requires expertise and substantial human and financial resources.[5]

On the one hand, the term "monitoring" is more specific than "surveillance" to describe the scientific and technical epidemiological activity of assessing population health, and this is why the notion of "population health monitoring" is used in many settings.[6] On the other hand, canceling the word "surveillance" for "monitoring" risks shifting the focus to data collection and analysis, downplaying the critical role of dissemination. This is concerning as reporting of surveillance findings is deficient in many jurisdictions. Reporting is a highly complex, value-laden process, shaped by political and administrative influences in the dialogue with decision-makers (public health authorities, politicians, stakeholders, and the public) who ultimately provide the legitimacy to disseminate monitoring information.

Another defining feature of public health surveillance not captured by the term "monitoring" is the built-in accountability of this activity, which is institutionalized and often legally constrained.[5] In many countries, population health monitoring is conducted partly by public health researchers in academic institutions. This might be necessary for high-level expertise and methodology but is not optimal for public health reporting as most researchers are not used to dialogue with decision-makers to produce actionable information, the overarching goal of surveillance.[7] Unlike many public health researchers without a surveillance duty, surveillance people, as civil servants, are accountable to the populations and the public health authorities they serve. Their mission is to disseminate the results of population health monitoring through easily accessible and understandable public health reports with actionable content and recommendations, following good health reporting practices.[7]

And this is why I suggest keeping "public health surveillance" as an umbrella term that encompasses both "population health monitoring" and "public health reporting." Most importantly, whatever the terminology, we must allocate more resources to surveillance and monitoring efforts to enable evidence-based public health decision-making.[8] AJPH

CORRESPONDENCE

Correspondence should be sent to Prof. Arnaud Chiolero, MD, PhD, Population Health Laboratory, University of Fribourg, Route des Arsenaux 41, 1700 Fribourg, Switzerland (e-mail: achiolero@gmail.com). Reprints can be ordered at https://www.ajph.org by clicking the "Reprints" link.

PUBLICATION INFORMATION

Full Citation: Chiolero A. Monitoring is not enough. *Am J Public Health*. 2025;115(5):656–657.

Acceptance Date: February 16, 2025.

DOI: https://doi.org/10.2105/AJPH.2025.308085

ORCID iD:
Arnaud Chiolero https://orcid.org/0000-0002-5544-8510

CONFLICTS OF INTEREST

The author reports no conflicts of interest.

REFERENCES

1. Morabia A, Dasgupta N, Thorpe L. Public health surveillance, monitoring, or data? Time to decide. *Am J Public Health*. 2024;114(7):661–662. https://doi.org/10.2105/AJPH.2024.307709
2. Thacker SB, Berkelman RL. Public health surveillance in the United States. *Epidemiol Rev*. 1988;10(1):164–190. https://doi.org/10.1093/oxfordjournals.epirev.a036021

3. Chiolero A, Buckeridge D. Glossary for public health surveillance in the age of data science. *J Epidemiol Community Health*. 2020;74(7):612–616. https://doi.org/10.1136/jech-2018-211654
4. Brownson RC, Fielding JE, Maylahn CM. Evidence-based public health: a fundamental concept for public health practice. *Annu Rev Public Health*. 2009;30(1):175–201. https://doi.org/10.1146/annurev.publhealth.031308.100134
5. Verschuuren M, Van Oers H. *Population Health Monitoring: Climbing the Information Pyramid*. Cham, Switzerland: Springer; 2019. https://doi.org/10.1007/978-3-319-76562-4
6. Verschuuren M, van Oers H. Population health monitoring: an essential public health field in motion. *Bundesgesundheitsblatt Gesundheitsforschung Gesundheitsschutz*. 2020;63(9):1134–1142. https://doi.org/10.1007/s00103-020-03205-9
7. Starke D, Tempel G, Butler J, Starker A, Zühlke C, Borrmann B. Good practice in health reporting—guidelines and recommendations. *J Health Monit*. 2017;2(suppl 1):2–19. https://doi.org/10.17886/RKI-GBE-2017-013
8. Brownson RC, Burke TA, Colditz GA, Samet JM. Reimagining public health in the aftermath of a pandemic. *Am J Public Health*. 2020;110(11):1605–1610. https://doi.org/10.2105/AJPH.2020.305861

Changing Ecosystems and the Role of One Health: Engaging Public Health Professionals

Helena J. Chapman, MD, PhD, MPH, Muge Akpinar-Elci, MD, MPH, Laura H. Kahn, MD, MPH, MPP, and Thomas J. Doker, DVM, MPH, CPH

ABOUT THE AUTHORS

Helena J. Chapman is with the Milken Institute School of Public Health, George Washington University, Washington, DC. Muge Akpinar-Elci is with the School of Public Health, University of Nevada, Reno. Laura H. Kahn is with the One Health Initiative, Washington, DC. Thomas J. Doker is with the One Health Commission, Washington, DC.

Note. The views expressed herein are those of the authors and do not reflect the official policy or position of George Washington University; University of Nevada, Reno; One Health Initiative; or One Health Commission.

AJPH May 2025, Vol. 115, No. 5

Public health professionals lead collaborative efforts across health systems to respond to diverse challenges, ranging from environmental stressors to infectious and chronic disease risks, and support established goals of the Healthy People 2030 and the 2030 Agenda for Sustainable Development.[1] Extreme climate and weather events and infectious disease outbreaks underscore the delicate balance of the global ecosystems and the influence of the social and structural determinants of health on physical and mental health and well-being. Increasing temperatures, which can affect crop production and yield, can influence heat stress responses and food access and availability, which compounds the prevalence of chronic conditions such as diabetes or other metabolic diseases.[2] Infodemic management, namely the rapid spread of misinformation and disinformation in daily practice, however, remains a significant hurdle to sharing timely and accurate health messages and calls to action for community engagement.

The One Health concept, which recognizes the dynamic interdependence of human, animal, and environmental health, provides an innovative framework for examining complex global challenges in a concise, systematic, and comprehensive manner. It promotes the urgent need for the 4Cs (coordination, communication, collaboration, capacity building) across disciplines and sectors, in efforts to protect, promote, and improve health.[3] Notably, the launch of the One Health Joint Plan of Action 2022–2026 highlighted six action tracks to direct global priorities toward strengthening health systems capacity, reducing risks from emerging zoonotic diseases, controlling endemic infectious diseases, enhancing food safety risk assessment and communication, combatting antimicrobial resistance, and integrating environmental factors into initiatives.[4] Understanding the impact of ecosystem changes through a One Health approach will be essential for developing comprehensive strategies of multidisciplinary and multisectoral actions to mitigate emerging risks and protect global health for all communities.

As environmental disturbances like wildfires and deforestation alter ecological niches, animals must adapt to new habitats that may encroach on human populations. This proximity may lead to the emergence of novel pathogen transmission from animals (zoonoses), as an estimated 60% of emerging human infectious diseases are reportedly of zoonotic origin.[4] Increased land surface temperatures can expand the geographic distribution of vector and disease hotspots, influence urban heat island effects, and alter animal migratory patterns. As marine and freshwater ecosystems adapt to increasing water temperatures, it can alter water chemistry, drive thermal stress on coral reefs, and modify oxygen exchange that can lead to the accumulation of algal blooms. Harmful air pollution, like greenhouse gases, aerosols, tropospheric ozone, and particulate matter, can alone exacerbate respiratory conditions, but when combined with increasing temperatures, heat can be trapped and worsen air quality conditions.[5]

ONE HEALTH AT THE APHA ANNUAL MEETING

Bringing this topic to the APHA audience, the authors organized a One Health session at the APHA 2023 Annual Meeting and Expo, which had the third highest average attendance of all APHA sections. During a panel discussion, veterinary medicine, medicine, public health and policy, and meteorology experts offered perspectives about how their disciplines collaborate with scientists and community stakeholders. They also described the role of data integration, community connectedness, and ethics, to leverage expertise, drive scientific advancement, and safeguard population health amid the changing Earth's systems through the One Health approach. The open discussion presented an interactive period of direct engagement between panelists and audience members on operationalizing the One Health approach to encourage the integration of new technologies and analytical approaches related to food safety, disease surveillance and risk assessment, and air quality management.

Examining Food Systems and Agriculture

As we live in a microbial world, the One Health framework can help us examine the microbial connections between climate, agriculture, antimicrobial resistance, and food safety and security, as well as improve our efforts to live more healthily and sustainably on our planet. These elements can be visualized as a multidimensional matrix involving four dimensions depending on the users' needs: (1) One Health factors (humans, animals, plants, environments, ecosystems); (2) scale and complexity factors (microbial/cellular, individuals, populations); (3) political, social, and economic factors (political borders at local, regional, national, and international levels); and (4) time factors (days, weeks, months, years, decades). By integrating these four dimensions in a holistic manner, researchers can investigate and analyze these emerging health challenges as well as discover previously unrecognized connections related to human, animal, and environmental health.[6]

Our microbiome is impacted by the microbes in our environments and ecosystems. Waste management practices influence the density of microbial burdens in the environments and ecosystems that impact health, particularly our consumption of liquid and solid nourishment. Global human and animal fecal wastes are analyzed at the population level, noting that 8 billion humans and 30 billion domesticated food animals constitute approximately 96% to 98% of the total global terrestrial biomass.[6,7] Collectively, humans and their domesticated terrestrial food animals produce more than 4 trillion kilograms of fecal wastes that contaminate soils and waterways and emit potent greenhouse gases including methane and nitrous oxide.[8] These fecal wastes contribute to food- and waterborne illnesses and food insecurity, serve as a reservoir for antimicrobial-resistant microbes, and jeopardize civilization through exacerbating climate conditions. Increasing global demand for animal proteins, including meat and dairy products, hinders the political will needed to address these issues.

Enhancing Disease Surveillance

As an essential component of health systems, public health surveillance represents the systematic data collection, analysis, interpretation, and reporting measures of disease and injury prevention to assist informed decision-making activities.[9,10] Identifying unusual events of public health importance is the first step to mitigating disease transmission as close as possible to the outbreak source. Over the past two decades, diverse disease outbreaks of epidemic or pandemic potential have been reported, including avian influenza virus, chikungunya virus, coronaviruses (including COVID-19), dengue fever, mpox, Oropouche fever, Nipah virus, and West Nile virus, demonstrating direct links to globalization and One Health. If these disease threats are detected as potential epidemic agents, especially with strong links to changing environmental conditions or zoonotic transmission, then public health mitigation efforts can accelerate the delivery of adequate resources and risk communication to surrounding populations and limit disease spread.

Public health disease surveillance systems are crucial to determining the county, city, tribal, territorial, and state health needs and priorities, yet many do not operate using a One Health framework. Understanding the role of state and federal agencies in operational surveillance and response as well as efforts to connect human and animal health surveillance systems can help identify practice gaps and align ongoing efforts. Incorporating stakeholder engagement must ensure that the ethical concepts of social beneficence, respect, justice, and transparency are built into the data sharing systems.[11] Developing key operational disease surveillance systems for sharing resources and disseminating reporting in an ethical manner can help accelerate health system preparedness and response efforts for the next global health emergency.

Integrating Earth Science Applications

Remote sensing and other geospatial data offer real-time information that can monitor environmental parameters from Earth's orbit that illustrate the dynamic processes of the aquatic, atmospheric, and terrestrial ecosystems. As National Aeronautics and Space Administration (NASA) Earth-observing satellites and sensors collect terabytes of these environmental data of public health importance each day (https://www.earthdata.nasa.gov), researchers can examine the temporal and spatial information to better understand how the natural and anthropogenic changes to the planetary ecosystems are influencing global health.[12] For example, environmental observations can monitor concentrations of atmospheric emissions (e.g., nitrogen dioxide, particulate matter) from power plants, wildfires, or prescribed burns, as well as surface temperatures coupled with precipitation levels that can influence vector suitability and risk of vector-borne disease transmission. Moreover, they can measure vegetation indices that depict land use changes (including deforestation activities) leading to potential animal encroachment on human habitats and risk of zoonotic spillover, and increased sea levels and temperatures influencing sea salinity, marine and other aquatic ecosystem health (e.g., accumulation of algal blooms), and pathogen survival (e.g., *Vibrio cholerae*). Together with traditional knowledge, or how local communities perceive the changing landscapes over time, researchers can expand their collective understanding of these ecological changes and design a tangible pathway to sustainable solutions.

Novel Earth science applications have streamlined how researchers observe the changing Earth's systems, providing a more comprehensive depiction of the current status of the environment. The NASA Tropospheric Emissions: Monitoring of Pollution (TEMPO) mission (https://tempo.si.edu), launched to geostationary orbit in April 2023. As the first Earth Venture instrument mission, TEMPO measures tropospheric pollution every daylight hour across greater North America. The NASA Plankton, Aerosol, Cloud, Ocean Ecosystem mission (https://pace.gsfc.nasa.gov), launched in February 2024, has hyperspectral and polarimetric instruments that observe ocean color, aerosols, and clouds, noting phytoplankton communities and carbon dioxide exchange between the ocean and atmosphere. An upcoming mission, the NASA Multi-Angle Imager for Aerosols (https://maia.jpl.nasa.gov), will offer the first partnership with epidemiologists on a satellite mission to study how particulate pollution affects human health. By incorporating satellite and in situ observations, including historical disease or vector counts from surveillance systems, researchers can develop disease early warning systems, as robust mathematical algorithms and models (e.g., ArboMAP, CHIKRisk, Vibrio Prediction Hub) that can predict higher exposure risks to specific geographic areas.

RECOMMENDATIONS

Addressing these complex and multifactorial ecosystem risks requires innovative approaches that integrate remote sensing, geospatial information, public

TABLE 1— Selected Strategies to Incorporate the 4Cs (Coordination, Communication, Collaboration, Capacity Building) Into Initiatives That Promote Operationalizing the One Health Approach

Recommendation	Description	Actions
Coordination	Working together with stakeholders toward a common goal	• Identifying synergies between stakeholders from public and private sectors and forming partnerships • Collectively developing relevant policies and guidelines to address gaps
Communication	Sharing information with community members and decision-makers	• Preparing case studies to help visualize challenges • Strengthening community preparedness and response efforts • Crafting ethically and culturally appropriate messaging with scientific visualizations, animations, and infographics
Collaboration	Bringing together diverse disciplines and stakeholders for joint efforts	• Organizing roundtable discussions and webinars • Forming multidisciplinary and multisectoral collaborations, of different training levels, for the preparation of publications • Establishing communities of practice to leverage expertise, enhance networking, and offer problem-solving
Capacity building	Enhancing skills, resources, and infrastructure to effectively address health challenges	• Defining the One Health concept • Promoting training opportunities on using and interpreting remote sensing, geospatial, and public health surveillance data • Offering internships and continuing education opportunities for learners of all ages

Source. Based on Chapman and Dunham[15] and Chapman and Judd.[16]

health surveillance, and qualitative data, including traditional knowledge. These approaches are essential to advancing scientific inquiry and strengthening connections between researchers and community stakeholders. Understanding the multidimensional elements of One Health, ranging from socioeconomic and political factors to time scale, can provide a deeper lens to identify implementation gaps, decipher nuances, and mark the next steps for action.[13] Health surveillance systems are powerful tools to examine health needs and inform decision-making activities, specifically to reduce risk of acute or chronic exposure to a pathogen or environmental hazard. In addition to satellite data, citizen science activities, including the NASA Global Learning and Observations to Benefit the Environment Program, can help expand data collection, validate satellite observations, and encourage science, technology, engineering, and mathematics engagement for learners across all age groups. Health professionals can identify knowledge and practice gaps and incorporate this insight into the development of relevant policies and guidelines as well as ethically and culturally appropriate health messaging to protect population health.[14] Implementing the One Health approach calls for designing both educational and community measures aligned with the guiding principles of coordination, communication, collaboration, and capacity building (4Cs). Table 1 presents key examples of applying the 4Cs to further advance our One Health initiatives on diverse topics and across communities.[15,16]

CONCLUSION

Health professionals are the driving force to lead timely educational interventions with public health messaging that incorporate agricultural and food safety, public health surveillance, and environmental topics, as well as highlight the power of scientific visualizations to display historical and emerging trends. With an estimated 10 million global health workforce shortage by 2030, building a robust workforce is imperative to meet local and national health needs, but limited resources and work-related stressors (workplace safety and burnout) cannot be ignored.[17] The One Health multidimensional matrix represents an important educational and policy tool for health professionals, enabling them to closely examine, analyze, interpret, and develop sustainable solutions to address environmental health challenges. Together with this matrix, robust surveillance systems and Earth science resources and tools can help operationalize the One Health concept through policy development and risk mitigation to support established indicators of the Healthy People 2030 and the 2030 Agenda for Sustainable Development. AJPH

CORRESPONDENCE

Correspondence should be sent to Helena Chapman, 950 New Hampshire Ave NW, Washington, DC 20052 (e-mail: hjchapman@gwu.edu). Reprints can be ordered at https://www.ajph.org by clicking the "Reprints" link.

PUBLICATION INFORMATION

Full Citation: Chapman HJ, Akpinar-Elci M, Kahn LH, Doker TJ. Changing ecosystems and the role of one health: engaging public health professionals. *Am J Public Health*. 2025;115(5):658–662.

Acceptance Date: December 16, 2024.

DOI: https://doi.org/10.2105/AJPH.2024.307982

ORCID iDs:
Helena J. Chapman https://orcid.org/0000-0003-1999-6453

Thomas J. Doker https://orcid.org/0000-0001-8920-4912

CONTRIBUTORS

All authors had substantial contributions to the preparation and completion of the article drafts.

ACKNOWLEDGMENTS

The authors thank the leadership of the APHA One Health section for their support of this scientific session held during the 2023 APHA Annual Meeting and Expo.

CONFLICTS OF INTEREST

The authors have no conflicts of interest to disclose.

REFERENCES

1. Lucero-Prisno DE, Oluwaseun Shomuyiwa D, Kouwenhoven MBN, et al. Top 10 public health challenges to track in 2023: shifting focus beyond a global pandemic. *Public Health Chall.* 2023;2(2):e86. https://doi.org/10.1002/puh2.86
2. Ratter-Rieck JM, Roden M, Herder C. Diabetes and climate change: current evidence and implications for people with diabetes, clinicians and policy stakeholders. *Diabetologia.* 2023; 66(6):1003–1015.
3. One Health High-Level Expert Panel, Adisasmito WB, Almuhairi S, et al. One Health: a new definition for a sustainable and healthy future. *PLoS Pathog.* 2022;18(6):e1010537.
4. One Health joint plan of action (2022–2026): working together for the health of humans, animals, plants and the environment. Geneva, Switzerland: World Health Organization, Food and Agriculture Organization of the United Nations, World Organisation for Animal Health, United Nations Environment Programme; 2022. Available at: https://www.who.int/publications/i/item/9789240059139. Accessed November 2, 2024.
5. Fuller R, Landrigan PJ, Balakrishnan K, et al. Pollution and health: a progress update. [erratum in *Lancet Planet Health.* 2022;6(7):e553]. *Lancet Planet Health.* 2022;6(6):e535–e547. https://doi.org/10.1016/S2542-5196(22)00090-0
6. Kahn LH. Developing a One Health approach by using a multi-dimensional matrix. *One Health.* 2021;13:100289. https://doi.org/10.1016/j.onehlt.2021.100289
7. Zeller U, Starik N, Göttert T. Biodiversity, land use and ecosystem services—an organismic and comparative approach to different geographical regions. *Glob Ecol Conserv.* 2017;10:114–125. https://doi.org/10.1016/J.GECCO.2017.03.001
8. Berendes DM, Yang PJ, Lai A, et al. Estimation of global recoverable human and animal faecal biomass. *Nat Sustain.* 2018;1(11):679–685. https://doi.org/10.1038/s41893-018-0167-0
9. Lee LM, Thacker SB. Public health surveillance and knowing about health in the context of growing sources of health data. *Am J Prev Med.* 2011;41(6):636–640. https://doi.org/10.1016/j.amepre.2011.08.015
10. Chiolero A, Buckeridge D. Glossary for public health surveillance in the age of data science. *J Epidemiol Community Health.* 2020;74(7):612–616. https://doi.org/10.1136/jech-2018-211654
11. Edelstein M, Lee LM, Herten-Crabb A, Heymann DL, Harper DR. Strengthening global public health surveillance through data and benefit sharing. *Emerg Infect Dis.* 2018;24(7):1324–1330. https://doi.org/10.3201/eid2407.151830

12. Seltenrich N. Remote-sensing applications for environmental health research. *Environ Health Perspect*. 2014;122(10):A268–A275. https://doi.org/10.1289/ehp.122-A268
13. Pepin KM, Carlisle K, Anderson D, et al. Steps towards operationalizing One Health approaches. *One Health*. 2024;18:100740. https://doi.org/10.1016/j.onehlt.2024.100740
14. Chapman HJ, Veras-Estévez BA. Integrating One Health topics to enhance health workers' leadership in health promotion activities. *Glob Health Promot*. 2023;30(2):40–45. https://doi.org/10.1177/17579759221126143
15. Chapman HJ, Dunham B. Engaging with 'One Health' audiences. *Clin Teach*. 2020;17(3):332–335. https://doi.org/10.1111/tct.13107
16. Chapman HJ, Judd LM. Adding satellite data to health curricula. *Clin Teach*. 2022;19(2):183. https://doi.org/10.1111/tct.13454
17. Samet J, Brownson RC. Reimagining public health: mapping a path forward. *Health Aff (Millwood)*. 2024;43(6):750–758. https://doi.org/10.1377/hlthaff.2024.00007

The Murder of Black Women in the United States: A Public Health Crisis

Tameka L. Gillum, PhD, Alexis Sheffield, MS, Antonia Drew Norton, and Clarice J. Hampton, MA

ABOUT THE AUTHORS

Tameka L. Gillum is with the College of Population Health and Alexis Sheffield is with the Department of Psychology, University of New Mexico, Albuquerque. Antonia Drew Norton is with The Asha Project, Milwaukee, WI. Clarice Hampton is with the Department of Psychology, University of Maryland, Baltimore County, Baltimore.

The murder of Black women in the United States is an urgent, yet neglected, public health crisis. In the United States, most homicides of women are committed by someone they know, most often a current or former intimate partner.[1–4] Existing data identified that in 2020, a total of 2059 women were murdered by a male.[3] A more comprehensive study of female homicide in the United States identified 31 627 homicides of women between the years 1999 and 2020.[2] Of note, data over the years have demonstrated significant disparities in homicides experienced by Black women in the United States. Most recently, using data from the Centers for Disease Control and Prevention, Waller et al.[5] identified persistent racial disparities in female homicides from 1999 to 2020. For the year 2020 specifically, the authors identified a homicide rate of 11.6 per 100 000 for Black women compared with 3 per 100 000 for their White counterparts.[5] The nature and magnitude of this disparity varies by state, as Black women in Wisconsin were 20 times more likely to die by homicide than White women. In addition, firearm deaths were disproportionately concentrated among Black women.[5] Other studies have identified similar disparities in homicides of Black women over the years, including but not limited to intimate partner homicides and homicides by police.[1,2,4,6–11] The sheer magnitude and persistence of these disparities point to the murder of Black women in the United States as a major public health crisis in need of urgent attention.

INTIMATE PARTNER HOMICIDE

One of the most documented contexts within which Black women are murdered is intimate relationships.[3,6,7,9,12,13] As noted, most homicides of women in the United States are perpetrated by someone the victim knew. According to homicide data from 2020, 90% of Black women killed by men knew their perpetrator.[3] In fact, 56% of murdered Black women were killed by current or former intimate partners (i.e., intimate partner homicide [IPH]).[3] In the only multistate study of IPH that evaluated victimization rates by race/ethnicity, non-Latina Black women were 2.22 times more likely to experience IPH than Latina women and 2.7 times more likely than White women.[12] One study calculated that Black women experience 7.3 more potential years of life lost due to intimate partner violence (IPV) than White women.[13]

Black women's heightened risk for IPH extends to the perinatal period.[6,7,9] McFarlane et al.[9] found that Black women were three times more likely to be victims of attempted or completed IPH during pregnancy than White women. A more recent study found that pregnant Black women were 8.1 times more likely to experience IPH than nonpregnant Black women.[7] From 2003 to 2007, although Black women represented only 17.7% of live births, they represented 37.3% of pregnant victims of IPH.[6]

Risk factors associated with structural inequalities, including structural racism, increase risk of IPH victimization for Black women and perpetration of IPH by Black men.[14–21] These include high rates of Black unemployment, problem drinking, illicit drug use, depression, posttraumatic stress disorder, and internalization of problematic stereotypes of Black women.[14–20]

An additional factor associated with increased risk for IPH among Black women is low use of social service and legal resources, including law enforcement.[21–24] A systematic review conducted by Waller et al.[25] found that Black women avoided use of social service resources as a result of barriers caused by structural racism, and they avoided use of police intervention because they believed they were better equipped to handle their situations than officers and feared that officers would mistreat their partners.[22]

AJPH May 2025, Vol. 115, No. 5

When they did engage law enforcement, they often encountered significant delays or inadequate help.[23] Indeed, officers have been less likely to arrest the perpetrator of IPV when Black women were the victims.[24] Such negative experiences of interacting with police officers reinforce Black women's avoidance of legal resources, such that they may not engage with the legal system until IPV has escalated in severity.[19,21]

HOMICIDE BY POLICE

Yet another reason for deferring use of police intervention is Black women's disproportionate risk for homicide by police officers.[8,10] Research demonstrates that Black women are at least 1.4 times more likely to be killed by police than White women.[8] One study estimated that between 2.4 and 5.4 Black women and girls per 100 000 will be killed by police in their lifetime.[8] Since 2015, Black women, who represent only 13% of the US female population, have constituted 20% of women shot and killed by police and 28% of unarmed deaths by police.[10] In fact, in a study conducted by Johnson et al.,[11] 57.2% of Black women were unarmed when killed, the only subgroup with such a pattern.

The higher risk of lethal violence by police may be partially explained by greater contact with police, related to the overpolicing of Black communities.[26] A study by the Prison Policy Initiative[27] found that Black women are at increased risk for police-initiated traffic stops, arrests, and use of force relative to White and Latina women.

Stereotypes of Black women may also magnify their risk for homicide by police officers. Shinde[28] theorizes that police brutality against Black women likely arises from a belief of the stereotype of the "angry black woman." Therefore, officers may be primed to observe indicators of perceived disrespect in interactions with Black women and react to perceived threats to their masculinity with disproportionate violence.[28,29] This is consistent with research supporting that police are more likely to use force, including lethal force, against Black people, including Black women, during "routine" encounters than they are against their White counterparts.[27,30–32] Relatedly, Crenshaw et al.[33] identified themes of police killings that overlap with negative stereotypes of Black women. The authors also noted that Black women experiencing mental health crises have been perceived by police officers as dangerous despite their vulnerability and level of distress.[33] It is possible that officers' insufficient training in mental health crisis intervention, paired with the perceived bias that Black women are dangerous, prevent the processing of cues that alert the observer to mental health symptoms. Research supports that police recruits seldom receive adequate training on engaging with individuals experiencing mental health crises and that, among people with mental illness in all racial/ethnic groups, Black individuals experience the highest death rate in police interactions.[34–36] Additionally, a recent study found that Black women were more likely to be killed by police when Black women held more political positions in the state where they resided.[37] This suggests that officers' use of lethal force may be partially motivated by perceived threat to gender and racial hierarchies.

Despite these existing disparities, the killing of Black women by police officers receives minimal attention and limited accountability from the legal system. An article by Dzhanova et al.[38] identified 50 Black women killed by police between 2015 and 2021. Of the 100 officers involved in the fatal shootings, only nine were fired, five were charged, and none were convicted.[38] Such inaction reinforces the message that Black women's deaths are inconsequential.

CONTRIBUTING FACTORS

In addition to factors identified thus far, other factors related to systemic racism also increase the risk of homicide for Black women.[21,26,39] Structural disadvantage experienced by Black people in the United States disproportionately places them, through residential segregation, in socioeconomically disadvantaged communities that experience increased rates of violent crime.[26] Pervasive poverty, disproportionately experienced by Black people in America, has also been identified as a contributing factor to violence in Black communities.[39] Increased gun access in these communities also increases risk for homicide.[26] Hence, structural inequalities experienced by Black people generally, and by Black women in particular, contribute to great disparities in the loss of Black female lives in the United States.

IMPACT

Violence in all its forms has a significant impact on the health and well-being of individuals and communities, particularly when the most severe consequence, fatality, is considered. The impact of the murders of Black women is monumental and extends far beyond individual loss of life. The murder of Black women is felt across family systems as well as at the community level. Disproportionate rates of IPH among Black women during the perinatal period further complicates this public health crisis. Although not often mentioned in literature on maternal mortality, IPH has a significant impact on rates of maternal mortality, particularly among Black women.[6,7] Ultimately, this contributes to decreased numbers of live births among Black women, affecting the health and well-being of Black families.[6,7] Relatedly, the high rates of murder of Black women mean the devastating loss of many daughters, mothers, partners and wives, sisters, nieces, grandmothers, aunts, cousins, and friends in Black communities, eroding support systems and imparting the psychological trauma of loss.

Gun violence, a public health crisis of extensive magnitude, has significant overlap with the murder of Black women in the United States. As previously noted, Black women are significantly more likely to be killed by a firearm.[5] At the systems level, historically limited prevention strategies that are focused on individual-level solutions alone are inherently unable to generate lasting change or address existing disparities. Violence is a systemic problem that extends beyond individual behavior affecting families and communities, often reinforced by systemic abuses.[26,39] With little faith in existing systems of reporting and seeking support, including the legal system, Black women are left without systematic ways of obtaining support and preventing victimization.[5]

EFFORTS TO RAISE AWARENESS

Efforts to raise awareness of this public health crisis have been limited, reflecting the low value placed on Black women's lives. In response, the African American Policy Forum released the "Say Her Name: Resisting Police Brutality Against Black Women" report in 2015,[33] following the launch of the #SayHerName social media campaign the previous year that brought attention to the issue of Black women being killed by police.[40] However, this movement is specifically focused on homicide by police officers rather than Black women's elevated homicide rate more generally. Despite the campaign, an analysis of the narratives in news coverage of Breonna Taylor's murder in 2020 shows that work is still needed to shift public discourse on this topic.[41]

IMPLICATIONS FOR PROGRAMS, SERVICES, AND INTERVENTIONS

The information presented here has significant implications for designing intervention services that target Black communities. The complex stressors experienced by Black men increase their risk for substance abuse and mental health concerns, which have been linked to perpetration of violence against women.[15–17,26,39] Hence, culturally informed substance abuse treatments and mental health services could prove helpful.

Programming such as that offered by The Asha Project, based in Milwaukee, Wisconsin, could serve as a model for such efforts.[42,43] Such programming includes the Ujima Men's Program and its most recent initiative, the SOS (Saving Our Selves/Saving Our Sisters) Project, launched in 2022.

SOS employs a two-pronged approach: awareness of services targeting Black men and the nature of those services. The first approach raises awareness through use of authentic credible messengers with messaging designed to destigmatize help-seeking by Black men, with information on where help is available in the community. Services include the provision of culturally responsive, trauma-informed mental health care and other community-based, noncarceral services that support the emotional and psychological health of Black men. Results of the pilot study indicate that 59 Black men challenged by mental and emotional struggles contacted the project through its social media sites, website, and office telephone number.

Data also suggest that women are at greater risk of IPV when their partners experience job instability.[44] Given the high unemployment rates experienced by Black men, initiatives that facilitate employment opportunities for Black men could prove helpful as well. Black women's substantial increase in risk for IPH during pregnancy and the perinatal period suggests that this may be a particularly important time to intervene.

Given the limited awareness identified here, efforts to increase awareness of this public health crisis could also prove informative and may increase resources dedicated to addressing this concern. Further, given that similar structural factors underlie all violence disparities experienced by Black communities,[26,39] culturally informed community violence intervention and homicide prevention programs, such as BrotherlyACT,[45] could also serve to reduce the risk of murder experienced by Black women. In addition, early intervention for Black boys could serve to foster positive youth development and shift social norms that foster violence against women.

IMPLICATIONS FOR POLICY

Beyond individual- and community-level prevention strategies such as those mentioned here, systemic change must occur to truly address violence against women generally and the murder of Black women specifically. Despite ample documentation that the murder of Black women reflects a public health crisis, the evidence continues to be met with invisibility in the media and little to no political action. Given stark disparities reflected in both national and state data, it is necessary to create relevant policy at both the state and national levels. For example, Minnesota established the first Missing and Murdered African American Women and Girls task force, with similar legislation being proposed in other states such as Wisconsin.[46] In addition, the US Congress introduced a similar bill at the national level. Although these are indeed steps in the right direction, ways to further address the vulnerability of Black women will need to be carefully considered and accompanied by financial resources to fund related initiatives.

As shown in this article, existing literature cites systemic racism as a significant contributing factor to existing disparities in rates of homicide of Black women.[5,46] Systemic racism has facilitated structural conditions in Black communities that increase the vulnerability of Black women.[26] Consequently, it is imperative that legislation be created to establish ongoing resources allocated specifically for the development and advancement of Black communities disenfranchised by centuries of inequality. In addition, it is critically important to interrogate the ways in which racism and the perpetuation of stereotypes of Black women influence the behaviors and perceptions of police officers and service providers. Given the decreased likelihood of Black women utilizing formal systems of support that heavily rely on carceral ideologies and have the potential to cause more harm,[21–25] identification of alternative responses that do not include carceral systems is imperative to meet the needs of the Black community generally, but particularly for Black women's safety.

One of the most contentious yet necessary steps to address the murder of Black women is stricter firearm legislation, particularly among individuals with reported histories of IPV. Recently, Congress passed the first piece of firearm legislation in 30 years, the Bipartisan Safer Communities Act (BPSCA). One of the major advancements in this legislation is increased restrictions on access to firearms for individuals with IPV-related convictions.[26] However, although the BPSCA includes legislation to restrict firearm access federally, state policies regarding reporting and tracking of protective orders and misdemeanors vary. Consequently, this inconsistency provides access to individuals who should be deemed ineligible. Although the BPSCA is progress, more needs to be done regarding the accessibility of firearms to keep our communities safe.

CONCLUSION

Data demonstrate that the murder of Black women is a clear and urgent public health crisis. Yet awareness of, attention to, and action toward addressing this issue is limited. Here, we shed light on this issue and the many factors contributing to its manifestation and place an urgent call to action to value and save the lives of Black women in the United States. AJPH

CORRESPONDENCE

Correspondence should be sent to Tameka L. Gillum, College of Population Health, MSC 09 5070 1, University of New Mexico, Albuquerque, NM 87131 (e-mail: tlgillum@salud.unm.edu). Reprints can be ordered at https://www.ajph.org by clicking the "Reprints" link.

PUBLICATION INFORMATION

Full Citation: Gillum TL, Sheffield A, Norton AD, Hampton CJ. The murder of Black women in the United States: a public health crisis. *Am J Public Health*. 2025;115(5):663–667.

Acceptance Date: December 24, 2024.

DOI: https://doi.org/10.2105/AJPH.2025.308010

ORCID iDs:

Tameka L. Gillum https://orcid.org/0009-0003-0171-809X

Alexis Sheffield https://orcid.org/0009-0000-5030-2638

Antonia Drew Norton https://orcid.org/0009-0003-8209-6658

Clarice J. Hampton https://orcid.org/0000-0002-9341-4020

CONTRIBUTORS

T. L. Gillum contributed to and facilitated the overall production of the manuscript, including conceptualization of the manuscript, production of the manuscript outline, and organization of the content; contributed to writing of all sections, edited content for all sections, and took the lead in revisions of the manuscript. A. Sheffield contributed content to multiple sections of the manuscript, including the introduction, the sections on intimate partner homicide, homicide by police, contributing factors, and efforts to raise awareness, and assisted with manuscript revisions. A. D. Norton contributed to the conceptualization of the manuscript and was a major contributor to the section related to implications for programs/services/intervention. C. J. Hampton was a major contributor to the sections related to impact and implications for policy.

CONFLICTS OF INTEREST

The authors have no conflicts of interest to disclose.

REFERENCES

1. Catalano S, Smith E, Snyder H, Rand M. *Female Victims of Violence*. Washington, DC: Bureau of Justice Statistics; September 2009. NCJ 228356.
2. Petrosky E, Blair JM, Betz CJ, Fowler KA, Jack SPD, Lyons BH. Racial and ethnic differences in homicides of adult women and the role of intimate partner violence—United States, 2003–2014. *MMWR Morb Mortal Wkly Rep*. 2017;66:741–746. https://doi.org/10.15585/mmwr.mm6628a1
3. Violence Policy Center. When men murder women: an analysis of 2020 homicide data. September 27, 2021. Available at: https://vpc.org/when-men-murder-women. Accessed June 12, 2024.
4. Violence Policy Center. When men murder women: a review of 25 years of female homicide. October 2023. Available at: https://www.vpc.org/studies/wmmw2023.pdf. Accessed December 14, 2024.
5. Waller BY, Joseph VA, Keyes KM. Racial inequities in homicide rates and homicide methods among black and white women aged 25–44 years in the USA, 1999–2020: a cross-sectional time series

study. *Lancet.* 2024;403(10430):935–945. https://doi.org/10.1016/S0140-6736(23)02279-1

6. Palladino CL, Singh V, Campbell J, Flynn H, Gold KJ. Homicide and suicide during the perinatal period: findings from the National Violent Death Reporting System. *Obstet Gynecol.* 2011;118(5):1056–1063. https://doi.org/10.1097/AOG.0b013e31823294da
7. Kivisto AJ, Mills S, Elwood LS. Racial disparities in pregnancy-associated intimate partner homicide. *J Interpers Violence.* 2022;37(13-14):NP10938–NP10961. https://doi.org/10.1177/0886260521990831
8. Edwards F, Lee H, Esposito M. Risk of being killed by police use of force in the United States by age, race–ethnicity, and sex. *Proc Natl Acad Sci USA.* 2019;116(34):16793–16798. https://doi.org/10.1073/pnas.1821204116
9. McFarlane J, Campbell JC, Sharps P, Watson K. Abuse during pregnancy and femicide: urgent implications for women's health. *Obstet Gynecol.* 2002;100(1):27–36.
10. Iati M, Jenkins J, Brugal S. Nearly 250 women have been fatally shot by police since 2015. *Washington Post.* September 2020. Available at: https://www.washingtonpost.com/graphics/2020/investigations/police-shootings-women. Accessed July 1, 2024.
11. Johnson O, Gilbert K, Ibrahim H. Race, gender, and the contexts of unarmed fatal interactions with police. Fatal Interactions with the Police Study (FIPS). 2018. Available at: https://cpb-us-w2.wpmucdn.com/sites.wustl.edu/dist/b/1205/files/2018/02/Race-Gender-and-Unarmed-1y9md6e.pdf. Accessed February 19, 2025.
12. Sabina C, Swatt M. Summary report: Latino intimate partner homicide. National Criminal Justice Reference Service. 2015. Available at: https://www.ncjrs.gov/pdffiles1/nij/grants/248887.pdf. Accessed July 1, 2024.
13. Graham LM, Ranapurwala SI, Zimmer C, et al. Disparities in potential years of life lost due to intimate partner violence: data from 16 states for 2006. *PLoS One.* 2021;16(2):e0246477. https://doi.org/10.1371/journal.pone.0246477
14. Campbell J, Campbell DW, Gary F, et al. African American women's responses to intimate partner violence: an examination of cultural context. *J Aggress Maltreat Trauma.* 2008;16(3):277–295. https://doi.org/10.1080/10926770801925684
15. Sharps PW, Campbell J, Campbell D, Gary F, Webster D. The role of alcohol use in intimate partner femicide. *Am J Addict.* 2001;10(2):122–135. https://doi.org/10.1080/105504901750227787
16. Lipsky S, Caetano R, Field CA, Bazargan S. The role of alcohol use and depression in intimate partner violence among black and Hispanic patients in an urban emergency department. *Am J Drug Alcohol Abuse.* 2005;31(2):225–242.
17. Hampton R, Oliver W, Magarian L. Domestic violence in the African American community: an analysis of social and structural Factors. *Violence Against Women.* 2003;9(5):533–557. https://doi.org/10.1177/1077801202250450
18. Gillum TL. Exploring the link between stereotypic images and intimate partner violence in the African American community. *Violence Against Women.* 2002;8(1):64–86.
19. Sabri B, Stockman JK, Campbell JC, et al. Factors associated with increased risk for lethal violence in intimate partner relationships among ethnically diverse black women. *Violence Vict.* 2014;29(5):719–741. https://doi.org/10.1891/0886-6708
20. Monterrosa AE. How race and gender stereotypes influence help-seeking for intimate partner violence. *J Interpers Violence.* 2021;36(17-18):NP9153–NP9174. https://doi.org/10.1177/0886260519853403
21. Waller BY, Bent-Goodley TB. "I have to fight to get out": African American women and intimate partner violence survivors' construction of agency. *J Interpers Violence.* 2022;38(3-4):4166–4188. https://doi.org/10.1177/08862605221113008
22. Anyikwa VA. The intersections of race and gender in help-seeking strategies among a battered sample of low-income African American women. *J Hum Behav Soc Environ.* 2015;25(8):948–959.
23. Few AL. The voices of black and white rural battered women in domestic violence shelters. *Fam Relat.* 2005;54(4):488–500.
24. Hirschel D, McCormack PD, Buzawa E. A 10-year study of the impact of intimate partner violence primary aggressor laws on single and dual arrest. *J Interpers Violence.* 2021;36(3-4):1356–1390. https://doi.org/10.1177/0886260517739290
25. Waller BY, Harris J, Quinn CR. Caught in the crossroad: an intersectional examination of African American women intimate partner violence survivors' help seeking. *Trauma Violence Abuse.* 2022;23(4):1235–1248. https://doi.org/10.1177/1524838021991303
26. Gillum TL, Hampton CJ, Coppedge C. Using the socio-ecological model to understand increased risk of gun violence in the African American community. *Psychol Rep.* 2025;128(1):126–148. https://doi.org/10.1177/00332941241256635
27. Prison Policy Initiative. Race and gender disparities in police stops, searches, and use of force. 2019. Available at: https://www.jstor.org/stable/resrep27309. Accessed July 1, 2024.
28. Shinde R. Black women, police brutality, and the Violence Against Women Act: how pro-arrest policies facilitate racialized and gendered police violence. *Georget J Gend Law.* 2021. Available at: https://www.law.georgetown.edu/gender-journal/wp-content/uploads/sites/20/2021/01/Final_Black-Women-and-VAWA_Rhea-Shinde_Issue-2.pdf. Accessed July 1, 2024.
29. Jacobs MS. The violent state: black women's invisible struggle against police violence. *Wm & Mary J Women & L.* 2017;24(1):39–100.
30. Ferrandino J. Minority threat hypothesis and NYPD stop and frisk policy. *Crim Justice Rev.* 2015;40(2):209–229. https://doi.org/10.1177/0734016814564989
31. Morrow WJ, Berthelot ER, Vickovic SG. Police use of force: an examination of the minority threat perspective. *Crim Justice Stud.* 2018;31(4):368–387. https://doi.org/10.1080/1478601X.2018.1513837
32. Ross CT. A multi-level Bayesian analysis of racial bias in police shootings at the county-level in the United States, 2011–2014. *PLoS One.* 2015;10(11):e0141854. https://doi.org/10.1371/journal.pone.0141854
33. Crenshaw KW, Ritchie AJ, Anspach R, Gilmer R, Harris L. Say her name: resisting police brutality against black women. African American Policy Forum. 2015. Available at: https://scholarship.law.columbia.edu/faculty_scholarship/3226. Accessed July 1, 2024.
34. Bailey RK, Barker CH, Grover A. Confluence of law enforcement, mental health, and race. *Behav Sci Law.* 2022;40:532–539. https://doi.org/10.1002/bsl.2567
35. Hacker RL, Horan JJ. Policing people with mental illness: experimental evaluation of online training to de-escalate mental health crises. *J Exp Criminol.* 2019;15:551–567. https://doi.org/10.1007/s11292-019-09380-3
36. Saleh AZ, Applebaum PS, Liu X, Stroup TS, Wall M. Deaths of people with mental illness during interactions with law enforcement. *Int J Law Psychiatry.* 2018;58:110–116. https://doi.org/10.1016/j.ijlp.2018.03.003
37. Boyle KM, Jones PT, Mancik AM. Racialized backlash: a state-level analysis of black women's homicide victimization by black men, white men, and police. *Crime Delinq.* 2024;70(5):1516–1540. https://doi.org/10.1177/00111287221134922
38. Dzhanova Y, Taylor A, Cranley E, Beckler H, Grant B. Black women have been killed by US police since 2015. *Business Insider.* 2021. Available at: https://www.businessinsider.com/black-women-killed-by-police-database-2021-6. Accessed July 1, 2024.
39. Gillum TL. The intersection of intimate partner violence and poverty in black communities. *Aggress Violent Behav.* 2019;46:37–44. https://doi.org/10.1016/j.avb.2019.01.008
40. Brown M, Ray R, Summers E, Fraistat N. #SayHerName: a case study of intersectional social media activism. *Ethn Racial Stud.* 2017;40(3):1836–1846. https://doi.org/10.1080/01419870.2017.1334934
41. Cecil DK. Saying her name: gendered narratives in news coverage of Breonna Taylor's death. *Race Justice.* 2024;14(3):423–439. https://doi.org/10.1177/21533687211070552
42. Vann A. Developing culturally relevant responses to domestic abuse: Asha Family Services, Inc. NRCDV. 2003. Available at: https://vawnet.org/material/developing-culturally-relevant-responses-domestic-abuse-asha-family-services-inc. Accessed July 16, 2024.
43. Gillum TL. The benefits of a culturally specific intimate partner violence intervention for African American survivors. *Violence Against Women.* 2008;14(8):917–943. https://doi.org/10.1177/1077801208321982
44. Benson ML, Fox GL. *When Violence Hits Home: How Economics and Neighborhood Play a Role.* Washington, DC: US Dept of Justice, National Institute of Justice; 2004. NCJ 205004.
45. Emezue C, Dan-Irabor D, Froilan A, et al. Evaluating an app-based intervention for preventing firearm violence and substance use in young black men and boys: usability evaluation study. *JMIR Form Res.* 2024;8:e60918. https://doi.org/10.2196/60918
46. Wilson RF, Blair JM. Racial inequities in homicide rates: black women in the USA. *Lancet.* 2024;403(10430):882–883. https://doi.org/10.1016/S0140-6736(23)02585-0

Mitigating Medical Debt as a Public Health Equity Issue: Challenges and Opportunities in New York City

Duncan Maru, MD, PhD, Rachel E. Schwartz, MPA, Judy Fordjuoh, MPH, Ellen Weiss Wiewel, DrPH, MHS, Rishi K. Sood, MPH, Emma Clippinger, JD, Jenai Jackson, MPH, Adeola Ayedun, MPH, Deirdre Flynn, MBA, Ashwin Vasan, MD, PhD, and Michelle Morse, MD, MPH

ABOUT THE AUTHORS

At the time of writing, all authors were with the New York City Department of Health and Mental Hygiene, New York, NY.

AJPH May 2025, Vol. 115, No. 5

Despite improvements in health insurance coverage since the implementation of the Affordable Care Act, high health care costs continue to be a top concern for Americans.[1] The total burden of medical debt in the United States is estimated at $220 billion. More than 14 million people owe more than $1000 and more than 3 million owe more than $10 000.[2] People with medical debt are more likely to be uninsured, living with low incomes, and from communities of color.[3] Medical debt is also a leading cause of personal bankruptcy,[4,5] contributing to more than half of bankruptcies between 2013 and 2016.[6] There is, increasingly, public discourse, justifiable outrage,[7] and community organizing[8] related to rising costs of health care. Here, we discuss avenues to address medical debt as a public health and health equity issue, specific to our work at the New York City (NYC) Health Department. In applying public health principles and tools to the problem of medical debt, we aim to develop infrastructure and strategies to (1) monitor, (2) mitigate, and (3) prevent medical debt and its negative health, social, and economic impacts in the nation's largest city, with more than 8 million residents.

MONITOR: ASSESS THE SCOPE AND HARMS OF MEDICAL DEBT

In establishing monitoring and surveillance capabilities for medical debt, we are leveraging existing public health data infrastructure, including the NYC Health Opinion Poll (HOP)[9] and qualitative research expertise. The HOP is a recurring population-based survey conducted by the NYC Health Department, in which 1200 adult respondents are recruited from existing online opt-in panels. Through this poll, we are able to characterize the prevalence of unpaid health care bills totaling $500 or more, the health care services or treatments contributing to these bills, and respondents' strategies for addressing these debts. We inquire about debt at the household level and use it to report on debt prevalence among NYC adults, consistent with national approaches such as the Kaiser Family Foundation's Health Care Debt Survey.[10] The relatively quick timeframe from NYC's survey question development to data availability has permitted us to share the April 2023 survey findings in local conferences, policy briefs, and community conversations about debt alleviation, as well as internal planning about NYC government strategies to offer debt relief.

These data showed that almost one million NYC adults owe at least $500 in unpaid health care bills. Medical debt of over $500 in unpaid bills exceeds the 13% citywide prevalence among most communities of color (25% of multiracial persons, 18% of Latinos, and 16% of Blacks, vs 10% among Whites), low-income households (17%, vs 11% among medium- and high-income households), and persons without health insurance (29%, vs 11% among insured persons). Although debt was more common among uninsured persons, over three quarters of New Yorkers with debt did have health insurance. These patterns and inequities are consistent with national patterns.[11]

In the 2024 HOP survey, we included the same medical debt questions to identify changes over time and incorporate new inquiries. We added questions to explore the extent to which acute or chronic conditions contribute to unpaid medical bills, reasons for individuals' inability to fully pay their medical bills upon receipt, and the broader impact of medical debt on their well-being. Results from this 2024 HOP survey will be available in 2025.

We also asked about medical debt in a large, diverse sample of NYC residents participating in a wealth and health survey in 2024, which is currently being analyzed, and will do so again in 2025 in a population representative sample. This work builds off our analysis relating to the racial wealth gap[12] as a driver of health inequities and source of injustice. These new survey items will enable us to measure medical debt prevalence among key racial and ethnic groups; and to connect medical debt with other measures of wealth and health.

Qualitative monitoring methods are equally important. We are currently conducting approximately 20 in-depth interviews with adult NYC residents who have or had medical debt about how they incur it, how they address it, how it affects their health care utilization and choices, their experiences with debt collection agencies, and their suggestions for improvements in hospital and insurance company practices to mitigate medical debt. Direct outreach to individuals at health fairs, community-based organizations' events, and within neighborhoods is in progress across the city. We will also conduct key informant interviews with hospital and insurance company leadership about hospital financial assistance programs, billing administrative procedures, and relevant staff training. Key informants will be recruited via e-mail outreach to hospital administrators and insurance representatives across for-profit and nonprofit clinics, hospitals, and organizations that provide health care services in NYC, including but not limited to Health Department partners. We will work collaboratively with community members, giving them access to data to help with interpretation and eliciting their support to disseminate findings to enhance real-world impact.

MITIGATE: IMPROVE THE LIVES OF THOSE BURDENED BY MEDICAL DEBT

Abolishing existing medical debt is one mitigation strategy that over a dozen US jurisdictions have begun to implement, at times coupled with efforts to prevent its accrual and address systemic health care issues.[13] NYC began pursuing this approach in 2023, based in part on the experiences of other jurisdictions.

In 2022, Cook County, Illinois launched its Medical Debt Relief Initiative in partnership with the nonprofit Undue Medical Debt (formerly known as RIP Medical Debt) to forgive medical debt, purchased from secondary markets at concessional prices, for low-income residents. Using $12 million in federal funds from the American Rescue Plan Act, the county has acquired and abolished $281 million in medical debt as of October 2023, benefiting over 150 000 Cook County residents.[14]

A number of localities have proposed or implemented similar programs in partnership with Undue Medical Debt. For example, in 2024, Los Angeles County, California announced an initial $5 million investment from its Board of Supervisors to forgive $500 million in medical debt.[15] This investment enhances the broader plan of the county's Medical Debt Coalition, to address the challenge of medical debt. For them, this includes eventually forgiving $2 billion in medical debt using funds from philanthropic partners, hospitals, and health plans, maintaining the online consumer resources that they compiled to prevent and address debt, and more.[16]

Based on the experiences of these and other jurisdictions, in 2024, NYC announced a partnership with Undue Medical Debt[17] to use $18 million in city funds over three years to purchase and forgive $2 billion of medical debt, the largest program of its kind to date in the nation. The program is designed to assist low- and middle-income New Yorkers (at or below 400% of the federal poverty level based on the US Census Bureau) and those whose debts total more than 5% of their total income. Eligible NYC residents will be identified by Undue Medical Debt starting in 2025 and do not need to take any action to have their debt forgiven. They will be notified when their debt has been purchased directly from a participating hospital and forgiven.

Although the effects of medical debt and other household debt on health and well-being are well-established,[18] evidence from two randomized controlled trials conducted in 2018 to 2020, involving over 80 000 people living with medical debt in the United States, suggests that debt abolishment programs alone are unlikely to improve public health. These programs, which prompted updates to Undue Medical Debt's debt cancelation approach, did not increase access to credit or improve mental well-being, and may have even unintentionally harmed the mental health of certain participants.[19] These findings support the implementation of the following approaches in debt abolishment programs: (1) tie such programs to, and use them to amplify, comprehensive debt prevention measures such as expanding access to health insurance; (2) prioritize individuals and communities suffering disproportionate harms, by neighborhood and in a race-conscious way; (3) address hospital and systems-level accountability to medical debt rather than framing the work as "charity," including in communication to participants; and (4) conduct implementation science research to understand how best to abolish medical debt. Given public health's historic work integrating prevention and cure measures, findings such as these provide motivation to improve medical debt mitigation programs, and to tie such measures to prevention, which we now discuss.

PREVENT: ELIMINATE MEDICAL DEBT AS A PUBLIC HEALTH THREAT

A primary role the NYC Health Department plays in prevention is in partnership with advocacy and consumer groups, community organizations, and New York State through policy memos, data analytics, and, ideally, identifying creative means at a local level to improve the enforcement of state laws. With medical debt, our role will likely largely be in monitoring and supporting enforcement of state law. Since 2022, New York State has taken steps to combat aggressive debt collection practices that disproportionately hurt low-income communities of color. The state banned hospitals and other health care facilities from garnishing wages[20] or placing liens on primary residences for individuals because of a medical debt lawsuit and subsequently banned the practice of reporting medical debt[21] of any amount to credit agencies.

Most recently, in the New York State fiscal year 2025 enacted budget, the state took unprecedented action[22] to update and improve the state's Hospital Financial Assistance Law, making financial assistance both more robust and more accessible to a wider swath of New Yorkers in need. The new law also bans hospitals from suing patients earning less than 400% of the federal policy level for unpaid medical debt. These changes could not have occurred without the work of consumer advocates, who continue to urge lawmakers to create a more just system for all New Yorkers.

Finally, prevention of medical debt goes hand in hand with universal health insurance coverage. In 2023, 12% of NYC adults lacked health insurance,[23] largely because of constraints on coverage related to immigration status. For decades, New York State has covered children through Child Health Plus (the state's Children's Health Insurance Program [CHIP]) regardless of immigration status. New York State expanded coverage of undocumented New Yorkers aged 65 years and older through Medicaid in January 2024. The state was also granted a federal waiver to implement an expansion of New York State's Basic Health Program (known as the Essential Plan) to New Yorkers with higher incomes and those with Deferred Action for Childhood Arrival (DACA) status. However, despite this progress, state lawmakers failed to use the opportunity[24] to further expand access to coverage for undocumented New York State residents aged 19 to 64 years. We will continue to operate insurance enrollment programs to ensure that New Yorkers can take advantage of existing benefits and will support enrollment in other health insurance as coverage opportunities expand. We will also continue to work with New York State to identify and address remaining coverage gaps.

Although fighting for universal health coverage is critical to addressing the harms of medical debt, this effort must be coupled with efforts to improve health insurance itself. High out-of-pocket costs, utilization management policies like prior authorization, and reports of widespread "red tape" mean insured patients are also at risk for accruing medical debt. Indeed, a majority of NYC residents with debt have health insurance. In a 2023 survey, 43% of US adults with private insurance reported that it was very or somewhat difficult to afford their health care. The percentage struggling to afford care was even higher for those with Medicaid (45%) and marketplace or individual market plans (57%.)[25] So in addition to expanding eligibility for insurance, it is also crucial to ensure that insurance is protective from high costs for those who have it.

It is impossible to ignore the reaction to the December 2024 premeditated murder of Brian Thompson, CEO of the for-profit American health insurance company UnitedHealthcare. His death has ignited a new wave of Americans expressing their justified anger and frustration at a system that often puts profit over patients' best interests.[26] Addressing the harms of a for-profit system will require action and cooperation at all levels of government, and necessitate an approach that acknowledges the harms of our current system. Significant policy action in this arena will also require the buy-in of nongovernmental actors like health systems and insurers, which profit from the current system and often serve as an impediment to large-scale change.

CONCLUSION

As we emerge from the COVID-19 emergency era, we can build bridges between public health and health care[27] by integrating public health's model of collective action and population impact with health care's focus on individual patients and the immediate communities in which they practice. Medical debt is a health care issue around which public health capacity must be built. Government public health in any jurisdiction focuses on whole-of-population approaches to improving health and its drivers, which includes economic and financial security. Following a United States presidential election that centered on the rising cost of living, including the burden of health care bills, public health institutions have an important role to play in identifying creative solutions to address the inequitable financial burdens created by our health care system. National debates around health care are necessary and can be bolstered by the work of local public health departments, whether regarding expanding access to insurance or lowering the cost of prescriptions. The public health approach to alleviating medical debt involves applying in new ways the core public health capabilities of monitoring, mitigation, and prevention, thus shifting the narrative of what governments can do about medical debt.

By developing routine monitoring systems of medical debt, operating debt abolishment programs, and developing new preventive policies, we can ultimately eradicate medical debt and the exacting toll it takes on health and well-being. AJPH

CORRESPONDENCE

Correspondence should be sent to Rachel Schwartz, 42-09 28th St, Long Island City, NY 11101 (e-mail: Rschwartz2@health.nyc.gov). Reprints can be ordered at https://www.ajph.org by clicking the "Reprints" link.

PUBLICATION INFORMATION

Full Citation: Maru D, Schwartz RE, Fordjuoh J, et al. Mitigating medical debt as a public health equity issue: challenges and opportunities in New York City. *Am J Public Health*. 2025;115(5): 668–672.

Acceptance Date: January 8, 2025.

DOI: https://doi.org/10.2105/AJPH.2025.308026

ORCID iDs:
Rachel E. Schwartz https://orcid.org/0009-0004-7547-9340

Ellen Weiss Wiewel https://orcid.org/0000-0002-5106-0500

Jenai Jackson https://orcid.org/0009-0008-0563-0008

Adeola Ayedun https://orcid.org/0000-0003-2440-984X

Deirdre Flynn https://orcid.org/0009-0009-6891-8241

CONTRIBUTORS

D. Maru conceptualized and contributed substantially to the development, design, drafting, and critical review of the work. R. Schwartz contributed substantially to the conceptualization, design, and development of the work, led policy interpretation and writing of the policy-focused sections for the work, and contributed to drafting and critical review of the other sections. J. Fordjuoh contributed substantially to the conceptualization, design, and development of the work; designed, analyzed, and interpreted quantitative data for the work; led writing of the sections about quantitative data; and contributed to drafting and critical review of the other sections. E. W. Wiewel contributed substantially to the conceptualization, design, and development of the work, contributed to the design and interpretation of quantitative data for the work, and contributed to drafting and critical review of the work. R. K. Sood contributed substantially to the conceptualization, design, and development of the work, contributed to the design and interpretation of quantitative data for the work, and provided critical review of the work. E. Clippinger contributed substantially to policy interpretation for the work and reviewed the piece critically for content. J. Jackson and A. Ayedun led writing of the section about qualitative research related to medical debt and reviewed the piece critically for content. D. Flynn provided editorial support and reviewed policy sections critically for content. A. Vasan and M. Morse contributed substantially to the conceptualization of the work and reviewed the piece critically for content.

CONFLICTS OF INTEREST

The authors have no conflicts of interest to report.

REFERENCES

1. Kearney A, Montero A, Valdes I, Kirzinger A, Hamel L. KFF health tracking poll February 2024: voters on two key health care issues: affordability and ACA. 2024. Available at: https://www.kff.org/affordable-care-act/poll-finding/kff-health-tracking-poll-february-2024-voters-on-two-key-health-care-issues-affordability-and-aca. Accessed October 8, 2024.
2. Rakshit S, Rae M, Claxton G, Amin K, Cox C. The burden of medical debt in the United States. 2024. Available at: https://www.healthsystemtracker.org/brief/the-burden-of-medical-debt-in-the-united-states. Accessed October 17, 2024.
3. Winger A, Claxton G, Rae M, Damico A, Rakshit S. How financially vulnerable are people with medical debt? 2024. Available at: https://www.healthsystemtracker.org/brief/how-financially-vulnerable-are-people-with-medical-debt. Accessed October 17, 2024.
4. Himmelstein DU, Thorne D, Warren E, Woolhandler S. Medical bankruptcy in the United States, 2007: results of a national study. *Am J Med.* 2009;122(8):741–746. https://doi.org/10.1016/j.amjmed.2009.04.012
5. Himmelstein DU, Warren E, Thorne D, Woolhandler S. Illness and injury as contributors to bankruptcy. *Health Aff (Millwood).* 2005;24(suppl 1):W5-63–W65-73. https://doi.org/10.1377/hlthaff.W5.63
6. Himmelstein DU, Lawless RM, Thorne D, Foohey P, Woolhandler S. Medical bankruptcy: still common despite the Affordable Care Act. *Am J Public Health.* 2019;109(3):431–433. https://doi.org/10.2105/AJPH.2018.304901
7. Johnson J. "Profiteering healthcare system" blamed as US medical debt surges to $140 billion. 2021. Available at: https://www.commondreams.org/news/2021/07/20/profiteering-healthcare-system-blamed-us-medical-debt-surges-140-billion. Accessed December 18, 2024.
8. Venkat M, Ozug M, Shapiro A. Before dying, she made a fund to cancel others' medical debt—now $60 million worth [podcast]. NPR. November 23, 2023. Available at: https://www.npr.org/2023/11/23/1215031473/before-dying-she-made-a-fund-to-cancel-others-medical-debt-now-60-million-worth. Accessed December 19, 2024.
9. New York City Dept of Health. NYC Health Opinion Poll. Available at: https://www.nyc.gov/site/doh/data/data-sets/health-opinion-poll.page. Accessed October 17, 2024.
10. Lopes L, Kearney A, Montero A, Hamel L, Brodie M. Health care debt in the US: the broad consequences of medical and dental bills. KFF. 2022. Available at: https://www.kff.org/report-section/kff-health-care-debt-survey-main-findings/#:~:text=Half%20of%20adults%20with%20health%20care%20debt%20say%20bills%20from,caused%20some%20of%20their%20debt. Accessed December 13, 2024.
11. Himmelstein DU, Dickman SL, McCormick D, Bor DH, Gaffney A, Woolhandler S. Prevalence and risk factors for medical debt and subsequent changes in social determinants of health in the US. *JAMA Netw Open.* 2022;5(9):e2231898. https://doi.org/10.1001/jamanetworkopen.2022.31898
12. Morse M, Anekwe A, Bloomstone S, Farquhar S, Darity WA Jr. Analyzing the racial wealth gap and implications for health equity. 2022. Available at: https://www.nyc.gov/assets/doh/downloads/pdf/cmo/racial-wealth-gap-health-equity.pdf. Accessed October 17, 2024.
13. Undue Medical Debt. Government partnerships in action. 2024. Available at: https://unduemedicaldebt.org/government-partnerships. Accessed December 23, 2024, 2024.
14. Cook County Government. Cook County Medical Debt Relief Initiative abolishes over $280 million in medical debt for Cook County residents. 2023. Available at: https://www.cookcountyil.gov/news/cook-county-medical-debt-relief-initiative-abolishes-over-280-million-medical-debt-cook-county. Accessed October 17, 2024.

15. County of Los Angeles Dept of Public Health. Public health launches Los Angeles County Medical Debt Relief Program—LA County and partners seek to relieve $2 billion in medical debt. 2024. Available at: http://publichealth.lacounty.gov/phcommon/public/media/mediapubhpdetail.cfm?prid=4905. Accessed December 19, 2024.
16. County of Los Angeles Dept of Public Health. Medical debt information for consumers. 2024. Available at: http://publichealth.lacounty.gov/hccp/medicalDebt/. Accessed December 19, 2024.
17. New York City Government. Canceling medical debt for New Yorkers. 2024. Available at: https://www.nyc.gov/content/getstuffdone/pages/canceling-medical-debt-for-new-yorkers. Accessed October 17, 2024.
18. American Public Health Association. The impacts of individual and household debt on health and well-being. 2021. Available at: https://www.apha.org/policies-and-advocacy/public-health-policy-statements/policy-database/2022/01/07/the-impacts-of-individual-and-household-debt-on-health-and-well-being#:~. Accessed October 17, 2024.
19. Kluender R, Mahoney N, Wong F, Yin W. The effects of medical debt relief. National Bureau Of Economic Research Working Paper Series. 2024. Available at: https://www.nber.org/papers/w32315. Accessed October 17, 2024.
20. An act to amend Section 5201 of the civil practice law and rules, in relation to protecting patients from certain penalties due to money judgments arising from actions brought by hospitals or health care professionals. NY Civil Practice Law §5201 (2024).
21. The Fair Medical Debt Reporting Act. NY Public Health Law §4926 (2024).
22. State of New York. Governor Hochul announces historic investments of FY 2025 New York State Budget. 2024; Available at: https://www.budget.ny.gov/pubs/press/2024/fy25-enacted-budget-highlights.html#:~:text=The%20FY25%20budget%20also%20includes,for%20a%20family%20of%20four. Accessed October 17, 2024.
23. New York City Dept of Health and Mental Hygiene. Community Health Survey 2019–2023. Available at: https://www.nyc.gov/site/doh/data/data-sets/community-health-survey-public-use-data.page. Accessed December 23, 2024.
24. Reisman N. Mayor Adams urges Hochul to back health insurance for more undocumented residents. 2023. Available at: https://spectrumlocalnews.com/nys/central-ny/ny-state-of-politics/2023/03/29/mayor-adams-backs-expanding-health-insurance-to-more-undocumented-residents. Accessed October 17, 2024.
25. Collins SR, Roy S, Relebohile M. Paying for it: how health care costs and medical debt are making Americans sicker and poorer. 2023. Available at: https://www.commonwealthfund.org/publications/surveys/2023/oct/paying-for-it-costs-debt-americans-sicker-poorer-2023-affordability-survey#:~:text=Among%20people%20in%20employer%20plans,to%20those%20with%20higher%20incomes. Accessed December 19, 2024, 2024.
26. Potter W. I was a health insurance executive. What I saw made me quit. *The New York Times.* December 19, 2024. Available at: https://www.nytimes.com/2024/12/18/opinion/health-insurance-united-ceo-shooting.html. Accessed December 20, 2024.
27. Wong C, Houry D, Cohen M. Integrating public health and health care—protecting health as a team sport. *N Engl J Med.* 2024;390(19):1739–1742. https://doi.org/10.1056/NEJMp2403274

Age Restricted Location Policies: A Potential Strategy for Advancing the Tobacco Endgame

Megan E. Roberts, PhD, Joseph G. Lee, PhD, Meghan E. Morean, PhD, Grace Kong, PhD, Amy K. Ferketich, PhD, Peter F. Craigmile, PhD, Rachel C. Ceasar, PhD, Vitoria Borges Spinola, DDS, and Micah L. Berman, JD

ABOUT THE AUTHORS

Megan E. Roberts, Amy K. Ferketich, and Vitoria Borges Spinola are with the College of Public Health, Ohio State University, Columbus. Joseph G. Lee is with the College of Health and Human Performance, East Carolina University, Greenville, NC. Meghan E. Morean and Grace Kong are with the Department of Psychiatry, Yale University School of Medicine, New Haven, CT. Peter F. Craigmile is with the Department of Mathematics and Statistics, Hunter College, CUNY, New York, NY. Rachel C. Ceasar is with the Keck School of Medicine, University of Southern California, Los Angeles. Micah L. Berman is with the College of Public Health and the Mortiz College of Law, Ohio State University, Columbus.

Tobacco use is responsible for more than 480 000 US deaths per year, making it the leading cause of preventable death for the country.[1] For the last decade, a popular topic of discussion among tobacco control researchers seeking to reduce tobacco-related morbidity and mortality has been "the tobacco endgame." This term refers to the goal of phasing out the sale of commercial tobacco products to near-zero levels. Though once considered an idealistic goal, there is an emerging consensus that tobacco endgame scenarios could be achieved through a combination of continued implementation of established measures, complemented by new and innovative policies.[2–5] Age restricted location (ARL) policies are an innovative strategy that advances this goal.

ARL policies are regulations that would restrict the sale of all tobacco products to adult-only establishments. Specifically, under an ARL policy, tobacco could only be sold in stores like tobacco shops and vape shops that bar entry to those under the minimum age of sale (age 21 years in the United States). Tobacco retailers like convenience stores, dollar stores, gas stations, grocery stores, and pharmacies (which, collectively, constitute more than 80% of tobacco retailers[6,7]) would no longer be permitted to sell tobacco, as they allow children and young people on their premises. An ARL policy would, in many ways, mirror how both cannabis (where legal) and liquor sales are restricted in many US states. And it could have a major impact on US tobacco retailer density, which is currently estimated at over 1.22 retailers per 1000 persons.[8] This value goes up to 16.7 retailers per capita when examining historically marginalized areas, such as neighborhoods with a greater composition of racially or ethnically minoritized residents.[8] To provide some global context, Finland reports 1.0 retailers per 1000 persons,[9] Scotland 7.5 per 1000 persons,[10] and New Zealand 1.6 per 1000 adults.[11]

Support for ARL policies is motivated by the extensive literature indicating the role that tobacco retailers play in perpetuating the tobacco epidemic by providing ready access to tobacco products.[12,13] Retailers are also a major source of exposure to the tobacco industry's marketing, with more than 50% of youths reporting frequent tobacco marketing exposures at retailers[14] (marketing exposure has been found to promote tobacco initiation and inhibit cessation[15–18]). Concerningly, these issues of access and marketing exposure are often greatest in historically marginalized communities, where there are, on average, both more retailers and more marketing per retailer.[19–24] There is, likewise, strong evidence that reducing access to tobacco retailers would reduce youth use and support people who use tobacco and want to quit.[25–27]

Perhaps through growing attention on the tobacco retail environment, ARL policies have received more consideration in the literature over the last few years, often in the context of reviewing endgame policies.[28–32] But ARL policies are not just a hypothetical tobacco prevention strategy. Recently, the Netherlands became the first country in the world to enact an ARL policy.[33,34] The multiphase implementation plan was intended to be gradual. In 2022, cigarette vending machines (previously allowed outside, as free-standing entities) were banned. Beginning July 1, 2024, tobacco sales in grocery stores were prohibited. By 2032, sales of tobacco in gas stations and convenience

AJPH May 2025, Vol. 115, No. 5

stores also will be prohibited. With the Netherlands blazing a trail for ARL policies, it is an excellent time for other countries, including the United States, to follow suit.

WHAT COULD AN AGE RESTRICTED LOCATION POLICY DO?

Likely benefits of an ARL policy include the following.

1. Reducing tobacco initiation among youths and improving cessation among youths and adults. Research has established that greater tobacco retailer density is associated with greater youth tobacco use[13] and fewer successful quit attempts among adults who smoke.[16,27] Conversely, policies that reduce access—such as restricting cigarette vending machines to adult-only facilities in the United States—is associated with reduced youth use.[35] Among youths aged 18 years and older who use tobacco, 56.4% purchase it directly from brick-and-mortar stores and 34.5% buy or borrow it from someone who made a purchase.[36] As previously stated, an ARL policy would prohibit the sale of tobacco products at an estimated 80% of existing US tobacco retailers. Thus, an ARL policy would drastically reduce the number and density of tobacco retailers, thereby reducing access to tobacco products. Further, retailers no longer selling tobacco would gradually remove their tobacco advertisements and promotions, thereby reducing exposure to tobacco marketing.
2. Reducing tobacco-related health disparities. Tobacco retailer density is typically greater in historically marginalized communities,[20–23,37] contributing to tobacco use disparities based on neighborhood income, racial and ethnic composition, and rurality[38–44] (which have, in turn, been linked to tobacco-related health disparities). Convenience stores and dollar stores are also more prevalent in historically marginalized communities.[7,45–47] For example, our work in Ohio found that, when we looked at the percentage of tobacco retailers that were convenience stores, the prevalence was 62.3% for urban areas with high prevalences of poverty and people of color, 60.1% for rural areas with a high prevalence of poverty, and only 52.6% for urban areas with low prevalences of poverty and people of color.[7] As tobacco sales from these types of stores would be eliminated by an ARL policy, the policy may potentially have the greatest impact for individuals living in historically marginalized communities, rendering it an equity-enhancing policy.
3. Complementing existing age-of-sale policies. Tobacco 21 laws in the United States prohibit tobacco sales to people aged younger than 21 years but do not restrict where tobacco can be sold or who can enter such locations. Under an ARL policy, tobacco sales would only be allowed in retailers that prohibit individuals younger than 21 years from entering, thus reducing the potential for illegal sales to minors. Currently, noncompliance with Tobacco 21 (i.e., sales to minors) is poor in some locations[48] and would remain a concern under an ARL policy. However, with considerably fewer retailers selling tobacco, retailer inspections will become more manageable, allowing retailers with repeat violations to receive more attention. This, in turn, could contribute to improvements in Tobacco 21 enforcement.

FUTURE CONSIDERATIONS

As with any new policy, important considerations are warranted. Because ARL policies are so new, there is not yet rigorous evidence concerning their effectiveness. Evaluations of the ARL policy in the Netherlands[49] and of other jurisdictions that adopt ARL policies in the future will be eagerly anticipated. In the meantime, simulation studies that model changes to observed tobacco retailer density data may also answer important questions about how ARL policies might unfold in various social, legal, and geographic contexts. For example, an ARL policy might complement and enhance the impact of some tobacco policies, such as licensing law strategies,[50,51] but could conflict with other endgame approaches, such as pharmacy-only policies (that would permit tobacco sales only in pharmacies).[52] It will also be important to determine how low tobacco retailer density must become to have a meaningful impact on tobacco use behavior.

Another important consideration is the drafting of the ARL policies themselves, which will need to be carefully written to avoid loopholes or unintended consequences. In the Netherlands, for example, there are concerns that, in response to their ARL policy, the number of specialist tobacco shops may increase.[49] To maximize the effectiveness of ARL policies, language can be added to limit the total number of licenses available for adult-only stores (e.g., caps on retail licenses); this could help prevent compensatory market responses such as new tobacco or vape shops opening—especially in historically marginalized areas. In addition, language can be added to prevent retailers from designating separate areas ("store within a store") as adult-only; this lesson was learned in the United States, when retailers sought loopholes to local flavor bans with adult-only exemptions.[53–55]

Meaningfully reducing tobacco-related morbidity and mortality and related inequities requires innovative policies. The time has come to seriously consider ARL policies as part of a tobacco endgame strategy. There will undoubtedly be challenges. In the United States, for example, there are 27 tobacco retailers for every one McDonald's fast-food establishment (the nation's largest fast-food chain),[56] and, on average, cigarettes generate more than $500 000 in annual sales for each convenience store (though far less in profit). Thus, tobacco retailers and tobacco companies more broadly would have a strong incentive to oppose ARL policies. But this is not an insurmountable obstacle. Economic analyses have found that US declines in cigarette sales have not negatively affected business; in fact, the number of retailers, revenues, and profits have risen[57] and are expected to continue rising, as money previously spent on tobacco shifts to other services or merchandise.[58] Moreover, the tobacco industry has been on notice for more than 60 years that they are selling an addictive and deadly product, and there is now strong public support for more aggressive tobacco policies.[3,59,60]

When we envision a world nearing the end of commercial tobacco sales, what does that look like? An ARL policy depicts a feasible scenario: just a small number of stores where adults who are unable or unwilling to quit retain their ability to legally purchase tobacco products. In this world, the preponderance of tobacco sales and point-of-sale marketing will be muted, perhaps most drastically in historically marginalized communities. It is a scenario worth real consideration. Achieving it will require the concerted and coordinated efforts of many strategies, including the continued implementation of established prevention and cessation measures. But the incorporation of ARL policies could bring us closer to that endgame. AJPH

CORRESPONDENCE

Correspondence should be sent to Megan E. Roberts, The Ohio State University College of Public Health, Columbus, OH 43210 (e-mail: Roberts.1558@osu.edu). Reprints can be ordered at https://www.ajph.org by clicking the "Reprints" link.

PUBLICATION INFORMATION

Full Citation: Roberts ME, Lee JG, Morean ME, et al. Age restricted location policies: a potential strategy for advancing the tobacco endgame. *Am J Public Health*. 2025;115(5):673–677.

Acceptance Date: January 8, 2024.

DOI: https://doi.org/10.2105/AJPH.2025.308031

ORCID iDs:

Megan E. Roberts https://orcid.org/0000-0003-4743-2145

Joseph G. Lee https://orcid.org/0000-0001-9698-649X

Meghan E. Morean https://orcid.org/0000-0003-4865-1155

Peter F. Craigmile https://orcid.org/0000-0002-9212-3950

Vitoria Borges Spinola https://orcid.org/0000-0003-4738-1202

Micah L. Berman https://orcid.org/0000-0002-0336-1317

CONTRIBUTORS

M. E. Roberts conceptualized the article and wrote the initial draft. All coauthors provided substantiative feedback to the draft and subsequent revisions. All authors approved the final version of the manuscript.

ACKNOWLEDGMENTS

Research reported in this publication was supported by the National Cancer Institute of the National Institutes of Health (award no. R01CA273206).

Note. The contents are solely the responsibility of the authors and do not necessarily represent the official views of the National Institutes of Health.

CONFLICTS OF INTEREST

The authors have no conflicts of interest to report.

REFERENCES

1. Centers for Disease Control and Prevention. The health consequences of smoking—50 years of progress. A report of the surgeon general, 2014. Available at: https://www.ncbi.nlm.nih.gov/books/NBK179276. Accessed February 1, 2025.
2. Nip J, Thornley L, Schwartz R, et al. Commercial tobacco endgame goals: early experiences from six countries. *Nicotine Tob Res.* 2024;26(10):1322–1330. https://doi.org/10.1093/ntr/ntae069
3. Kim H, Gartner C, Edwards R, et al. Public support for tobacco endgame policies: a systematic review and meta-analysis. Published online 2024. https://doi.org/10.1101/2024.01.07.24300815
4. Smith EA, McDaniel PA, Malone RE. California advocates' perspectives on challenges and risks of advancing the tobacco endgame. *J Public Health Policy.* 2020;41(3):321–333. https://doi.org/10.1057/s41271-020-00230-5
5. Kong AY, King BA. Boosting the tobacco control vaccine: recognizing the role of the retail environment in addressing tobacco use and disparities. *Tob Control.* 2021;30(e2):e162–e168. https://doi.org/10.1136/tobaccocontrol-2020-055722
6. Golden SD, Baggett CD, Kuo TM, et al. Trends in the number and type of tobacco product retailers, United States, 2000–2017. *Nicotine Tob Res.* 2022;24(1):77–84. https://doi.org/10.1093/ntr/ntab150
7. Jenkins C, Craigmile PF, Schwartz E, Onnen N, Roberts ME. Variations in tobacco retailer type across community characteristics: place matters. *Prev Chronic Dis.* 2022;19:E49. https://doi.org/10.5888/pcd19.210454
8. Mills SD, Kong AY, Reimold AE, Baggett CD, Wiesen CA, Golden SD. Sociodemographic disparities in tobacco retailer density in the United States, 2000–2017. *Nicotine Tob Res.* 2022;24(8):1291–1299. https://doi.org/10.1093/ntr/ntac020
9. Pätsi SM, Toikka A, Ollila H, Ruokolainen O. Area-level sociodemographic differences in tobacco availability examined with nationwide tobacco product retail licence data in Finland. *Tob Control.* 2024;33(e2):e158–e164. https://doi.org/10.1136/tc-2022-057798
10. Caryl FM, Pearce J, Reid G, Mitchell R, Shortt NK. Simulating the density reduction and equity-impact of potential tobacco retail control policies. *Tob Control.* 2021;30(e2):e138–e143. https://doi.org/10.1136/tobaccocontrol-2020-056002
11. Marsh L, Doscher C, Robertson LA. Characteristics of tobacco retailers in New Zealand. *Health Place.* 2013;23:165–170. https://doi.org/10.1016/j.healthplace.2013.07.003

12. Lee JGL, Kong AY, Sewell KB, et al. Associations of tobacco retailer density and proximity with adult tobacco use behaviours and health outcomes: a meta-analysis. *Tob Control.* 2022;31(e2):e189–e200. https://doi.org/10.1136/tobaccocontrol-2021-056717
13. Finan LJ, Lipperman-Kreda S, Abadi M, et al. Tobacco outlet density and adolescents' cigarette smoking: a meta-analysis. *Tob Control.* 2019;28(1):27–33. https://doi.org/10.1136/tobaccocontrol-2017-054065
14. Papaleontiou L, Agaku IT, Filippidis FT. Effects of exposure to tobacco and electronic cigarette advertisements on tobacco use: an analysis of the 2015 National Youth Tobacco Survey. *J Adolesc Health.* 2020;66(1):64–71. https://doi.org/10.1016/j.jadohealth.2019.05.022
15. Paynter J, Edwards R. The impact of tobacco promotion at the point of sale: a systematic review. *Nicotine Tob Res.* 2009;11(1):25–35. https://doi.org/10.1093/ntr/ntn002
16. Carter OBJ, Mills BW, Donovan RJ. The effect of retail cigarette pack displays on unplanned purchases: results from immediate postpurchase interviews. *Tob Control.* 2009;18(3):218–221. https://doi.org/10.1136/tc.2008.027870
17. Levy DT, Lindblom EN, Fleischer NL, et al. Public health effects of restricting retail tobacco product displays and ads. *Tob Regul Sci.* 2015;1(1):61–75. https://doi.org/10.18001/TRS.1.1.7
18. Setodji CM, Martino SC, Gong M, et al. How do tobacco power walls influence adolescents? A study of mediating mechanisms. *Health Psychol.* 2018;37(2):188–193. https://doi.org/10.1037/hea0000558
19. Yerger VB, Przewoznik J, Malone RE. Racialized geography, corporate activity, and health disparities: tobacco industry targeting of inner cities. *J Health Care Poor Underserved.* 2007;18(4 suppl):10–38. https://doi.org/10.1353/hpu.2007.0120
20. Rodriguez D, Carlos HA, Adachi-Mejia AM, Berke EM, Sargent JD. Predictors of tobacco outlet density nationwide: a geographic analysis. *Tob Control.* 2013;22(5):349–355. https://doi.org/10.1136/tobaccocontrol-2011-050120
21. Yu D, Peterson NA, Sheffer MA, Reid RJ, Schnieder JE. Tobacco outlet density and demographics: analysing the relationships with a spatial regression approach. *Public Health.* 2010;124(7):412–416. https://doi.org/10.1016/j.puhe.2010.03.024
22. Kong AY, Herbert L, Feldman JM, Trangenstein PJ, Fakunle DO, Lee JGL. Tobacco and alcohol retailer availability and neighborhood racialized, economic, and racialized economic segregation in North Carolina. *J Racial Ethn Health Disparities.* 2023;10(6):2861–2871. https://doi.org/10.1007/s40615-022-01463-8
23. Adibe C, Craigmile PF, Onnen N, Schwartz E, Roberts ME. The relationship between tobacco retailer density and neighborhood demographics in Ohio. *Ohio J Public Health.* 2019;2(1)12–18.
24. Lee JGL, Henriksen L, Rose SW, Moreland-Russell S, Ribisl KM. A systematic review of neighborhood disparities in point-of-sale tobacco marketing. *Am J Public Health.* 2015;105(9):e8–e18. https://doi.org/10.2105/AJPH.2015.302777
25. Henriksen L, Feighery EC, Schleicher NC, Cowling DW, Kline RS, Fortmann SP. Is adolescent smoking related to the density and proximity of tobacco outlets and retail cigarette advertising near schools? *Prev Med.* 2008;47(2):210–214. https://doi.org/10.1016/j.ypmed.2008.04.008
26. Mennis J, Mason M, Way T, Zaharakis N. The role of tobacco outlet density in a smoking cessation intervention for urban youth. *Health Place.* 2016;38:39–47. https://doi.org/10.1016/j.healthplace.2015.12.008
27. Reitzel LR, Cromley EK, Li Y, et al. the effect of tobacco outlet density and proximity on smoking cessation. *Am J Public Health.* 2011;101(2):315–320. https://doi.org/10.2105/AJPH.2010.191676
28. McDaniel PA, Smith EA, Malone RE. The tobacco endgame: a qualitative review and synthesis. *Tob Control.* 2016;25(5):594–604. https://doi.org/10.1136/tobaccocontrol-2015-052356
29. Bhatnagar A, Whitsel LP, Blaha MJ, et al. New and emerging tobacco products and the nicotine endgame: the role of robust regulation and comprehensive tobacco control and prevention: a presidential advisory from the American Heart Association. *Circulation.* 2019;139(19):e937–e958. https://doi.org/10.1161/CIR.0000000000000669
30. Friedman AS, Warner KE. The e-cigarette flavor debate—promoting adolescent and adult welfare. *N Engl J Med.* 2022;386(17):1581–1583. https://doi.org/10.1056/NEJMp2119107
31. Warner KE, Kiessling KA, Douglas CE, Liber AC. A proposed policy agenda for electronic cigarettes in the US: product, price, place, and promotion. *Health Aff (Millwood).* 2022;41(9):1299–1306. https://doi.org/10.1377/hlthaff.2022.00187
32. Malone RE, McAfee T. Birthdate-based commercial tobacco sales restrictions: will "tobacco-free generation" policies advance or delay the endgame? *Tob Control.* 2024;tc-2024-058716. https://doi.org/10.1136/tc-2024-058716
33. van Deelen TRD, Kunst AE, van den Putte B, Veldhuizen EM, Kuipers MAG. Ex ante evaluation of the impact of tobacco control policy measures aimed at the point of sale in the Netherlands. *Tob Control.* 2023;32(5):620–626. https://doi.org/10.1136/tobaccocontrol-2021-057205
34. van Lier B, de Kanter W. Netherlands: move to phase out tobacco sales in supermarkets and petrol stations. *Tob Control.* 2020;29(3). https://tobaccocontrol.bmj.com/content/29/3/247
35. Bonnie RJ, Stratton K, Kwan LY. Restrictions on youth access to tobacco products. In: *Public Health Implications of Raising the Minimum Age of Legal Access to Tobacco Products.* Washington, DC: National Academies Press; 2015:chap 5. https://doi.org/10.17226/18997
36. Creamer MR, Everett Jones S, Gentzke AS, Jamal A, King BA. Tobacco product use among high school students—Youth Risk Behavior Survey, United States, 2019. *MMWR Suppl.* 2020;69(1):56–63. https://doi.org/10.15585/mmwr.su6901a7
37. Lee JGL, Sun DL, Schleicher NM, Ribisl KM, Luke DA, Henriksen L. Inequalities in tobacco outlet density by race, ethnicity and socioeconomic status, 2012, USA: results from the ASPiRE Study. *J Epidemiol Community Health.* 2017;71(5):487–492. https://doi.org/10.1136/jech-2016-208475
38. Jamal A, Homa DM, O'Connor E, et al. Current cigarette smoking among adults—United States, 2005–2014. *MMWR Morb Mortal Wkly Rep.* 2015;64(44):1233–1240. https://doi.org/10.15585/mmwr.mm6444a2
39. Roberts ME, Doogan NJ, Stanton CA, et al. Rural versus urban use of traditional and emerging tobacco products in the United States, 2013–2014. *Am J Public Health.* 2017;107(10):1554–1559. https://doi.org/10.2105/AJPH.2017.303967
40. Scarinci IC, Robinson LA, Alfano CM, Zbikowski SM, Klesges RC. The relationship between socioeconomic status, ethnicity, and cigarette smoking in urban adolescents. *Prev Med.* 2002;34(2):171–178. https://doi.org/10.1006/pmed.2001.0967
41. Reid JL, Hammond D, Boudreau C, Fong GT, Siahpush M. Socioeconomic disparities in quit intentions, quit attempts, and smoking abstinence among smokers in four western countries: findings from the International Tobacco Control Four Country Survey. *Nicotine Tob Res.* 2010;12(suppl 1):S20–S33. https://doi.org/10.1093/ntr/ntq051
42. Roberts ME, Colby SM, Lu B, Ferketich AK. Understanding tobacco use onset among African Americans. *Nicotine Tob Res.* 2016;18(suppl 1):S49–S56. https://doi.org/10.1093/ntr/ntv250
43. Vidrine JI, Reitzel LR, Wetter DW. The role of tobacco in cancer health disparities. *Curr Oncol Rep.* 2009;11(6):475–481. https://doi.org/10.1007/s11912-009-0064-9
44. Glasser AM, Onnen N, Craigmile PF, Schwartz E, Roberts ME. Associations between disparities in tobacco retailer density and disparities in tobacco use. *Prev Med.* 2022;154:106910. https://doi.org/10.1016/j.ypmed.2021.106910
45. Powell LM, Slater S, Mirtcheva D, Bao Y, Chaloupka FJ. Food store availability and neighborhood characteristics in the United States. *Prev Med.* 2007;44(3):189–195. https://doi.org/10.1016/j.ypmed.2006.08.008
46. Shannon J. Dollar stores, retailer redlining, and the metropolitan geographies of precarious consumption. *Ann Assoc Am Geogr.* 2021;111(4):1200–1218. https://doi.org/10.1080/24694452.2020.1775544
47. Raskind IG, Vishwakarma M, Schleicher NC, Andersen-Rodgers E, Henriksen L. The changing retail landscape for tobacco: dollar stores and the availability of cheap cigarettes among tobacco-related priority populations. *Tob Control.* 2022;31(e2):e140–e147. https://doi.org/10.1136/tobaccocontrol-2020-056389
48. Hrywna M, Kong AY, Ackerman C, Hudson SV, Delnevo CD. retailer compliance with Tobacco 21 in New Jersey, 2019–2020. *JAMA Netw Open.* 2022;5(10):e2235637. https://doi.org/10.1001/jamanetworkopen.2022.35637
49. Nagelhout GE, Poole NL, Metze M, Willemsen MC, Vermeulen W, van den Brand FA. Reducing the number and types of tobacco retail outlets in the Netherlands: study protocol for a comprehensive mixedmethods policy evaluation. *Tob Prev Cessat.* 2023;9:08. https://doi.org/10.18332/tpc/161825
50. Glasser AM, Roberts ME. Retailer density reduction approaches to tobacco control: a review. *Health Place.* 2021;67:102342. https://doi.org/10.1016/j.healthplace.2020.102342
51. Marsh L, Doscher C, Iosua E, Quigg R, Tomintz M. What impact would tobacco retailer proximity limit have on tobacco availability in New Zealand. *Tob Control.* 2024;33(2):215–220. https://doi.org/10.1136/tc-2022-057462
52. Kang H, Steadman KJ, Hoek J, Hall WD, Gartner CE. Restricting supply of tobacco products to pharmacies: a scoping review. *Tob Control.* 2024:tc-2023-058486. https://doi.org/10.1136/tc-2023-058486
53. Chen JC, Green KM, Chen J, Hoke KS, Borzekowski DLG. Restricting the sale of flavored e-cigarettes in

the US: an examination of local regulations. *Tob Regul Sci.* 2018;4(4):32–40. https://doi.org/10.18001/TRS.4.4.4

54. Bosma LM, D'Silva J, Moze J, Matter C, Kingsbury JH, Brock B. Restricting sales of menthol tobacco products: lessons learned from policy passage and implementation in Minneapolis, St. Paul, and Duluth, Minnesota. *Health Equity.* 2021;5(1):439–447. https://doi.org/10.1089/heq.2020.0137
55. California Tobacco Endgame Center for Organizing and Engagement. Case study: City of Oakland closes loophole in flavored tobacco products policy, strengthens enforcement. 2021. Available at: https://countertobacco.org/wp-content/uploads/2021/08/Case-Study-City-of-Oakland-Flavors-Policy-Enforcement-June-2021.pdf. Accessed July 2024.
56. ASPIRE. Tobacco retail policy trends in 2019: insights from the field. 2019. Available at: https://aspirecenter.org/wp-content/uploads/2020/07/TobaccoRetailPolicyTrends_2019.pdf. Accessed July 2024.
57. Tauras JA, Chaloupka FJ. The economic effects of cigarette sales and flavor bans on tobacco retail businesses. *Tobacconomics.* 2023. Available at: https://www.tobacconomics.org/research/the-economic-effects-of-cigarette-sales-and-flavor-bans-on-tobacco-retail-businesses. Accessed July 2024.
58. Ribisl KM, Evans WN, Feighery EC. Falling cigarette consumption in the US and the impact upon tobacco retailer employment. In: Bearman P, Neckerman K, Wright L, eds. *Social and Economic Consequences of Tobacco Control Policy.* New York, NY: Columbia University Press; 2011.
59. Blake KD, Gaysynsky A, Mayne RG, et al. US public opinion toward policy restrictions to limit tobacco product placement and advertising at point-of-sale and on social media. *Prev Med.* 2022;155:106930. https://doi.org/10.1016/j.ypmed.2021.106930
60. Czaplicki L, Perks SN, Liu M, et al. Support for e-cigarette and tobacco control policies among parents of adolescents. *Nicotine Tob Res.* 2020;22(7):1139–1147. https://doi.org/10.1093/ntr/ntz222

Forging Radical Hope: Waiting for the World to Change, or Changing the World?

Robert J. Kim-Farley, MD, MPH

ABOUT THE AUTHOR

The author is with the Departments of Epidemiology and Community Health Sciences, Fielding School of Public Health, University of California, Los Angeles, and is an associate editor of the American Journal of Public Health.

See also Zaragoza, p. 681, and Bradeanu, p. 682.

AJPH May 2025, Vol. 115, No. 5

> Learn from yesterday, live for today, hope for tomorrow. The important thing is not to stop questioning.
>
> —Albert Einstein

Public health students, much like in the lyrics of John Mayer's song "Waiting on the World to Change" ("One day our generation/Is gonna rule the population/So we keep on waiting/Waiting on the world to change"),[1] often find themselves in a state of anticipation, yearning for the systemic shifts needed to address the pressing health challenges of our time. Yet, they are learning that true change requires active engagement and creativity, which are powerful forces for community-driven solutions.

As noted in the *AJPH* Think Tank Call for Papers, the need for radical hope has never been more urgent in this era marked by unprecedented challenges. We are living through times of great uncertainty in which the threat of future pandemics, the ongoing impact of climate change, and the enduring legacies of colonialism loom large. Public health students feel the weight of these challenges as they enter a profession tasked with the monumental responsibility of improving community health with often inadequate resources. The traditional tools of public health are no longer sufficient to address the complexities of today's world.

HOPE AS AN ACTIVE PROCESS

Hope is not a passive state of mind; it is a process that requires committed effort, imagination, and resilience. In the face of today's problems, hope must be forged through deliberate actions and innovative thinking. Public health students are uniquely positioned to lead this challenge, as they bring fresh perspectives and a deep commitment to social justice. By embracing hope as an active process, they can inspire and mobilize communities to take charge of their health and well-being.

CREATIVITY AS A KEY CHARGE OF PUBLIC HEALTH

Creativity is essential in addressing the multifaceted challenges of public health. Traditional approaches often fall short in the face of complex and evolving issues. Public health students and professionals must harness the power of creativity to develop innovative solutions that are responsive to the needs of diverse communities. This involves thinking outside of the box, confronting conventional wisdom, and embracing new technologies and methodologies that enhance equity, diversity, inclusion, and justice.

One example of creativity in public health is the use of digital storytelling to raise awareness about health issues. By leveraging the power of narrative, public health students and professionals can engage communities in meaningful conversations about their health and well-being. Digital storytelling "addresses health inequities by combining technology with the voices of members of vulnerable, often underrepresented populations"[2(p793)]; allows people to share perspectives and experiences; fosters empathy; and promotes understanding. This creative approach can be particularly effective in reaching marginalized populations that may be overlooked by traditional public health campaigns.

THE NECESSITY OF COMMUNITY BUILDING

Community building is at the heart of effective public health practice. Strong, resilient communities are better equipped to address health challenges and promote well-being. Public health professionals must prioritize community engagement and collaboration, recognizing that the most effective solutions are often those that are co-created with the people they serve.

An example of an approach that helps community building is community-based participatory research (CBPR), a powerful, culturally relevant tool for building community capacity, fostering collaboration, and addressing community needs. CBPR involves partnering with community members to identify health priorities, develop interventions, and evaluate outcomes. "CBPR challenges researchers to listen to, learn from, solicit and respect the contributions of, and share power, information and credit for accomplishments with the groups they are trying to learn about and help."[3(p2634)] By involving community members in the research process, CBPR empowers individuals and promotes a sense of ownership and agency.

REIMAGINING PUBLIC HEALTH WITHOUT BORDERS

To truly address the global health challenges of our time, we must radically reimagine public health without borders. This means breaking down the silos that separate different disciplines, sectors, and communities. Public health students and professionals must be holistic in their approach and consider the social, economic, and environmental determinants of health. This requires collaboration across sectors, including education, housing, transportation, and the environment. One example of a borderless approach to public health is the One Health initiative.

> One Health recognizes that the health of humans, animals and ecosystems are interconnected. It involves applying a coordinated, collaborative, multidisciplinary and cross-sectoral approach to address potential or existing risks that originate at the animal-human-ecosystems interface.[4(p88)]

The One Health initiative seeks to address complex health challenges such as zoonotic diseases, antimicrobial resistance, and climate change. This holistic approach is essential for building a healthier, more equitable future for all.

THE ROLE OF PUBLIC HEALTH STUDENTS

Public health students play a crucial role in shaping the future of the field. Their perspectives on hope, creativity, and community work are invaluable in driving innovation and change. Through their education and training, public health students are exposed to a wide range of theories, methodologies, and practices. The Council on Education for Public Health's 2024 accreditation criteria for schools of public health and public health programs call for "systematic, coherent, and long-term efforts to incorporate elements of diversity and cultural humility. . .bridging the cultural gap between public health professionals and communities to promote culturally sensitive and population-centric strategies."[5] Advancing public health training through incorporating a diverse knowledge base will better equip students with the tools they need to address the complex health challenges of today and tomorrow.

Public health students understand that hope is not a passive state but an active process that requires effort and imagination. They recognize the importance of creativity in developing innovative solutions and the necessity of community building in promoting health and well-being. By embracing these principles, public health students can inspire and mobilize communities to take charge of their health and work together to achieve a healthier future.

CONCLUSION

Forging radical hope through creativity and community is essential for addressing the complex health challenges of our time. Public health students and professionals must embrace hope as an active process, harness the power of creativity, and prioritize community building. By reimagining public health without borders, we can develop innovative solutions that are responsive to the needs of diverse communities. Together, we can change the world—actively build a healthier, more equitable future for all and not passively be "waiting on the world to change."

> We must accept finite disappointment but never lose infinite hope.
>
> —Martin Luther King, Jr.

AJPH

CORRESPONDENCE

Correspondence should be sent to Robert J. Kim-Farley, MD, MPH, UCLA Department of Epidemiology, Room 71-279A CHS, 650 Charles E. Young Dr S, Los Angeles, CA 90095 (e-mail: robert@kimfarley.org). Reprints can be ordered at https://www.ajph.org by clicking the "Reprints" link.

PUBLICATION INFORMATION

Full Citation: Kim-Farley RJ. Forging radical hope: waiting for the world to change, or changing the world? *Am J Public Health*. 2025;115(5):678–680.

Acceptance Date: December 24, 2024.

DOI: https://doi.org/10.2105/AJPH.2025.308006

ORCID iD:

Robert J. Kim-Farley https://orcid.org/0000-0003-3022-6548

ACKNOWLEDGMENTS

I acknowledge the outstanding work of the members of the Student Think Tank in preparing this *AJPH* special section and for their kind review of this editorial.

CONFLICTS OF INTEREST

The author reports no conflicts of interest.

REFERENCES

1. Mayer J. Waiting on the world to change. Available at: https://www.songfacts.com/lyrics/john-mayer/waiting-on-the-world-to-change. Accessed November 4, 2024.
2. Briant KJ, Halter A, Marchello N, Escareño M, Thompson B. The power of digital storytelling as a culturally relevant health promotion tool.

Health Promot Pract. 2016;17(6):793–801. https://doi.org/10.1177/1524839916658023

3. Horowitz CR, Robinson M, Seifer S. Community-based participatory research from the margin to the mainstream: are researchers prepared? *Circulation.* 2009;119(19):2633–2642. https://doi.org/10.1161/CIRCULATIONAHA.107.729863
4. Mackenzie JS, Jeggo M. The one health approach—why is it so important? *Trop Med Infect Dis.* 2019;4(2):88. https://doi.org/10.3390/tropicalmed4020088
5. Council on Education for Public Health. Accreditation criteria for schools of public health and public health programs. Available at: https://media.ceph.org/documents/2024.Criteria.pdf. Accessed December 21, 2024.

A Love Letter to Hope

Michelle Zaragoza, MSW, LCSW

ABOUT THE AUTHOR

The author is a doctoral student at the School of Social Welfare, University of California, Berkeley.

See also Kim-Farley, p. 678, and Bradeanu, p. 682.

Dear Hope,

You were the silent force that initiated my family's journey from Mexico, guiding them as they crossed borders and navigated the unknown in pursuit of a better future. Amid the uncertainties that lined their path, you were their anchor. Eventually, you became the spark that set my transformation into motion. When a high school counselor doubted my capacity for an advanced psychology course, your voice echoed "sí se puede," infusing me with the strength to defy expectations. With that whispered assurance, you empowered me to become the first in my family to graduate from college. Over the years, you have cultivated in me, in us, a collective spirit of resistance and strength to carve out new trajectories for our future.

However, there have been times when your power seemed to fade, slipping beyond my grasp. When the world shut down and my inner world crumbled under the weight of depression and anxiety, you became elusive. Where were you for the immigrant families I served, those striving to secure shelter, access food, and find refuge from the threat of deportation? Your presence felt intangible, powerless against the stark realities of a deepening complex society. I questioned your whereabouts in those moments, hoping you were still there.

Even amid my fears and uncertainties, the thought of your existence was enough to keep me resisting your opposite.[1] Although often overlooked, your power undeniably shapes the world around you. With every action, you are crafting a reality that reflects a vision and determination. If not for you, my journey to who I am today would never have happened: you guided a family journey from Mexico to Southeast Los Angeles and supported an immigrant single mother in raising her daughter, who has become the Latina scholar and mental health practitioner I am today.

Upon reflection, you have always been here, even in my (and our) darkest moments. The only thing I can think of that binds us is love—the love we share for our families, communities, and world. This love inspires us to envision the world we long for and unlocks your transformative potential to address the challenges before us today. I see clearly how the power to change the world (and with it) resides within me through you.

I turn to you once more to inspire how we—individually and collectively—envision and shape the future of public health. I can already hear your guiding words. As a practitioner, navigating the world's growing complexity demands your informed vision, fueling movement, resistance, and advocacy for accountability within unjust systems.[2] As a scholar, I know this involves embracing creativity and generating alternatives to adaptability[3] by exploring diverse approaches to finding solutions and overcoming the limitations of conventional methods. Hope, through our love, we have the power to create a healthier and more equitable future for our communities and the world. You have illuminated this truth for me. Can you share it with the world, too?

With love,

A hopeful public health professional AJPH

CORRESPONDENCE

Correspondence should be sent to Michelle Zaragoza, MSW, LCSW, School of Social Welfare, University of California, Berkeley, Haviland Hall, Berkeley, CA 94709 (e-mail: michellezaragoza@berkeley.edu). Reprints can be ordered at https://www.ajph.org by clicking the "Reprints" link.

PUBLICATION INFORMATION

Full Citation: Zaragoza M. A love letter to hope. *Am J Public Health.* 2025;115(5):681.

Acceptance Date: December 8, 2024.

DOI: https://doi.org/10.2105/AJPH.2024.307977

ORCID iD:

Michelle Zaragoza https://orcid.org/0009-0008-5424-5499

CONFLICTS OF INTEREST

The author has no conflicts of interest to disclose.

REFERENCES

1. Govier T. Hope and its opposites. *J Soc Philos.* 201;42(3):239-253. https://doi.org/10.1111/j.1467-9833.2011.01532.x
2. French BH, Lewis JA, Mosley DV, et al. Toward a psychological framework of radical healing in communities of color. *Couns Psychol.* 2020;48(1):14-46. https://doi.org/10.1177/0011000019843506
3. Macy J, Johnstone C. *Active Hope: How to Face the Mess We're in Without Going Crazy.* Novato, CA: New World Library; 2012.

We Don't Give Hope, We Build It Together

Iulia I. Bradeanu

ABOUT THE AUTHOR

The author is with the Department of Medicine, Morehouse School of Medicine, Atlanta, GA.

See also Kim-Farley, p. 678, and Zaragoza, p. 681.

As the focus group was about to start, the air was heavy with a sense of reluctance and skepticism. A wave of discouragement settled over me. There we were, a spirited team of first-year medical students, eager to invest time, energy, and resources to collaborate with this community of senior citizens, and we were facing cynicism from the most unexpected source: the intended recipients of our partnership. Why were our attempts to engage these seniors met with such resistance? "Why should we care?" demanded a focus group participant in a stern voice. Although I did not immediately understand, their attitude was the result of chronic frustration and hopelessness caused by countless unmet promises in their facility. In that awkward silence, their words pierced my idealism, revealing a hard truth—hope is not something we give but something we build together.

The seniors' skepticism was understandable. Many of their complaints extended beyond what we were able to address. They reside in an independent senior living facility nestled within a neighborhood marked by contradictions. This community has assets and resources, including numerous houses of worship, a major sports arena, higher education institutions, and a network of public transportation. Yet, the legacy of systemic neglect is evident in stark disparities: higher rates of chronic disease, lower standards of living, and increased poverty, violence, and mental health distress relative to other areas of the county.[1–3] These inequities disproportionately affect the area's predominantly Black residents.[4,5]

As part of a required service learning community health course, we completed a community assets and needs assessment that underscored this contrast, revealing how social determinants of health such as age, food insecurity, limited transportation, and lack of social support profoundly shape the residents' lives. The seniors we met lived many of these realities. Their initial reluctance revealed that hope is an active process that must be fostered through genuine connection and tangible action.

We embarked on this course with idealism and theoretical knowledge. The seniors' initial skepticism served as a humbling reminder that public health extends far beyond academia; it requires building trust and recognizing systemic inequities. The Healthy People 2030 initiative mirrors this perspective, emphasizing community engagement and tackling social determinants of health to achieve health equity.[6] For seniors, Healthy People 2030 promotes increasing access to preventive services, promoting physical activity and healthy eating, and reducing social isolation.[6] Guided by this framework, we searched the literature for evidence-based models developed by public health professionals for addressing similar needs while actively listening to residents' perspectives to ensure that our efforts reflected their priorities.

Partnering with local and state organizations enhanced our impact. Our interventions included chair yoga, nutrition education workshops, and a health fair. The residents played a central role in outlining the interventions. For example, during our focus groups and key informant interviews, the issue of access to nutritious food was raised multiple times. This led us to tailor the nutrition workshops with a focus on affordable meal options and resources. The health fair included stations based on their input: blood pressure screenings, chronic disease management, and cognitive health, areas identified as important for their community. We scheduled activities at times residents requested and accommodated their mobility limitations.

Implementing these interventions required adapting theoretical concepts to fit our limited budget, complicated schedules, and community needs. Each component was approached with creativity, from tailoring yoga poses and interactive nutrition activities to coordinating a robust health fair. These evidence-based interventions, coupled with our weekly visits, fostered social connection and encouraged the seniors to prioritize their well-being.

We made community building the cornerstone of our approach, aiming to create a space where voices are heard, trust is earned, and genuine relationships are forged. Research underscores the importance of social connection, particularly for older adults, linking loneliness to cognitive decline and highlighting the benefits of strong social ties for well-being.[7,8] As we painted, laughed during games, and shared conversations,

AJPH May 2025, Vol. 115, No. 5

skepticism gave way to trust, transforming us from students with a project to community members. Participating residents reported increased happiness, purpose, and a desire for continued engagement.

In a quiet moment between Bingo rounds, Mrs. D confided in me about her struggles with loneliness. "It's the silence that's the hardest," she said with a broken voice. "Sometimes I don't talk to anyone all week until I come down to meet you guys." Her words reminded me that our involvement is meaningful—it filled a void and offered companionship. At the end of our last chair yoga session, Mrs. B expressed how much practicing yoga increased her confidence in her abilities to exercise and regain flexibility, highlighting the potential of community-based interventions to affect more than physical health and sparking hope and a sense of possibility.

These moments fundamentally revealed that hope is not a passive state but an active force that must be forged through the collective efforts of people working together to create a better future. We were surprised to discover just how invested the residents became in our education and well-being. Their eagerness to share words of wisdom, their expressed desire to be present at our graduation, and their nurturing support were expressions of their faith in us, the next generation of healers. The ripple effects of their trust were profound, as it became clear that our genuine connections fostered hope, not just for the present but for the future.

The transformation was not one-sided. As future physicians, this experience taught us that patients are much more than a collection of symptoms—they are individuals with complex needs and valuable perspectives. The project deepened our empathy and understanding of the social determinants of health. It equipped us with the tools necessary for understanding health care through the lived experiences of the community we serve, not merely through the lens of textbooks and clinical guidelines. Witnessing the seniors' inspiring resilience highlighted the importance of collaborating with patients as partners in their care. We learned that healing often requires more than medication; it may be critically linked to fostering hope, connections, and community building.

What began as a course assignment evolved into a deeply personal experience that taught me the value of community and connection. The seniors I met became much more than participants in a project—they became friends, and their stories continue to inspire me. I remain in regular contact with several of them and visit whenever I can. This experience showed me an unexpected facet of medicine: building relationships that offer hope and support is as fundamental to health care as clinical knowledge and skills. I also came to understand just how much one can learn through genuine listening. As I move forward in my medical career, I will work to build trust and partnership with the communities I serve.

I observed that the challenges faced by this senior living facility mirror broader systemic issues. Understanding the complex interplay between systemic challenges and social determinants of health allows us to view the residents' focus group reflections through a wider lens. "Going to the bank, going to the store, going anywhere, is not like it was before COVID," one of them said. Another resident pleaded for access to assisted living services at the facility, emphasizing their importance in supporting residents' well-being. Their laments highlight the impact of inequities, the difficulties of navigating a world that neglects their needs, and the vulnerability that comes with feeling isolated and unsupported. In this challenging reality, the aging population is particularly susceptible to losing motivation and hope.

The outcomes of our interventions call for strategies that can achieve lasting, beneficial effects in other communities. Medical schools can lead such efforts by integrating more community-centered training to prepare students to identify and partner with local resources and community leaders, by strengthening collaborations with local organizations to ensure continuity, and by encouraging students to engage in long-term service learning to foster deep relationships for strong collaborations and sustained benefits. Establishing such programs where they do not yet exist could be truly impactful in advancing health equity.

This transformative experience revealed to me implications with far-reaching significance for the field of public health. Building trust, engaging members, and fostering hope within a community are essential not just for patient care but for creating a more inclusive and equitable health care system. A patient's health encompasses much more than a properly working biology; achieving well-being is dependent on the symbiosis between social, emotional, and environmental factors—the very determinants that public health strives to address.

Our work highlighted the importance of a multicollaborative approach, bringing together academia, nonprofit organizations, and local and state agencies to implement focused interventions. Above all, we learned that prioritizing the voice of the community we serve is paramount. Our senior friends redefined hope for us: not a fleeting feeling but a resilient force fostered within a community. As future physicians, we are dedicated to nurturing this hope, both in our patients and within the health care system. Our vision is a health care landscape that prioritizes not just the absence of disease but the presence of hope, connection, and well-being for all. AJPH

CORRESPONDENCE

Correspondence should be sent to Iulia I. Bradeanu, 146 Highway 81, Oxford, GA 30054 (e-mail: ibradeanu@msm.edu). Reprints can be ordered at https://www.ajph.org by clicking the "Reprints" link.

PUBLICATION INFORMATION

Full Citation: Bradeanu II. We don't give hope, we build it together. *Am J Public Health*. 2025; 115(5):682–684.

Acceptance Date: December 8, 2024.

DOI: https://doi.org/10.2105/AJPH.2024.307975

ORCID iD:

Iulia I. Bradeanu https://orcid.org/0009-0009-7483-6170

ACKNOWLEDGMENTS

I express my gratitude to and acknowledge the invaluable contributions of the residents and staff at Oasis at Scholars Landing, my fellow classmates in the Leadership Learning Community Class of 2027, and the Morehouse School of Medicine community health course. The interventions and routine engagements that played a pivotal role in the progress and achievements of our community project were founded by the Morehouse School of Medicine Department of Community Health and Preventive Medicine. A special thank you goes to my mentors, Carla Durham Walker and Chima J. Ohuabunwo, for their unwavering support and guidance.

CONFLICTS OF INTEREST

The author has no conflicts of interest to disclose.

REFERENCES

1. Fulton County Board of Health. 2022 Fulton County Community Health Assessment. Available at: https://www.fultoncountyhealthcenter.org/wp-content/uploads/2022/12/Fulton-County-2022-Community-Health-Needs-Assessment.pdf. Accessed August 18, 2024.
2. Atlanta Regional Commission. Metro Atlanta Racial Equity Atlas. Available at: https://opendata.atlantaregional.com/documents/GARC:metro-atlanta-racial-equity-atlas/explore. Accessed August 10, 2024.
3. Fulton County Board of Health. Fulton County Community Health Assessment 2020. Available at: https://fultoncountyga.gov/-/media/Departments/Board-of-Health/ FCBOH20202020CHA20Report FINAL20Reduced20Size.pdf. Accessed August 10, 2024.
4. Fulton County. Environmental Scan Public Health: major cardiovascular disease. Available at: https://sharefulton.fultoncountyga.gov/stories/s/Environmental-Scan_PublicHealth/c53k-xkkw. Accessed August 10, 2024.
5. Fulton County Board of Health. Fulton County health: leading causes of death. Available at: https://data.fultoncountyga.gov/download/w2ur-vte3/application%2Fpdf. Accessed August 10, 2024.
6. US Department of Health and Human Services, Office of Disease Prevention and Health Promotion. Healthy People 2030. Available at: https://health.gov/healthypeople. Accessed August 12, 2024.
7. Lara E, Martín-María N, De la Torre-Luque A, Gil-Salmerón A. Does loneliness contribute to mild cognitive impairment, dementia, and mortality in older people? A systematic review and meta-analysis of longitudinal observational studies. *J Gerontol B Psychol Sci Soc Sci*. 2019;74(5):803–812.
8. Kuiper JS, Zuidersma M, Oude Voshaar RC, Zuidema SU, van den Heuvel W. Social relationships and cognitive decline in healthy older adults: a systematic review and meta-analysis of longitudinal cohort studies. *J Am Geriatr Soc*. 2016;64(10): 2086–2095.

"We Who Believe in Freedom Cannot Rest": Affirming the Call to Critically Engage Public Health

Lisa Bowleg, PhD

ABOUT THE AUTHOR

Lisa Bowleg is with the Department of Psychological and Brain Sciences, The George Washington University, Washington, DC, and the Intersectionality Training Institute, Philadelphia, PA.

See also Parmet, p. 687.

"We who believe in freedom cannot rest
We who believe in freedom cannot
rest until it comes."

—Bernice Johnson Reagon,
Ella's Song: We Who Believe in Freedom Cannot Rest[1]

People committed to public health and health equity have had little rest in recent weeks. Freedom to access federal public health data and resources, conduct federally funded research, and publish it have all been disrupted by a flurry of authoritarian and ideological executive orders. It is from this tumultuous and monumentally dangerous era in our history that I write. I have two objectives: one, to congratulate *AJPH* on its 115th anniversary; two, to affirm that the Perspectives From the Social Sciences Section's interest in critically engaging public health has not wavered.

In 2019, when I assumed editorship of this laudable section, I defined critical perspectives as those that "interrogate, expose, and challenge assumptions about policies, institutions, and practices that obscure power relations that foster inequality and oppression and conceal how dominant groups construct knowledge, facts, and problems."[2(p15)] Observing the new administration erase public health data and resources, particularly those relevant to gender, racial group, sexual and gender minority status, and disability; diversity, equity, and inclusion; and health equity, all underscore author Linda Tuhiwai Smith's observation that "research exists within a system of power."[3(p226)]

This current torrent of abuse of power on public health science is extreme. Yet, even before it, public health research existed within systems of power. Which populations and topics are worthy of research and publication? Who is funded to do the research? Which methodologies and methods are deemed legitimate? Which styles of writing, sources, and words are considered scholarly? Which theories and theoretical frameworks are sanctioned? Whose knowledge counts? What counts as knowledge? Who benefits from research? Which dissemination sources are valued? Who has access to the knowledge produced by research? In their quest to make novel and transformative contributions to advance public health and reduce health inequities, critical researchers engage these types of questions about power and research.

This 19-year-old section's goal to "promote high-quality public health research from the social and behavioral sciences; multi-disciplinary and transdisciplinary research; and a variety of research methods, including qualitative and multiple methods . . . as well as synthesis"[4(p1537)] and review articles remains unchanged. As for the critical perspectives that I advocated back in 2019, they too remain unchanged. I can't recall a time when these have been more vital and timely. You? Submissions on those topics and populations remain welcome, with one caveat: no capitulation to the current zeitgeist with euphemisms or linguistic subterfuge, please!

Additionally, I invite submissions that courageously meet the demands of this moment. This includes, but is not limited to, articles that

- Assess and document the public health consequences of the administration's policies in areas such as reproductive justice and rights, and for oppressed groups such as people who are gender minority, undocumented, or both;
- Highlight preliminary results from interrupted social and behavioral science (SBS) health and health equity research;
- Introduce novel or advance qualitative, quantitative, and mixed methods research for designing, conducting, and analyzing structural

AJPH May 2025, Vol. 115, No. 5

and multilevel determinants of health inequities;

- Envision the "art of the possible" to continue or develop new individual-, community-, and structural-level research and interventions in the absence of state and federal support;
- Document new or nontraditional research collaborations and alliances (e.g., researchers and local policymakers) to advance public health knowledge and practice; and
- Highlight community-led, community-engaged or citizen-science projects that seek to democratize health equity research and practice.

Freedom to conduct and disseminate research without the government's ideological interference. This is a new and dire public health need. One hundred and fifteen years hence, when we're all long gone and this era has been rendered a dreadful blip of history, SBS researchers and practitioners may have earned rest. But for those of us in the here and now, those committed to SBS research and practice that fosters freedom from health inequities, there is no rest. We await your submissions. AJPH

CORRESPONDENCE

Correspondence should be sent to Lisa Bowleg, Department of Psychological and Brain Sciences, The George Washington University, 2013 H St, NW, Washington, DC 20006 (e-mail: lbowleg@gwu.edu). Reprints can be ordered at https://www.ajph.org by clicking the "Reprints" link.

PUBLICATION INFORMATION

Full Citation: Bowleg L. "We Who Believe in Freedom Cannot Rest": affirming the call to critically engage public health. *Am J Public Health*. 2025;115(5):685–686.

Acceptance Date: February 19, 2025.

DOI: https://doi.org/10.2105/AJPH.2025.308088

ORCID iD:
Lisa Bowleg https://orcid.org/0000-0003-4677-8195

CONFLICTS OF INTEREST

The author has no conflicts of interest to disclose.

REFERENCES

1. Sweet Honey in the Rock. *Ella's Song: We Who Believe in Freedom Cannot Rest* [CD]. Rounder Records; 1988.
2. Bowleg L. Perspectives from the social sciences: critically engage public health. *Am J Public Health*. 2019;109(1):15–16. https://doi.org/10.2105/AJPH.2018.304825
3. Smith LT. *Decolonizing Methodologies: Research and Indigenous Peoples*. London, UK: Zed Books; 1999.
4. McLeroy K, Holtzman D. Framing health matters? *Am J Public Health*. 2006;96(9):1537. https://doi.org/10.2105/AJPH.2006.096180

Protecting Public Health in the Courts

Wendy E. Parmet, JD

ABOUT THE AUTHOR

Wendy E. Parmet is with the Center for Health, Policy & Law, Northeastern University, Boston, MA.

See also Bowleg, p. 685.

The fate of public health interventions often rests with courts. Until recently, the judiciary was a relatively hospitable terrain for public health. Although courts sometimes struck measures that violated constitutional rights or exceeded statutory requirements, more often than not, judges accepted the importance of protecting the public's health and granted health officials a significant degree of deference.

Today, that deference is waning. In the last several years, across a wide span of doctrinal areas (e.g., religious liberty[1] and administrative law[2]) and diverse subject matters (e.g., vaccines[3] and warning labels[4]), the Supreme Court and many lower courts have replaced deference with skepticism.[5] They have overturned or narrowed precedent, discounted public health expertise, and empowered individuals and businesses that wish to undermine public health orders, often to the detriment of socially vulnerable populations. Taken together, such decisions make it increasingly difficult for health officials at all levels of government to know what they can and cannot do.[6] When long-established precedents are unstable and courts give little weight to the scientific conclusions of public health experts, officials may be forgiven for concluding that inaction is safer than action. In the face of a new pandemic and ongoing health threats, such inaction may be deadly.

Although public health has unquestionably contributed to its own legal woes, the roots of the current crisis go back more than 50 years. In 1971, Lewis F. Powell, who was later elevated to the Supreme Court by President Nixon, wrote a famous memo to the US Chamber of Commerce arguing that "the judiciary may be the most important instrument for social, economic and political change."[7] Citing this "opportunity," Powell called upon the Chamber to employ "a highly competent staff of lawyers," who could "appear as counsel amicus in the Supreme Court." He also urged the Chamber to take "the greatest care . . . in selecting the cases in which to participate, or the suits to institute," and underscored that the "opportunity merits the necessary effort." In short, he urged the Chamber to develop and carry out a court-focused strategy to advance the interests of the Chamber and its allies.

In the years that followed, business interests and their allies heeded Powell's call and implemented a well-coordinated and richly funded plan to alter American jurisprudence and reduce government's regulatory capacity. At the center of the strategy was the Federalist Society, which has nurtured generations of law students, scholars, and judges who developed and canonized a conservative jurisprudence that utilizes a variety of legal theories, from originalism to the unitary executive, that have transformed the contours of American law, leading to the overturning of *Roe v Wade*[8] and affirmative action,[9] new threats to vaccine mandates, and novel limits on the Centers for Disease Control and Prevention's ability to respond to a pandemic,[5] among other changes. The Federalist Society and its cochair, Leonard Leo, who oversees a dark money network of more than $1 billion,[10] also wielded extraordinary influence over judicial nominations during the first Trump administration and can be expected to exercise similar influence during Trump's second term. Importantly, these judges will, for the most part, continue to serve and rule on public health cases in the decades to come.

In the face of these challenges, public health needs a similar multifaceted, long-term legal strategy that looks behind today's legal battles and seeks to restore the traditional relationship between the judiciary and public health. To begin that process, in May 2024, a group of public health professionals, legal and public health academics, representatives of foundations, and public and private lawyers with different specialties met at Northeastern University to devise an action plan designed to protect public health in the courts. The plan that emerged identified seven broad goals (Box 1) and multiple concrete steps that can be taken to realize each of those goals in the near, medium, and long term.

Among the key goals is doctrinal research toward the development of a new jurisprudence that can "push back against the hyper-individualism ascendant in much of American law."[11] To be effective, this jurisprudence must

AJPH May 2025, Vol. 115, No. 5

BOX 1— Goals From the Action Plan for Protecting Public Health in the Courts

Create the Operational Structure for Coordinated Activities
Conduct doctrinal research and development
Implement a coordinated litigation strategy
Engage with the judicial selection/election process
Educate the legal profession/establishment
Develop messaging content and outreach plans
Develop a sustained funding strategy

resonate with American legal traditions and transcend specific cases and doctrines. It should also offer an intellectually and ethically compelling alternative to originalism, one that future generations of law students, lawyers, and judges will find convincing.

Another critical goal is greater engagement with the judicial selection and nomination process. As the Federalist Society has shown, the fate of public health cases, especially before the Supreme Court and other "apex courts," can depend as much if not more on who is on the bench as on the clarity of the precedent or the quality of the lawyering. To ensure a judiciary that is open to well-supported public health interventions, public health advocates (to the extent permitted by law) need to become educated about and engaged in judicial nominations and elections (most state court judges are elected). They should also nurture law students and young lawyers who will be the judges of tomorrow. To do that, public health must reach out to students, young lawyers, and judges, educating them about population health and its relationship to law, and providing the type of opportunities for interaction, exchange, and career development that the Federalist Society has fostered over the past 50 years.

Finally, the effort to protect public health in the courts requires a long-term, sustained funding stream. Public health law efforts will never be able to match the resources available to those who seek to weaken it. But the funds could go further if they were consistent and sustained, and not dependent on two- or three-year grant or electoral cycles.

In this moment when public health faces innumerable threats, it is worth remembering that, to echo Martin Luther King Jr, "the arc of the moral universe is long, but it bends toward health." But to achieve a healthier tomorrow, the public health community needs to recognize the central role played by courts and begin the long and hard work of repairing its relationship with the judiciary. AJPH

CORRESPONDENCE

Correspondence should be sent to Wendy E. Parmet, Northeastern University School of Law, 416 Huntington Ave, Boston, MA 02115 (e-mail: w.parmet@northeastern.edu). Reprints can be ordered at https://www.ajph.org by clicking the "Reprints" link.

PUBLICATION INFORMATION

Full Citation: Parmet WE. Protecting public health in the courts. *Am J Public Health*. 2025;115(5): 687–688.

Acceptance Date: February 19, 2025.

DOI: https://doi.org/10.2105/AJPH.2025.308087

ORCID iD:
Wendy E. Parmet https://orcid.org/0000-0002-5797-0863

ACKNOWLEDGMENTS

This work was funded in part by a grant from ChangeLab Solutions as part of the Act for Public Health partnership, which is funded by the Robert Wood Johnson Foundation.

Many thanks to Linda Tvrdy for her work on the convening and action plan described in the editorial and her comments on an earlier draft of this editorial, and to the members of the Act for Public Health Partnership for their support for this work.

CONFLICTS OF INTEREST

This work was funded in part by a grant from ChangeLab Solutions. The author is also the co-Principal Investigator on grants from the Robert Wood Johnson and W. K. Kellogg Foundations to support a judicial education program.

REFERENCES

1. *Tandon v Newson*, 593 US 61 (2021).
2. *Loper Bright Enterprises v Raimondo*, 603 US 369 (2024).
3. *Bosarge v Edney*, 2023 WL 5598983 (SD Miss Aug 29, 2023).
4. *National Institute of Family & Life Advocates v Becerra*, 585 US 755 (2018).
5. Mello MM, Jiang DH, Parmet WE. Judicial decisions constraining public health powers during COVID-19: implications for public health policy making. *Health Aff (Millwood)*. 2024;43(6):759–767. https://doi.org/10.1377/hlthaff.2024.00073
6. Adler S, DH Briggs, Brownson RC, et al. The (un?)intended consequences of COVID-19-era judicial decisions and new public health-related laws. *Health Affairs Forefront*. 2023. Available at: https://www.healthaffairs.org/content/forefront/un-intended-consequences-covid-19-era-judicial-decisions-and-new-public-health-related. Accessed March 17, 2025.
7. The Lewis Powell Memo: a corporate blueprint to dominate democracy. 1971. Available at: https://www.greenpeace.org/usa/democracy/the-lewis-powell-memo-a-corporate-blueprint-to-dominate-democracy. Accessed March 3, 2025.
8. *Dobbs v Jackson Women's Health Org*, 597 US 215 (2022).
9. *Students for Fair Admissions, Inc v President and Fellows of Harvard College*, 600 US 181 (2023).
10. Przybla H. Leonard Leo used Federalist Society contact to obtain $1.6B donation. *Politico*. May 2, 2023. Available at: https://www.politico.com/news/2023/05/02/leonard-leo-federalist-society-00094761. Accessed March 11, 2025.
11. Report by Act for Public Health Partnership calls for court-centered strategy for protecting public health. January 15, 2025. Available at: https://law.northeastern.edu/aph-convening-report-action-plan/#:~:text=In%20%E2%80%9CA%20Plan%20for%20Action,nomination%20and%20election%20of%20judges. Accessed March 17, 2025.

Addressing Unsheltered Homelessness and Substance Use Disorder From Tent Encampment to Safe Spaces, Boston 2021–2022

Monica Bharel, MD, MPH, Michele N. Clark, DrPH, MPH, Daniel Dooley, and Bisola O. Ojikutu, MD, MPH

Increasing numbers of individuals experiencing unsheltered homelessness and substance use disorder are living in tent encampments in cities across the United States. In response, the City of Boston, Massachusetts employed a public health approach comprising four implementation components: centralized leadership with cross-agency collaboration, creation of low-threshold spaces, person-centered engagement, and stakeholder-driven long-term planning. These steps led to the equitable transition of unsheltered individuals into harm reduction spaces and formed the foundation for future planning and encampment response in the city. (*Am J Public Health*. 2025;115(5):689–692. https://doi.org/10.2105/AJPH.2025.308009)

AJPH May 2025, Vol. 115, No. 5

Cities throughout the United States have experienced a rise in the number of individuals who are unsheltered and living in places not intended for habitation.

INTERVENTION AND IMPLEMENTATION

To address these challenges in Boston, Massachusetts, the city employed a four-pronged, public health–led approach. This implementation experience demonstrates the importance of a public health strategy to address the encampment and navigate residents to safer indoor living spaces.

The implementation consisted of four components:

1. Establishing cross-agency collaboration with centralized leadership;
2. Developing a new low-threshold shelter (LTS) model;
3. Conducting a person-centered needs assessment and other outreach efforts to plan alternative shelter and housing accommodations; and
4. Creating a long-term public health strategy with multistakeholder input.

Cross-Agency Collaboration

Mayor Michelle Wu created a cabinet-level position and a Coordinated Response Team composed of members from various agencies (housing, public health, fire, police, public works, inspectional, neighborhood services, etc.) that met daily to discuss the safety needs of the encampment residents. This proved critical for aligning and prioritizing the response across city departments.

The City Encampment Protocol[1] used at the time outlined the regulatory and legal process for respectfully engaging individuals and offering indoor living options, storage solutions, housing navigation, clinical care, and social services. This fostered collaboration among previously siloed teams, including public health, housing, and health care.

Low-Threshold Shelter Model

LTS, based on the Housing First philosophy, provides temporary living spaces for individuals experiencing unsheltered homelessness and substance use disorder (SUD) prior to moving to permanent housing. Irrespective of readiness for recovery, individuals receive immediate harm reduction and housing services.[2] Boston's LTS model has shown effectiveness in providing safe and stabilizing environments resulting in increased engagement in clinical, treatment, and housing services.[3–5]

To prepare for the new LTS, the city developed LTS Practice Guidance[6] based on best practices. With funding from multiple sources, six LTS sites providing more than 200 beds were established through collaboration with state government partners, social service programs, clinical providers, homeless service providers, and community members. These included three noncongregate sites (two hotels and a pallet home community) and three emergency shelters that transformed existing congregate spaces to incorporate the LTS model.

Needs Assessment and Other Outreach Efforts

A comprehensive tent-to-tent survey (Table 1) was conducted over a two-day period in early December 2021, assessing the needs of all 145 identified individuals occupying 77 tents in the encampment. The results presented a clearer understanding of their individual and collective unmet social, primary care, and mental health service needs, providing much-needed documentation to inform a coordinated response.

Based on individualized assessments, outreach and engagement plans were deployed over four weeks, informing encampment residents of opportunities for indoor accommodation. Trusted outreach providers systematically matched individuals to the sites that best met their clinical and social service needs. Collected demographic information enabled overall monitoring of the equitable placement of encampment residents by race, ethnicity, gender, and age.

TABLE 1— Summary Characteristics of Individuals Living in Encampments From the Tent Census: Boston, MA, December 2021

Characteristic (No. of Responses)	%
Age, y (n = 138)	
24–34	28.3
35–44	47.8
45–60	23.9
Gender[a] (n = 145)	
Female	34.5
Male	65.5
Racial/ethnic group (n = 144)	
Non-Hispanic/Latinx Black	21.5
Hispanic/Latinx	36.8
Non-Hispanic/Latinx other/multi	3.5
Non-Hispanic/Latinx White	38.2
Primary language (n = 131)	
English	87.8
Spanish	12.2
Years living in tents (n = 87)	
< 1	21.8
1	20.7
2–3	34.5
4–9	16.1
≥ 10	6.9
No. of tent occupants (n = 117)	
1	29.9
2	50.4
≥ 3	19.7
Had been incarcerated during past 2 y (n = 86)	18.6
Ever have disability diagnosis (n = 86)	45.4
Currently have a health care provider (n = 88)	53.4
Currently have a mental health care provider (n = 88)	22.7
No mental health provider but would like to have one (n = 67)	55.2

[a]Two individuals also identified as transgender.

Long-Term Public Health Strategy

Following the closure of the encampments, a series of focus groups, listening sessions, and individual stakeholder interviews were conducted to inform development of a strategic plan. Participants included more than 250 individuals composed of community members with lived experience, clinical partners, neighborhood associations, community health centers, shelter and housing partners, faith-based organizations, outreach teams, city and state legislative partners, and criminal justice partners. The resulting Long-Term Public Health Strategic Outlook[7] outlined mid- and long-term strategies to further address and sustain the public health–led approach to unsheltered homelessness and SUD in the city.

To foster community support and decrease stigma, city officials engaged with community members through meetings and outreach in the communities where LTS sites were established. A public-facing dashboard was created to improve transparency by sharing real-time data pertaining to LTS placements and other city services.[8]

PLACE, TIME, AND PERSONS

Between 2020 and 2021, Boston experienced a 25.6% increase in its unsheltered population[9] and an unsanctioned encampment in the "Mass & Cass" area (named after intersecting streets). This was fueled by pandemic-related factors such as reduced access to SUD treatment and shelter beds. In November 2021, Mayor Wu declared homelessness a public health emergency,[10] thus accelerating a citywide response to relocate encampment residents by mid-January 2022 to safer indoor accommodations to avoid winter weather risks.

PURPOSE

In 2022, 40% of people experiencing homelessness were unsheltered,[11] often residing in encampments—unofficial outdoor makeshift structures. Encampments are a visible reminder of society's inability to meet the needs of people experiencing unsheltered homelessness, including housing, safety, food, and health care.[12] National studies have documented high rates of SUD, mental health conditions, and other comorbidities among unsheltered individuals.[13] This multipronged public health–led approach is necessary to address this complex issue.

EVALUATION AND ADVERSE EFFECTS

Of the 145 encampment residents, 108 (74.5%) transitioned to an indoor space and 37 (25.5%) voluntarily left the area and were considered lost to follow-up on the date of the encampment closure. Eighty-seven individuals (60%) were placed in LTS, 14 (9.7%) were permanently housed, and six (4.1%) were placed in emergency shelter. Equitable placement into alternative accommodations was assessed, revealing similar rates of LTS or permanent placement across race/ethnicity and age groups, but with a higher rate of placement for females compared with males ($P < .05$). Six months following the encampment closure, among those from the encampment who moved into LTS, 65% were still living in LTS and 22% were placed in permanent housing. Among those living in LTS at six months, percentages of self-reported access to clinical services were 64% for primary care engagement, 53% for medication for opioid use disorder, and 30% for mental health services.

Despite demonstrated early success, limitations exist. Time constraints, geographic area of focus, and the chaotic nature of conducting the census led to missed individuals. Additionally, about a quarter of the surveyed encampment residents were lost to follow-up. These challenges underscore the need for additional time, expanded and continued outreach, and additional accommodations for future responses.

SUSTAINABILITY

Boston's public health approach established systems to address co-occurring unsheltered homelessness and SUD.[14] Although promising outcomes were observed, long-term evaluation is critical. Identifying long-term funding and reimbursement for LTS and housing programs is critical for sustaining this system-level change. Evolving data systems, cross-agency collaboration, and ongoing engagement are essential for equitable person-centered approaches. When an encampment returned, these implementation steps provided a foundation for aligning public health and public safety approaches identified through the strategic planning process.

PUBLIC HEALTH SIGNIFICANCE

A public health approach to addressing chronic unsheltered homelessness and SUD is based on the understanding that structural barriers and systematic gaps in our systems of care have resulted in increased numbers of encampments across the country. The foundational elements leading to equitable access to services, shelter, and housing require working across silos, person-centered planning with trusted outreach teams, and creation of new shelter models. Boston's experience navigating individuals from a tent encampment demonstrates that focusing on the root causes of encampments and offering alternatives that are amenable to the individuals' circumstances can provide a pathway to supportive shelter and housing. All four components of this cross-sector coordinated approach are required to build systems that effectively address this complex public health issue facing so many cities and towns. AJPH

ABOUT THE AUTHORS

At the time of this study, Monica Bharel was with the City of Boston and Daniel Dooley was with the Boston Public Health Commission, Boston, MA. Michele Clark is with the Boston Public

Health Commission and Bisola Ojikutu is with the Boston Public Health Commission and Mass General Brigham, Boston, MA.

CORRESPONDENCE

Correspondence should be sent to Monica Bharel, 355 Main St, Cambridge MA 02142 (e-mail: mobharel@gmail.com). Reprints can be ordered at https://www.ajph.org by clicking the "Reprints" link.

PUBLICATION INFORMATION

Full Citation: Bharel M, Clark MN, Dooley D, Ojikutu BO. Addressing unsheltered homelessness and substance use disorder from tent encampment to safe spaces, Boston 2021–2022. *Am J Public Health*. 2025;115(5):689–692.

Acceptance Date: December 23, 2024.

DOI: https://doi.org/10.2105/AJPH.2025.308009

CONTRIBUTORS

M. Bharel and B. O. Ojikutu contributed to the conceptualization and design of the work, acquisition, analysis, and interpretation of data, drafting and revisions of the work, and final approval. M. N. Clark contributed to analysis and interpretation of data, drafting and revisions of the work, and final approval. D. Dooley contributed to the analysis and interpretation of data and revisions of the work.

ACKNOWLEDGMENTS

We thank the Mayor's Office for leadership and strategic direction; Boston Public Health Commission Recovery Services and Homeless Services Bureau leadership and outreach teams for providing trusted, compassionate outreach and services to support clients; the Boston Mayor's Office of Housing for providing low-threshold shelter and housing services; Boston City Department agency members of the Coordinated Response team; the Massachusetts Department of Public Health for establishing and funding temporary and permanent low-threshold housing programs; the Massachusetts Executive Office of Health and Human Services for leadership and funding; the clinical, housing, homeless services, and outreach providers who provided frontline health and social services; the Low Threshold Site provider partners for implementing novel programs; and the clients for sharing their experiences to help shape the program.

CONFLICTS OF INTEREST

M. Bharel is currently with Google, LLC. This work represents M. Bharel's opinion and not the position of Google, LLC.

HUMAN PARTICIPANT PROTECTION

The tent/survey data presented here were collected for program planning purposes and thus exempt from institutional review board approval.

REFERENCES

1. Fact sheet: Boston homeless encampment liaison protocol. Mayor's Office, City of Boston. Updated October 29, 2021. Available at: https://www.boston.gov/news/fact-sheet-boston-homeless-encampment-liaison-protocol. Accessed May 30, 2024.
2. Homeless and Housing Resource Center, Substance Abuse and Mental Health Services Administration. Low-barrier shelter: policies into practice. 2024. Available at: https://hhrctraining.org/system/files/paragraphs/download-file/file/2024-03/HHRC_Low_Barrier_Shelter_Policies_508.pdf. Accessed May 30, 2024.
3. Beaugard CA, Khudairi F, Yesufu O, Farina A, Laks J. "I don't think of it as a shelter. I say I'm going home": a qualitative evaluation of a low-threshold shelter for women who use drugs. *Harm Reduct J*. 2024;21(1):44. https://doi.org/10.1186/s12954-024-00930-1
4. Mayer M, Mejia Urieta Y, Martinez LS, Komaromy M, Hughes U, Chatterjee A. Encampment clearings and transitional housing: a qualitative analysis of resident perspectives. *Health Aff (Millwood)*. 2024;43(2):218–225. https://doi.org/10.1377/hlthaff.2023.01040
5. Komaromy M, Stone A, Peterson A, Gott J, Koenig R, Taylor JL. Facilitating exit from encampments: combining low-barrier transitional housing with stabilizing treatment for substance related problems. *Addict Sci Clin Pract*. 2023;18(1):66. https://doi.org/10.1186/s13722-023-00420-y
6. City of Boston Recovery Services. Overnight low-threshold spaces practice guidance. 2021. Available at: https://www.boston.gov/sites/default/files/file/2021/07/OLTS%20Practice%20Guidance.pdf. Accessed May 30, 2024.
7. City of Boston. Long-term public health strategic outlook: serving the Mass & Cass area and unsheltered individuals in Boston, updates and strategic direction. 2022. Available at: https://www.boston.gov/sites/default/files/file/2023/07/Strategic%20Outlook.pdf. Accessed May 30, 2024.
8. City of Boston. Mass/Cass Dashboard. Available at: https://app.powerbigov.us/view?r=eyJrIjoiYTI3NTZkNGQtNDA5OS00MmNjLWFjODQtNWE5Yjk3ZGI1ZmU4IiwidCI6Ijg1NTI4ODdjLWNiYzMtNGVlNS05ZmQzLWVhMjE3ZTMwMjZmYyJ9. Accessed May 30, 2024.
9. City of Boston. City of Boston 41st Annual Homeless Census. Department of Neighborhood Development. 2021. Available at: www.boston.gov/sites/default/files/file/2021/04/2021%20Census%20Memo.pdf. Accessed May 30, 2024.
10. City of Boston. Coordinated response team. Updated May 28, 2024. Available at: https://www.boston.gov/departments/mayors-office/coordinated-response-team. Accessed May 30, 2024.
11. De Sousa T, Andrichik A, Cuellar M, Marson J, Prestera E, Rush K. Abt Associates. The 2022 Annual Homelessness Assessment Report (AHAR) to Congress, Part 1: Point-in-Time Estimates of Homelessness. US Dept of Housing and Urban Development. 2022. Available at: https://www.huduser.gov/portal/sites/default/files/pdf/2022-ahar-part-1.pdf. Accessed May 30, 2024.
12. Richards J, Kuhn R. Unsheltered homelessness and health: a literature review. *AJPM Focus*. 2022;2(1):100043. https://doi.org/10.1016/j.focus.2022.100043
13. Cohen R, Yetvin W, Khadduri J. Abt Associates. Understanding encampments of people experiencing homelessness and community responses: emerging evidence as of late 2018. Office of Policy Development and Research, US Dept of Housing and Urban Development. 2019. Available at: https://www.huduser.gov/portal/sites/default/files/pdf/Understanding-Encampments.pdf. Accessed May 30, 2024.
14. Bharel M, Auerbach J. Using public health tools to alleviate homeless encampments. *J Public Health Manag Pract*. 2023;29(6):759–761. https://doi.org/10.1097/PHH.0000000000001811

Going Places: An Active Transportation Intervention to Increase Youth Physical Activity, Durham, North Carolina, 2023–2024

Emily M. D'Agostino, DPH, MS, MEd, MA, Cody D. Neshteruk, PhD, Tang Li, MS, Jeremiah Davis, MD, Isa Granados, PhD, MS, Advika Kumar, BS, Jeffrey Forde, BA, and Christoph P. Hornik, MD, PhD, MPH

Routine youth physical activity (PA) fosters healthy habits and lasting cardiometabolic benefits into adulthood; however, significant disparities in PA persist by race, ethnicity, and income. Active transportation is an optimal intervention target to promote youth PA equity by building transportation self-efficacy skills. Going Places, a multilevel transportation self-efficacy intervention, aims to increase underserved youth PA and cardiometabolic health. We demonstrate preliminary efficacy, based on increased levels of PA, improved transportation self-efficacy, and reduced barriers to transportation use and PA to support positive patterns for lifelong health. (*Am J Public Health*. 2025;115(5):693–697. https://doi.org/10.2105/AJPH.2025.308012)

AJPH May 2025, Vol. 115, No. 5

Youth physical activity (PA) supports healthy habits early in life, with lasting benefits into adulthood, including protection against cardiometabolic risk factors like high blood pressure, obesity, and diabetes. However, only 26% of White adolescents meet the World Health Organization's PA guidelines (60 minutes of daily moderate-to-vigorous PA [MVPA]), compared with just 21% of Black and Hispanic adolescents. Low-income youths are also less likely than high-income youths to meet PA guidelines.[1] Minoritized and low-income youths have fewer opportunities for PA through community-based programs, such as sports clubs and accessible, age-appropriate adolescent programs,[2] which may in part explain disparities in PA. Moreover, limited transportation is a major barrier for high-priority youths to access PA programs and spaces.[3] The American Academy of Pediatrics states that youth active transportation (e.g., walking, running, and biking) is an optimal target to increase MVPA[4] through improved access to youth programs and the activity required to reach recreation sites.[5] Given that active transportation accounts for less than 20% of total MVPA among US adolescents, there is a prime opportunity for programs to promote active transportation.[6] A key component of routine active transportation among minoritized adolescents is transportation self-efficacy skills,[3] or belief in one's ability to effectively use transportation systems. Although prior interventions have targeted youth self-efficacy skills more generally,[7] we are unaware of other programs targeting youth transportation self-efficacy.

INTERVENTION AND IMPLEMENTATION

Going Places is a multilevel transportation self-efficacy intervention (Appendix Table A, available as a supplement to the online version of this article at http://www.ajph.org) designed to increase PA among underserved youths and improve their cardiometabolic health. Going Places is informed by the Socioecological Framework and Bandura's Self-efficacy Theory and includes the following components: weekly workshops on navigating transportation systems (individual level), community field trips and participatory mapping activities (recreation center level), and local transportation advocacy (environment level).[8] Going Places was codeveloped under the joint leadership of Duke University and

Durham Parks and Recreation (DPR; Durham, NC).

Going Places was offered to individual youths as part of DPR's no-cost adolescent afterschool program for youths aged 13 to 19 years. Going Places provided weekly workshops co-led by Duke and DPR that aimed to promote transportation self-efficacy (e.g., how to use local transportation systems, including biking and walking path trail maps, acquiring a free bus pass, using the bus and rail system, pedestrian and biking safety). Workshops also included engaging in active games and recreation.

Monthly field trips organized with the recreation center provided opportunities for youth to navigate transportation systems and engage in PA, primarily in outdoor settings (Appendix Figure A). Youths also participated in a series of participatory mapping exercises[9] to identify safe routes to reach neighborhood sites for active recreation.

The intervention's environmental components focused on promoting equitable access to transportation and PA for youths. The Going Places study team, youth participants, and the program's Steering Committee collaborated with local organizations that oversee recreation and transportation programs and policy in Durham. These organizations are involved in ongoing advocacy to promote safe, affordable, and sustainable transportation and recreation, including park renovation and restoration projects, public mural contests, and social activism (web; social media).

PLACE, TIME, AND PERSONS

Going Places is offered in areas with high social vulnerability (Appendix Figure B).[10] The study was held at two DPR recreation centers in Durham, North Carolina during 2023 and 2024. In the last full year, DPR enrolled more than 1257 adolescents across its six centers in youth programs (55% Black, 18% Hispanic; $19 000 mean per capita household income). Going Places participants (n = 70) were enrolled by DPR staff through typical DPR recruitment methods (e.g., on-site information sessions and word-of-mouth). Neighborhood audits using the Microscale Audit of Pedestrian Streetscapes (MAPS) abbreviated tool[11] showed that built environment infrastructure at all six youth recreation centers is conducive to active transit, with access to sidewalks, public transit, and the extensive Durham trails system (Appendix Table B).

PURPOSE

This single-arm study aimed to demonstrate the preliminary efficacy of Going Places, based on PA, transportation self-efficacy, and reduced personal and environmental barriers to transportation use and PA. It was conducted January 2023 to June 2024.

Participants' demographics were collected with self-report surveys. Frequency, type, and location of MVPA were assessed using the Web-Survey of Physical Activity and Nutrition (Web-SPAN) and the Teen Environment and Neighborhood (TEAN) measures, as previously described.[12] Transportation self-efficacy and personal and environmental barriers to MVPA were assessed using the TEAN measure and the Physical Activity Neighborhood Environment Scale.[12] Three focus groups were conducted to understand barriers to transportation use and PA, and to generate feedback on the intervention from youth participants, parents and guardians, and Parks and Recreation staff. Youth participants also were provided with Garmin accelerometers (VivoFit 4, Garmin International, Olathe, KS) to monitor step data over seven consecutive days.[13] We used the threshold of 11 500 or more steps per day to evaluate whether participants met daily steps goals.[14]

EVALUATION AND ADVERSE EFFECTS

We enrolled 70 participants who completed all baseline surveys (Table 1). Community partner engagement was maintained with biweekly meetings held with four DPR staff and monthly Steering Committee meetings (shifting to quarterly meetings in January 2024).

TABLE 1— Pilot Participant Characteristics: Durham, NC, 2023–2024

Pilot Participant Characteristics	Participants (n = 70), % or Mean (SD)
Age at enrollment, y	15.2 (1.9)
Race	
Black	89
White	3
Other	8
Hispanic ethnicity	20
Male gender	78
Overweight or obese	50
Eligible for free/reduced price school meals	81

A total of 15 youth workshops were held approximately once per week. Six total field trips were offered once every one to two months.

Survey Findings

Baseline survey data indicated that most participants did not use active transportation, had low PA levels, and demonstrated low transportation self-efficacy. Thirty-eight percent reported that they never engaged in MVPA during school day leisure time. More than half (56%) indicated that the most common site for engaging in MVPA was their home and 39% did not participate in any additional community programs. Forty-one percent indicated that they never used public transportation, 61% never walked or biked to school, and 33% spent no time biking, using walking paths, or using public transit each week without their parents.

Regarding barriers to MVPA and transportation use, less than half (42%) of participants knew where to obtain a free bus pass (available for all Durham youths). Almost half (43%) of participants strongly agreed or somewhat agreed that there was too much traffic in their neighborhood, and 55% strongly agreed or somewhat agreed that traffic made it difficult to walk.

Focus Group and Accelerometer Findings

Focus group participants (n = 20; 100% Black, 80% males, 3 adults, 17 youths) described concerns, such as violence, traffic, and access to paths or trails. Other MVPA barriers included transportation limitations, safety, resource scarcity, time constraints, and peer influence. Participants perceived Going Places as a catalyst for enhancing mobility by teaching adolescents how to navigate transportation systems, fostering access to recreation and raising safety awareness.

Step data were collected for seven consecutive days from 86% of devices. Mean seven-day step count across the participants was 8170 (SD = 3099) steps per day. Mean PA was 30% lower than the PA guidelines threshold.[14]

Pre–Post Data Findings

Based on the Web-SPAN and TEAN measures,[12] participants (n = 70 preintervention; n = 58 postintervention) showed improvements on the Getting Around Your Neighborhood, Places for Physical Activity, and reduced Barriers to Walking and Biking subscales (Figure 1). For example, the percentages of participants who reported never using public transportation, never walking or biking to school, and never biking, walking, or using public transit without their parents decreased by 12% (41% to 36%), 26% (61% to 45%), and 18% (33% to 27%), respectively.

SUSTAINABILITY

Our long-standing community-engaged partnership with DPR has fostered this codesigned, co-led, park-based multilevel transportation self-efficacy

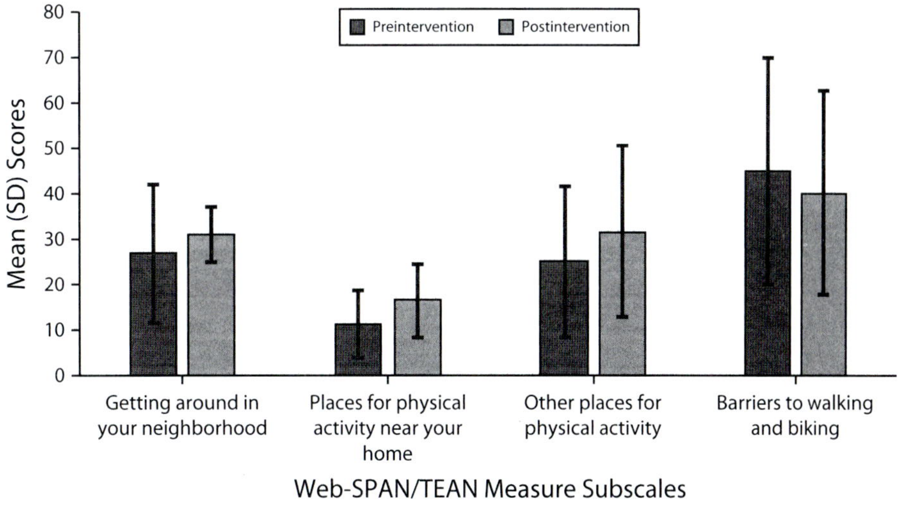

FIGURE 1— Pre- and Postintervention Web-SPAN and TEAN Group Mean (SD) Scores Across Subscale Questions for Participants: Durham, NC, 2023–2024

Note. Web-SPAN = Web-Survey of Physical Activity and Nutrition; TEAN = Teen Environment and Neighborhood. The number of participants was 70 preintervention and 58 postintervention. The mean value for pre- and postintervention scores was calculated by summing individual scores for all questions under each subscale and then taking the average score as the group mean.

intervention to increase PA and cardiometabolic health among underserved youths. This partnership provides a unique and necessary opportunity to comanage this program in an applied setting, and inform sustainability and future dissemination through national Parks and Recreation channels. Going Places provides Parks and Recreation organizations with a novel intervention that was codeveloped with Parks and Recreation to be integrated into an ongoing youth programs infrastructure. Also, the curriculum and field trips are modifiable and designed to be led by Parks and Recreation staff based on their youth programming expertise, contextual factors, and lived experience of engaging with the youth populations served by the organizations.

PUBLIC HEALTH SIGNIFICANCE

Promoting equitable access to active transportation for youths can reduce MVPA disparities, which otherwise pose a significant disease burden across the lifespan.[15] The Going Places multilevel transportation self-efficacy intervention aims to increase PA and cardiometabolic health among underserved youths. We demonstrate the preliminary efficacy of Going Places, based on PA, transportation self-efficacy, and reduced personal and environmental barriers to transportation use and PA. Next steps for this work include prospective trials to determine effectiveness to improve youth PA and blood pressure over 18 months and understand key implementation factors to promote the dissemination of Going Places. Given the urgent need for innovative solutions to address youth health disparities, this work will inform longer-term community-based cardiometabolic interventions and wider dissemination to promote access to PA programs and spaces for underserved youths. AJPH

ABOUT THE AUTHORS

Emily M. D'Agostino and Christoph P. Hornik are with the Duke Clinical Research Institute, Duke University School of Medicine, Durham, NC. Cody D. Neshteruk and Isa Granados are with the Department of Population Health Sciences, Duke University School of Medicine. Tang Li is with the Department of Public Health Science, Penn State College of Medicine, Hershey, PA. Jeremiah Davis is with the Department of Family Medicine, Duke University School of Medicine. Advika Kumar is with the Duke Global Health Institute, Duke University School of Medicine. Jeffrey Forde is with the Durham Parks and Recreation, Durham, NC.

CORRESPONDENCE

Correspondence should be sent to Emily M. D'Agostino, 311 Trent Dr, 2nd FL, Occupational Therapy Doctorate Division, Duke University School of Medicine, Durham, NC 27710 (e-mail: emily.m.dagostino@duke.edu). Reprints can be ordered at https://www.ajph.org by clicking the "Reprints" link.

PUBLICATION INFORMATION

Full Citation: D'Agostino EM, Neshteruk CD, Li T, et al. Going Places: an active transportation intervention to increase youth physical activity, Durham, North Carolina, 2023–2024. *Am J Public Health*. 2025;115(5):693–697.

Acceptance Date: December 31, 2024.

DOI: https://doi.org/10.2105/AJPH.2025.308012

ORCID iDs:

Emily M. D'Agostino https://orcid.org/0000-0003-0468-4836

Cody D. Neshteruk https://orcid.org/0000-0002-0516-6873

Tang Li https://orcid.org/0009-0001-2579-2433

Isa Granados https://orcid.org/0000-0002-2789-2040

Advika Kumar https://orcid.org/0009-0004-7932-3263

Christoph P. Hornik https://orcid.org/0000-0001-7056-8759

CONTRIBUTORS

E. M. D'Agostino and C. P. Hornik conceptualized and supervised the research. E. M. D'Agostino, J. Forde, J. Davis, and A. Kumar administered the project. E. M. D'Agostino, T. Li, and I. Granados curated the data and completed the analyses. E. M. D'Agostino, A. Kumar, C. D. Neshteruk, and C. P. Hornik wrote the original draft and edited the manuscript. All authors provided critical review.

ACKNOWLEDGMENTS

Funding for this study was provided by the Duke Clinical Research Institute and the Duke Global Health Institute. This research did not receive any specific grant from funding agencies in the public, commercial, or not-for-profit sectors.

We acknowledge the following individuals for their valuable contributions to the Going Places program: Cherise Hairston, Norwood Biggs, Cimarron Reed, Alexander Hurdle, Jason Jones, Brandon Reed, Shannon Teamer, Hiwot Zewdie, Sofia Massare, Kate Seneshen, Laura Brackett, Caitlin O'Reilly, Leah Topper, Andrew Yuan, Joseph Colosimo, Teah Bayless, Anne Berry, and participants of MyDurham, Durham Parks and Recreation, NC.

CONFLICTS OF INTEREST

The authors have no disclosures or competing interests to declare.

HUMAN PARTICIPANT PROTECTION

The study and all procedures were approved by the Duke University Health System institutional review board (Pro00106083).

REFERENCES

1. Physical Activity Alliance. The 2022 United States report card on physical activity for children and youth. Available at: paamovewithus.org/wp-content/uploads/2022/10/2022-US-Report-Card-on-Physical-Activity-for-Children-and-Youth.pdf. Accessed May 1, 2024.
2. Pelcher A, Rajan S. After-school program implementation in urban environments: increasing engagement among adolescent youth. *J Sch Health*. 2016;86(8):585–594. https://doi.org/10.1111/josh.12411
3. Piccone C, D'Agostino EM. Targeting youth transportation equity and self-efficacy to reduce youth physical activity disparities: a novel approach for a Public Health 3.0 agenda. *Am J Public Health*. 2021;111(5):795–798. https://doi.org/10.2105/ajph.2020.306143
4. Tester JM. The built environment: designing communities to promote physical activity in children. *Pediatrics*. 2009;123(6):1591–1598. https://doi.org/10.1542/peds.2009-0750
5. Chaix B, Kestens Y, Duncan S, et al. Active transportation and public transportation use to achieve physical activity recommendations? A combined GPS, accelerometer, and mobility survey study. *Int J Behav Nutr Phys Act*. 2014;11:124. https://doi.org/10.1186/s12966-014-0124-x
6. Moseley CA, Skinner AC, Perrin EM, Armstrong SC, Peterson ED, Wong CA. Adolescent and young adult recreational, occupational, and transportation activity: activity recommendation and weight status relationships. *J Adolesc Health*. 2019;65(1):147–154. https://doi.org/10.1016/j.jadohealth.2019.01.021
7. Cromer KD, D'Agostino EM, Hansen E, Alfonso C, Frasier S. After-school poly-strengths programming for urban teens at high-risk for violence exposure. *Transl Behav Med*. 2019;9(3):541–548.

8. Bandura A. *Social Foundations of Thought and Action: A Social Cognitive Theory*. Englewood Cliffs, NJ: Prentice-Hall; 1986.
9. Nykiforuk CI, Vallianatos H, Nieuwendyk LM. Photovoice as a method for revealing community perceptions of the built and social environment. *Int J Qual Methods*. 2011;10(2):103–124. https://doi.org/10.1177/160940691101000201
10. Centers for Disease Control and Prevention, Agency for Toxic Substances and Disease Registry. Social Vulnerability Index. Available at: https://www.atsdr.cdc.gov/place-health/php/svi/index.html. Accessed January 10, 2025.
11. Cain KL, Gavand KA, Conway TL, et al. Developing and validating an abbreviated version of the Microscale Audit for Pedestrian Streetscapes (MAPS-Abbreviated). *J Transp Health*. 2017;5:84–96.
12. Chung N, Ostbye T, Jones J, et al. Feasibility of a park-based active transportation intervention to promote youth physical activity and access to parks and recreation. *J Park Recreat Admi*. 2023;41(4):79–94. https://doi.org/10.18666/JPRA-2023-11830
13. Trost SG, Pate RR, Freedson PS, Sallis JF, Taylor WC. Using objective physical activity measures with youth: how many days of monitoring are needed? *Med Sci Sports Exerc*. 2000;32(2):426–431. https://doi.org/10.1097/00005768-200002000-00025
14. Adams MA, Johnson WD, Tudor-Locke C. Steps/day translation of the moderate-to-vigorous physical activity guideline for children and adolescents. *Int J Behav Nutr Phys Act*. 2013;10:49. https://doi.org/10.1186/1479-5868-10-49
15. Powell-Wiley TM, Martinez MF, Heneghan J, et al. Health and economic value of eliminating socioeconomic disparities in US youth physical activity. *JAMA Health Forum*. 2024;5(3):e240088. https://doi.org/10.1001/jamahealthforum.2024.0088

Public Health Enumeration in 2024: Who Is Keeping the Public Healthy?

Andrea C. Young, PhD, Christina L. Chung, MPH, and Leslie A. Dauphin, PhD

ABOUT THE AUTHORS

Andrea C. Young, Christina L. Chung, and Leslie A. Dauphin are with the National Center for State, Tribal, Local, and Territorial Public Health Infrastructure and Workforce, Centers for Disease Control and Prevention, Atlanta, GA.

See also Public Health Enumeration in 2024, pp. 701–725.

Public health workers are the backbone of the US public health system, protecting health and saving lives through the delivery of essential public health services in communities across the country. Yet we struggle to answer a seemingly simple question about this important national asset: How many governmental public health workers are there in the United States?

Workforce enumeration is the practice of counting workers and the means through which we acquire an understanding of the current size and composition of the nation's governmental public health workforce. This practice is foundational for strategic, evidence-based workforce planning and development. It serves as a crucial input into multiple workforce-related activities, such as recruitment and hiring, training, succession planning, and retention. Moreover, understanding current workforce supply is prerequisite to determining if the United States has enough workers to protect the health of the nation. The most recent attempt to enumerate the public health workforce is approximately 10 years old,[1] and limitations identified then still linger today; namely, the lack of a standard taxonomy of public health occupations and challenges with the completeness and specificity of workforce data (see Balio et al., p. 701).[2]

INVESTMENT IN THE WORKFORCE

Despite these challenges, federal and philanthropic investments spanning three decades have supported multiple initiatives that have contributed to today's enumeration efforts. Examples include the following.

Public Health Infrastructure Grant

This updated enumeration effort ("Enumeration 2024") is supported by the Centers for Disease Control and Prevention (CDC) through OE22-2203: Strengthening US Public Health Infrastructure, Workforce, and Data Systems Grant (hereafter referred to as the Public Health Infrastructure Grant, or PHIG). PHIG is a five-year grant supported in part by the American Rescue Plan Act of 2021 (ARPA) to strengthen the nation's public health infrastructure and systems related to the workforce, foundational capabilities, and data infrastructure, which includes a landmark investment of approximately $3 billion for its public health workforce component (ARPA Sec. 2501, Sec. 2404).[3] This enumeration will help further our understanding of how this investment contributes to changes in the public health workforce over time.

Public Health Workforce Research Center

In 2022, the CDC and the Health Resources and Services Administration (HRSA) partnered to establish the nation's first federally funded Public Health Workforce Research Center (PHWRC) through a five-year cooperative agreement (HRSA-22-054). From 2022 to 2024, the CDC and HRSA cofunded the University of Minnesota School of Public Health to conduct rigorous, state-of-the-art applied research that strengthens the evidence base for public health workforce planning, policymaking, and development. As the funded PHWRC, the University of Minnesota established the Consortium for Workforce Research in Public Health (CWORPH), a group of academic member institutions and practice-oriented partner organizations focused on strengthening the evidence base for public health workforce recruitment, retention, and development. Using PHWRC funding, CWORPH members have conducted research that complements today's enumeration work. This includes projects that examined variation in the public health workforce composition by geography, race, and ethnicity,[4] created comprehensive estimates of public health workforce supply,[5] and studied US Department of

Labor standard occupational classification codes and identified gaps in federal data regarding the public health workforce.[2] In the third year of the PHWRC, CWORPH members will continue to advance our understanding of the public health workforce and explore how to leverage various data sets for enumeration purposes.

ASTHO Profiles and NACCHO Profiles

The CDC and the Robert Wood Johnson Foundation have a deep-rooted association of provided funding and technical assistance through cooperative agreements and grants to the Association of State and Territorial Health Officials (ASTHO; 17 years) and the National Association of County and City Health Officials (NACCHO; 34 years) to systematically collect information about state, territorial, and local public health infrastructure.[6,7] Referred to as the ASTHO and NACCHO Profiles, these census surveys track state, territorial, and local health departments' activities, organizational characteristics, and resources, which include funding and workforce. Lacking access to direct counts of state and local public health workers, researchers have found the ASTHO and NACCHO Profiles to be an important source of data for enumeration studies. The authors of the enumeration work featured in this issue used data from the ASTHO 2022 Profile and the NACCHO 2022 Profile to estimate employee counts for an updated synthetic enumeration.

Public Health Workforce Interest and Needs Survey

Created in part to complement the ASTHO and NACCHO Profiles, which are administered at the agency level, the Public Health Workforce Interest and Needs Survey (PH WINS) is a survey of individual workers at government public health agencies. PH WINS collects demographic data from individual workers and captures their perspectives regarding crucial topics, such as training needs, employee morale, and worker engagement.[8] The survey was created by the de Beaumont Foundation in collaboration with ASTHO. First fielded in 2014, PH WINS was originated in partnership with organizations such as NACCHO, the HRSA, the CDC, and other public health organizations and practitioners. It draws heavily from previously used instruments, such as the Federal Employee Viewpoint Survey, the CDC Technical Assistance and Service Improvement Initiative: Project Officer Survey, the 2009 Epidemiology Capacity Assessment, and others.[9] Using data collected from PH WINS in 2021, the authors of articles featured in this issue were able to provide a fuller picture of the current governmental public health workforce, with demographic information regarding age, race/ethnicity, and education. For this 2024 synthetic enumeration, PH WINS data were also used to complement ASTHO- and NACCHO-derived counts for the local public health workforce.

ADVANCING WORKFORCE ENUMERATION

The enumeration work reflected in this issue, conducted by the Public Health Accreditation Board in partnership with CWORPH, builds on previous enumeration efforts and leverages existing data sets acquired through previously listed initiatives. This work advances our understanding of the size and composition of the governmental public health workforce in multiple ways, as follows:

1. It provides updated total counts of federal, state, and local governmental public health workers;
2. It examines current distribution, density, and demographics of public health workers at the state and local levels;
3. It highlights the importance of occupation-specific enumeration, and offers new insight into the distribution of public health nurses; and
4. It presents new enumeration methods and sources of data that help address missing and incomplete information about the US governmental public health workforce.

These articles highlight the challenges resulting from the lack of a standard taxonomy for public health occupations, which will continue to limit our ability to further refine and improve future enumerations. The authors of these articles echo recommendations from the President's Council of Advisors on Science and Technology[10] and the national Public Health Services & Systems Research agenda[11] that call for the establishment of federal occupational standards for public health.

CONCLUSIONS

At the heart of the US public health system lies the public health worker. They are the means through which essential public health services are delivered to communities across the country. The articles presented in this issue advance the practice of public health workforce enumeration by capitalizing on previous initiatives and making good use of available workforce data. The authors offer key insights into the total size, distribution, and specific occupations of the current public health workforce, and methodological considerations and recommendations for the practice of enumeration moving forward. Understanding how many public health workers there are, where they are, and the occupations they fill lays the foundation for future research and evidence-based workforce planning and development. AJPH

CORRESPONDENCE

Correspondence should be sent to Andrea C. Young, PhD, MS, Director, Division of Workforce Development, National Center for State, Tribal, Local, and Territorial Public Health Infrastructure and Workforce, Centers for Disease Control and Prevention, 2400 Century Center, MS-V24-5, Atlanta, GA 30345 (e-mail: acy2@cdc.gov).

PUBLICATION INFORMATION

Full Citation: Young AC, Chung CL, Dauphin LA. Public health enumeration in 2024: who is keeping the public healthy? *Am J Public Health*. 2025;115(5): 698–700.

Acceptance Date: November 5, 2024.

DOI: https://doi.org/10.2105/AJPH.2024.307924

ORCID iDs:

Andrea C. Young https://orcid.org/0000-0003-3176-1729

Christina L. Chung https://orcid.org/0000-0001-8980-0052

Leslie A. Dauphin https://orcid.org/0009-0009-2447-6365

CONTRIBUTORS

A. C. Young led the drafting of the manuscript. C. L. Chung and L. A. Dauphin provided substantive input and revisions throughout the writing process. All authors contributed to the conceptual design of the manuscript and reviewed and approved the final manuscript.

ACKNOWLEDGMENTS

We thank Paul Reid, Marion Carter, and Karen Mumford for their thoughtful suggestions.

Note. The findings and conclusions of this editorial are those of the authors and do not represent the official position of the Centers for Disease Control and Prevention.

CONFLICTS OF INTEREST

The authors have no conflicts of interest to declare.

REFERENCES

1. Beck AJ, Boulton ML, Coronado F. Enumeration of the governmental public health workforce, 2014. *Am J Prev Med.* 2014;47(5 suppl 3):S306–S313. https://doi.org/10.1016/j.amepre.2014.07.018
2. Krasna H, Venkataraman M, Robins M, Patino I, Leider JP. Standard occupational classification codes: gaps in federal data on the public health workforce. *Am J Public Health.* 2024;114(1):48–56. https://doi.org/10.2105/AJPH.2023.307463
3. Carter MW, Simone PM, Houry DE, et al. Centers for Disease Control and Prevention's Public Health Infrastructure Grant: a better approach to empowering more state and local decision making and strengthening the public health workforce and infrastructure. *J Public Health Manag Pract.* 2024;9900. https://doi.org/10.1097/PHH.0000000000002055
4. Balio CP, Leslie H, Meit MB. Racial and ethnic representation of the local public health workforce. *Am J Public Health.* Published online ahead of print December 19, 2024:e1–e11. https://doi.org/10.2105/AJPH.2024.307903.
5. Onal S, Martin S, Weiss NM, Leider JP. Exploring the geospatial variations in the public health workforce: implications for diversifying the supply of potential workers in governmental settings. *Health Aff Sch.* 2024;2(10):qxae116.
6. *ASTHO Profile of State and Territorial Public Health*, vol 6. Arlington, VA: Association of State and Territorial Health Officials; 2023.
7. Cunningham M, Patel K, McCall T, et al. *2022 National Profile of Local Health Departments.* Washington, DC: National Association of County and City Health Officials; 2024.
8. Robins M, Leider JP, Schaffer K, Gambatese M, Allen E, Hare Bork R. PH WINS 2021 methodology report. *J Public Health Manag Pract.* 2023; 29(suppl 1):S35–S44.
9. Leider JP, Bharthapudi K, Pineau V, Liu L, Harper E. The methods behind PH WINS. *J Public Health Manag Pract.* 2015;21(suppl 6):S28–S35. https://doi.org/10.1097/PHH.0000000000000285
10. *Report to the President Supporting the US Public Health Workforce.* Washington, DC: President's Council of Advisors on Science and Technology; 2023.
11. Froeb K, Weinberg S, Adam A, Cope E. *A Research Agenda for an Evolving Public Health System: Directions for the Field of Public Health Services and Systems Research.* Washington, DC: AcademyHealth; 2023.

Enumerating the US Governmental Public Health Workforce

Casey P. Balio, PhD, Nathan A. Dockery, BS, and Rachel Hogg-Graham, DrPH, MA

ABOUT THE AUTHORS

Casey P. Balio is with the Center for Rural Health and Research and the Department of Health Services Management & Policy, East Tennessee State University, Johnson City, and is a member of the Consortium for WOrkforce Research in Public Health (CWORPH), led by the University of Minnesota. Nathan A. Dockery is with the Center for Rural Health and Research and the Department of Biostatistics & Epidemiology, East Tennessee State University, Johnson City. Rachel Hogg-Graham is with the Department of Health Management & Policy, College of Public Health, University of Kentucky, Lexington.

See also Public Health Enumeration in 2024, pp. 698–725.

Enumeration of the governmental public health workforce is a crucial component of understanding and bolstering nationwide public health infrastructure, involving the systematic counting of all members that are a part of the US governmental public health workforce. Enumeration is difficult to execute, but it can provide vital information regarding the workforce that can be used for advocacy, recruitment, retention, training, and planning efforts. For example, having estimates of the total workforce, and by occupation, level, educational background, geography, and other characteristics may inform funding requests at the federal, state, and local level. It can also provide benchmarks to compare staffing levels and their impacts, and help to identify where there are or may be staffing shortages. Many iterations of public health workforce enumeration have occurred in recent history, each utilizing different methodologies and providing insights across the years. Physical enumeration with a "direct counting" methodology was conducted at the federal level in the early 20th century, with a switch to more data-driven, synthetic methods in the late 20th and early 21st centuries.[1–3] Since the most recent enumeration of the public health workforce in 2012 by Beck et al.,[4] significant changes have occurred in the workforce that warrant a reexamination, including departures related to the COVID-19 pandemic and an aging public health workforce.[4,5] These notable changes highlight the importance of an occupation-specific enumeration to inform policymakers and agency leadership.

THE NEED FOR OCCUPATION-SPECIFIC ENUMERATION

In response to the COVID-19 pandemic and growing recognition of the infrastructure needs in state and local public health, the Centers for Disease Control and Prevention awarded $4.35 billion through the Public Health Infrastructure Grant (PHIG).[6] PHIG provided funding to 107 state and local health departments to support their infrastructure needs, such as bolstering and retaining workers, supporting technological upgrades, and ensuring that staff are trained in foundational skills and services to meet the needs of the public, in addition to technical assistance and evaluation of the funding.[6] As a subgrantee of this funding, a team of researchers as part of the Consortium for Workforce Research in Public Health[7] was tasked with enumerating the governmental public health workforce as a foundation for evaluating PHIG, referred to as Enumeration 2024. Although there are many others doing work related to public health and social determinants of health in various sectors (including nonprofit organizations) and in Tribal and Territorial health departments, this project specifically focused on the federal, state, and local governmental public health workforce.

Enumeration 2024, a multipronged approach to enumerate and describe the governmental public health workforce, included three distinct objectives: (1) enumerate the full public health workforce, including those working at the federal, state, and local levels; (2) enumerate and describe specific occupation groups within the public health workforce; and (3) enumerate and describe public health nurses specifically using novel data sources and approaches.[8] This enumeration will serve as a baseline description of the workforce for planning for future needs and understanding the public health workforce nationally, and will be replicated at the end of PHIG to understand how the workforce has changed over time. Results from each of the objectives that are a part of Enumeration 2024 are described elsewhere in more detail[8]; however, this commentary aims to describe the limitations specific to enumerating and describing key occupations in public health (Enumeration 2024 objective 2).

Occupation-specific enumeration has been requested for many years to support a more detailed understanding of the public health workforce and to tailor efforts to support specific occupations and roles in public health. Although Enumeration 2024 builds upon what has been done previously, it is not without limitations. In this commentary, we describe the limitations that we encountered in conducting the 2024 occupation-specific enumeration, including limitations of the underlying data, and offer opportunities for advancement and potential strategies to improve these data moving forward. Having more robust data that are structured in a way to facilitate enumeration more readily, efficiently, and frequently is needed to be able to understand the ever-changing public health workforce and plan for future needs.

LIMITATIONS TO OCCUPATION-SPECIFIC ENUMERATIONS

Although there are considerable limitations to enumerating and describing key occupations in public health, we focus on the three areas of (1) data challenges, (2) differences in definitions and categories, and (3) differences in public health structures. Although these challenges are not new to the field, they remain pertinent to data collection and enumeration, and some of these challenges are changing over time. We discuss each of these challenges and changes, including the importance of these issues to understanding the workforce now and in the future.

Data Challenges

Primary public health workforce data sources include Association of State and Territorial Health Officials (ASTHO) Profiles, National Association of County and City Health Officials (NACCHO) Profiles, and the de Beaumont Public Health Workforce Interest and Needs Survey (PH WINS).[9–11] Each of these provides unique and valuable data, but even in combination, they do not provide a comprehensive census of all public health agencies or individuals in the public health workforce. Although these data sources were central to Enumeration 2024 because of their national scope and coverage of the full public health workforce, they are not specific to any occupation and have limitations both individually and collectively.

First, the most recent iterations of NACCHO Profiles and PH WINS have response rates of 38% and 32.5%, respectively.[10,11] This limits the comprehensiveness of the data available, which may result in estimates for specific areas or types of agencies that are not generalizable or may require modeling that is not without other limitations. For example, small and rural local health departments have historically been underrepresented in these data sets and there is no full directory of all local health departments nationwide, making the response rates presented here underestimates of all local health departments across the country. We also were unable to include Tribal and Territorial health departments. Additionally, not all states and agencies participate in PH WINS.

Second, national weights for NACCHO Profiles and PH WINS are invaluable for national-level estimates and overcoming some of the limitations described here, but they do not allow for a robust understanding of the workforce for all state and local areas. Finally, each of these data sources undertakes new data collection approximately every three years, making longitudinal and timely analyses difficult.

Other data sources, such as licensure or membership data and Bureau of Labor Statistics (BLS) data, may also be used for enumerating the workforce but have their own limitations. First, data from membership organizations, professional societies, and licensure or credentialing groups may offer insights into specific occupations; however, they are often optional, based on convenience sampling, and may be broader than those directly and actively working in governmental public health. For example, membership to these organizations and participation in their data collection are often available to trainees and retired individuals. Including them in counts of the workforce may overestimate the current supply.

The BLS also collects critical data on workers in all sectors by occupation type and industry, but its applicability to governmental public health is limited. First, occupations within BLS data are defined using Standard Occupational Classification (SOC) codes.[12,13] The existing schema classifies workers into categories based on job duties; however, there are no specific SOC codes for most public health occupations, and existing SOC codes do not align well with most public health occupations.[14] Second, there is not a specific state or local health department industry. An industry of state or local government, excluding schools and hospitals, may be useful, but it is still not specific to state or local health departments. Even the intersection of a more general SOC code with this setting may be insufficient. For example, the SOC code for nurses in a local government setting may still include nurses working in behavioral health agencies or within the criminal–legal system, not just those working in a local public health agency. These challenges of the BLS data limit their applicability specifically for public health, therefore increasing the reliance on other data sources that may not be as comprehensive.

Defining Occupations

There is no consistent way to define occupations within public health, although numerous taxonomies exist.[6,15,16] Further, key data sources described here do not largely align with any specific existing taxonomy, or each other. For example, ASTHO and NACCHO Profiles use the category "laboratory worker," whereas PH WINS includes numerous occupations that may fit into this category, such as laboratory aide or assistant, laboratory quality control worker, laboratory scientist/medical technologist, and laboratory technician.[9–11] The differences in these definitions of occupations across the commonly used data sources make it difficult to harmonize into specific occupations and instead often result in combining occupations into larger occupation groups or categories, which inherently represent a more heterogeneous group and are less useful for the purposes of enumeration activities. In addition to the lack of standardization of occupations and categories that exist across data sources, the occupations are often defined by titles, roles, education, and responsibilities, which are not synonymous or substitutes. For example, a count of registered nurses is based on credentialing, but not all registered nurses may be performing the same duties, or those that are specific to registered nurses. Further, individuals may serve in multiple occupations, titles, roles, and responsibilities, particularly in smaller and rural agencies, which are generally not well captured in these data sources. Lastly, roles, titles, and responsibilities within public health continue to evolve as the field changes and can be specific to individual states and agencies. These challenges may be difficult to overcome, and have implications for how comparable enumerations may be over time.

Definition and Structure of Public Health

The substantial heterogeneity in public health agency structure, function, and workforce that exists across the United States also affects the ability to generate robust, occupation-specific enumerations. Further, differences in state governance structure, regionalization, and resource sharing make it difficult to assess where specific workers are conducting their work. For example, using only ASTHO and NACCHO Profiles may not adequately capture workers in centralized or largely centralized states (e.g., Arizona, South Carolina, Rhode Island, and Virginia) that are assigned to a smaller geographic level.

DEFINING OCCUPATIONS IN ENUMERATION 2024

Although there are considerable challenges to the data needed to support occupation-specific enumerations in public health, Enumeration 2024 represents the most comprehensive analysis possible given the available data. Although it can and should be improved upon moving forward, it provides valuable insights that would otherwise be unavailable. To establish this baseline occupation enumeration, we developed a crosswalk to triangulate occupations from NACCHO, ASTHO, and PH WINS (Box 1). Although some occupations could map one-to-one, others were only present in one source. As such, we had to group some occupations together into categories, resulting in a loss of granularity across some individual occupations. The challenges in the underlying data affect the estimates provided, but do not preclude Enumeration 2024 from being the most timely and robust occupation-specific enumeration in recent years.

IMPROVING OCCUPATION ENUMERATION AND FUTURE STEPS

Throughout the process of generating estimates for the occupation-specific enumeration and working through the data challenges that exist, we identified two key areas for improvement that may facilitate stronger occupation enumerations in the future: alignment of occupation definitions across major data sources and development of new SOC codes that capture occupation data at the federal level. Although other solutions may exist to enhance data quality and generate meaningful, national, occupation-specific enumerations, the opportunities described here may be among the most feasible at this time and offer a practical path forward. First, creating standardized occupation titles, categories, and groupings would help substantially in occupation-specific enumeration. Having common categories across agencies and data sources would facilitate cleaner data collection and analysis, providing more robust and complete estimates of public health occupations.

Second, establishing SOC codes that align with public health occupation categories would enable the use of

BOX 1— Crosswalk of Occupations From ASTHO, NACCHO, and PH WINS

Occupation Type	PH WINS (2021)	ASTHO Profile (2019)	NACCHO Profile (2019)
Agency leadership	• Department/bureau director • Deputy director • Health officer • Public health agency director	• Executive leadership	• Agency leadership
Behavioral health professional	• Behavioral health professional • Peer counselor	• Behavioral health staff	• Behavioral health staff
Business support—financial and operations	• Business support—accountant/fiscal • Grants or contracts specialist	• Business and financial operations staff	• Business and financial operations staff
Community health worker	• Community health worker • Health navigator		• Community health worker
Disease intervention specialist	• Disease intervention specialist/contact tracer		
Environmental health worker	• Animal control worker • Environmental health worker • Sanitarian or inspector • Engineer	• Environmental health worker	• Environmental health worker • Animal control worker
Epidemiologists & statisticians	• Epidemiologist • Statistician	• Epidemiologist • Statistician	• Epidemiologist • Statistician
Health educator	• Health educator	• Health educator	• Health educator
Information systems manager/information technology specialist	• Information systems manager/information technology specialist • Public health informatics specialist	• Public health informatics specialist	• Information systems specialist
Laboratory workers	• Laboratory aide or assistant • Laboratory quality control worker • Laboratory scientist/medical technologist • Laboratory technician	• Laboratory worker	• Laboratory worker
Nutritionist or dietitian	• Nutritionist • Dietitian	• Nutritionist	• Nutritionist
Office and administrative support	• Clerical personnel—administrative assistant • Customer service/support professional • Clerical personnel—secretary • Business support services—administrative • Human resources personnel • Business support services—coordinator	• Office and administrative support	• Office and administrative support
Oral health professional	• Other oral health professional • Public health dentist	• Oral health professional	• Oral health professional
Emergency preparedness/management worker	• Emergency preparedness/management worker	• Preparedness staff	• Preparedness staff
Public/community health nurse	• Combination of profession and degree(s) to be consistent with other public health nurse research in the field Occupations: • Other nurse—clinical services • Registered nurse—public health or community health nurse • Nurse practitioner • Registered nurse—unspecified Degrees: • Associate's degree in nursing • Bachelor's degree in nursing • Master's degree in nursing • Doctorate degree in nursing	• Nurse practitioner • Public health nurse	• Registered nurse

Continued

BOX 1— Continued

Occupation Type	PH WINS (2021)	ASTHO Profile (2019)	NACCHO Profile (2019)
Public health physicians and other clinicians	• Public health/ preventive medicine physician • Pharmacist • Physical/occupational/rehabilitation therapist • Public health veterinarian • Physician assistant • Licensed practical or vocational nurse	• Public health physician	• Public health physician • Licensed practical or vocational nurse
Social worker/social services professional	• Social worker/social services professional		

Note. ASTHO = Association of State and Territorial Health Officials; NACCHO = National Association of County and City Health Officials; PH WINS = Public Health Workforce Interest and Needs Survey.

federal-level data for public health enumeration. Work is currently underway to propose new SOC codes for core public health professions, including for public health nurses and disease intervention specialists,[17,18] and the guidelines and mechanisms for establishing new codes are available for future use.[13] Further, a specific Public Health Major Domain may also facilitate better data collection to capture the unique roles of public health professionals. Having SOC codes specific to key public health occupations will increase the utility of federal BLS data to be used for future public health workforce enumeration efforts, but will take time to implement the codes and make them available.[14]

CONCLUSION

Enumerating key public health occupations as part of Enumeration 2024 highlighted the long described need for better data and tracking of the public health workforce. Although our methodology built on past occupation enumerations and created a baseline for future work, it is critical that public health partners at all levels come together and create consensus on how to define occupations and improve data collection to improve enumeration efforts in the future. Creating common definitions in practice and across data collection efforts, along with improving federal-level data collection for enumeration, have the potential to provide a powerful mechanism for public health workforce advocacy, recruitment, retention, training, and planning. AJPH

CORRESPONDENCE

Correspondence should be sent to Casey P. Balio, 2109 W Market St #127, Johnson City, TN 37604 (e-mail: balioc@etsu.edu). Reprints can be ordered at https://www.ajph.org by clicking the "Reprints" link.

PUBLICATION INFORMATION

Full Citation: Balio CP, Dockery NA, Hogg-Graham R. Enumerating the US governmental public health workforce. *Am J Public Health*. 2025;115(5):701–706.

Acceptance Date: December 8, 2024.

DOI: https://doi.org/10.2105/AJPH.2024.307981

ORCID iDs:

Casey P. Balio https://orcid.org/0000-0002-2987-4268

Nathan A. Dockery https://orcid.org/0009-0004-9398-9280

Rachel Hogg-Graham https://orcid.org/0000-0003-0555-4902

CONTRIBUTORS

C. P. Balio, N. A. Dockery, and R. Hogg-Graham all contributed to the development, editing, and final approval of this manuscript, as well as the analysis that is referenced.

ACKNOWLEDGMENTS

This work was supported by funds made available from the Centers for Disease Control and Prevention (CDC) of the US Department of Health and Human Services (HHS), National Center for State, Tribal, Local, and Territorial Public Health Infrastructure and Workforce, through OE22-2203: Strengthening US Public Health Infrastructure, Workforce, and Data Systems grant.

PH WINS data from this study were obtained from the Public Health Workforce Interests and Needs Survey, a project supported through a collaboration of the Association of State and Territorial Health Officials (ASTHO) and the de Beaumont Foundation. The use of the data does not imply ASTHO's or the de Beaumont Foundation's endorsement of the research, research methods, or conclusions contained in this report.

We thank the following data owners and contributors used in the underlying analysis referenced in this manuscript: the de Beaumont Foundation (Public Health Workforce Interests and Needs Survey), National Association of County and City Health Officials (NACCHO Profile), and Association of State and Territorial Health Officials (ASTHO Profile). We thank the Public Health Accreditation Board and the CDC for their partnership. We also thank members of the Consortium for Workforce Research in Public Health for their feedback and guidance, including J. P. Leider, Michael Meit, Heather Krasna, Beth Resnick, and Valerie Yeager.

Note. The contents are those of the authors and do not necessarily represent the official views of, nor an endorsement by, CDC/HHS or the US Government.

CONFLICTS OF INTEREST

The authors have no conflicts of interest to disclose.

HUMAN PARTICIPANT PROTECTION

The analysis referenced in this article was deemed non-human participant research by the East Tennessee State University institutional review board.

REFERENCES

1. *A Report on Public and Community Health Personnel.* Washington, DC: US Dept of Health, Education, and Welfare, Public Health Service; 1980.

2. Gebbie KM. The Public Health Work Force: Enumeration 2000. Health Resources and Services Administration, Bureau of Health Professions, National Center for Health Workforce Information and Analysis. 2000. Available at: https://books.google.com/books?hl=en&lr=&id=OFIDWF9Ee4kC&oi=fnd&pg=PA11&ots=mwqSpgrAyR&sig=F-3sBl0rVISZxM0-gdW4kMA04ks#v=onepage&q&f=false. Accessed February 25, 2025
3. Merrill J, Btoush R, Gupta M, Gebbie K. A history of public health workforce enumeration. *J Public Health Manag Pract.* 2003;9(6):459–470. https://doi.org/10.1097/00124784-200311000-00005
4. Beck AJ, Boulton ML, Coronado F. Enumeration of the governmental public health workforce, 2014. *Am J Prev Med.* 2014;47(5):S306–S313. https://doi.org/10.1016/j.amepre.2014.07.018
5. Leider JP, Castrucci BC, Robins M, et al. The exodus of state and local public health employees: separations started before and continued throughout COVID-19. *Health Aff (Millwood).* 2023;42(3):338–348. https://doi.org/10.1377/hlthaff.2022.01251
6. Centers for Disease Control and Prevention. Public Health Infrastructure Grant. May 16, 2024. Available at: https://www.cdc.gov/infrastructure-phig/about/index.html. Accessed November 19, 2024.
7. University of Minnesota. Consortium for Workforce Research in Public Health. 2021. Available at: https://cworph.umn.edu. Accessed November 19, 2024.
8. Leider J, Balio C, Hogg-Graham R, et al. An enumeration of the public health workforce in 2024. 2024. Available at: https://cworph.umn.edu/sites/cworph.umn.edu/files/2024-08/enumeration-2024.pdf. Accessed November 19, 2024.
9. Association of State and Territorial Health Officials. ASTHO profile of state and territorial public health. 2019. Available at: https://www.astho.org/topic/public-health-infrastructure/profile/previous-reports. Accessed April 12, 2024.
10. National Association of County and City Health Officials. NACCHO national profile of local health departments. 2019. Available at: https://www.naccho.org/uploads/downloadable-resources/Programs/Public-Health-Infrastructure/NACCHO_2019_Profile_final.pdf. Accessed April 12, 2024.
11. de Beaumont Foundation and Association of State and Territorial Health Officials. Public Health Workforce Interests and Needs Survey: 2021 Dashboard. 2022. Available at: https://debeaumont.org/phwins/2021-findings. Accessed April 5, 2024.
12. Bureau of Labor Statistics. Standard occupational classification. March 24, 2008. Available at: https://www.bls.gov/soc. Accessed November 19, 2024.
13. Executive Office of the President. Standard occupational classification manual. 2018. Available at: https://www.bls.gov/soc/2018/soc_2018_manual.pdf. Accessed November 19, 2024.
14. Krasna H, Venkataraman M, Robins M, Patino I, Leider JP. Standard occupational classification codes: gaps in federal data on the public health workforce. *Am J Public Health.* 2024;114(1):48–56. https://doi.org/10.2105/AJPH.2023.307463
15. Beck AJ, Coronado F, Boulton ML, Merrill JA. The public health workforce taxonomy: revisions and recommendations for implementation. *J Public Health Manag Pract.* 2018;24(5):E1–E11. https://doi.org/10.1097/PHH.0000000000000690
16. Boulton ML, Beck AJ, Coronado F, et al. Public health workforce taxonomy. *Am J Prev Med.* 2014;47(5):S314–S323. https://doi.org/10.1016/j.amepre.2014.07.015
17. Regulations.gov. Comment on FR Doc # 2024-12825. August 14, 2024. Available at: https://www.regulations.gov/comment/BLS-2024-0001-36911. Accessed November 20, 2024.
18. Comment on FR Doc # 2024-12825. August 14, 2024. Available at: https://www.regulations.gov/comment/BLS-2024-0001-37067. Accessed November 20, 2024.

Enumeration 2024: What We Know and What We Wish We Knew About the Governmental Public Health Workforce in a COVID-19 Recovery Landscape

Jonathon P. Leider, PhD, Casey P. Balio, PhD, Rachel Hogg-Graham, DrPH, Nicole M. Weiss, PhD, Abby Vogel, MS, Sezen O. Onal, PhD, Xiao Zang, PhD, Paula Kett, RN, PhD, MPH, Joyce Edmonds, RN, PhD, MPH, Harshada Karnik, PhD, Nathan Dockery, BS, Bibin Joseph, MPH, Morgan Pak, MPH, Amy Belflower Thomas, MHA, MSPH, and Betty Bekemeier, RN, PhD, MPH

See also Public Health Enumeration in 2024, pp. 698–725.

Objectives. To expand on previous enumerations by assessing the size and composition of the governmental public health workforce in the wake of the COVID-19 pandemic, identifying workforce trends, occupational distributions, and potential gaps in staffing.

Methods. From 2023 to 2024, using 2022 data in the United States, we conducted 3 distinct analyses: (1) estimating the total workforce size, (2) profiling occupation-specific distributions, and (3) evaluating the role and prevalence of public health nurses using novel data sources. For total counts, we used multiple imputation by chained equations to develop robust agency-level estimates and address missingness from multiple data sets.

Results. State and local public health agencies grew to approximately 239 000 staff in 2022, up from an estimated 206 500 in 2019. The largest occupation groups included office and administrative support workers (37 576) and public health or community health nurses (29 387). We found that 73 478 (1.8%) of registered nurses nationwide served in governmental public health roles.

Conclusions. The size of the workforce during the COVID-19 response has returned to 2008 levels although temporary staff largely constitute the increase.

Public Health Implications. An undersized workforce leaves the United States vulnerable to future disasters and current challenges. (*Am J Public Health*. 2025;115(5):707–715. https://doi.org/10.2105/AJPH.2024.307960)

AJPH May 2025, Vol. 115, No. 5

For decades, public health practitioners, policymakers, and, at times, the public, have asked how many people work in public health. Yet the federal government has never systematically answered this question; enumerations of the governmental public health workforce have long been left to nonprofits, academics, and others in the field.[1] The reasons for this are many but ultimately reduce to (1) lack of licensure data for public health officials, and (2) disagreement on how to define the taxonomies of public health workers.[2] The public health domain has attempted to resolve these 2 issues since 1908, when the first "limited enumeration" of the field was undertaken.[1]

In 1908, only 1 organization's employees were counted; by 1933, data for 569 organizations were collected.[1] These first enumerations, as well as the successive enumerations until 1964, were undertaken using a direct counting technique.[1] These were direct federal surveys that hand counted employees. As the field grew, continuing to use this method became impractical, and synthetic enumeration became the preferred method for counting employees.[1] Synthetic enumerations use questionnaire data from hundreds of agencies from multiple data sets to produce informed estimates. Relatively recent synthetic enumerations have estimated that the public health workforce declined by roughly 10% between 1980 and 2000, from about 500 000[3] to 448 254[4] individuals. It is possible that discrepancies in the taxonomies of public health worker definitions as well as actual decreases in the workforce contributed to this decline.[1] More recently, in 2012, Beck et al. conducted a synthetic enumeration and estimated that approximately 290 988 individuals worked in governmental public health.[5] They used 6 data sources, focusing on various hierarchical levels, such as local, state, and federal workers.[5]

Although such synthetic enumerations are more pragmatic for characterizing large workforces, they are associated with their own issues.[1] In their enumeration report, Beck et al. recommended developing a "consensus-driven taxonomy of occupations and disciplines."[5(p7)] Other scholars have made similar recommendations, such as defining public health's scope of work.[6] Scholars also warned against Band-Aid solutions to address decades of neglect of public health systems research.[6,7] More recently, Leider et al. argued that public health needed to reach a consensus on how to define its workforce.[8]

The latest effort, Enumeration 2024,[9] sought to build on recommendations for addressing data challenges. We aimed to expand on previous enumerations by providing 3 distinct enumeration efforts: (1) total counts enumeration of the full governmental public health workforce; (2) occupation-specific enumeration; and (3) using novel data, analyses, and enumeration of public health nurses (PHNs).

METHODS

In our total counts enumeration, we sought to estimate the number of staff and full-time equivalents (FTEs) in the local, state, and federal governmental public health workforce.

Total Counts and Occupational Profile

Owing to the lack of direct, census-style data on this subject and the excessive burden required to collect such data, we performed a synthetic enumeration[1] by triangulating primary data sources. We took state central office, regional office, and occasionally local estimates from the Association of State and Territorial Health Officials (ASTHO) Profile 2022 census.[10] We used FEDSCOPE[11] to estimate federal workforce size. And we used data from the National Association of County and City Health Officials (NACCHO) Profile survey 2022[12] to identify local staffing and FTE levels.

The NACCHO data representing the staffing and FTEs of local health departments were incomplete. Therefore, we used multiple imputation by chained equations,[13,14] treating NACCHO Profile 2022 employees and FTEs as the data of interest. To assist the imputation algorithm in developing robust agency-level estimates, we incorporated previous NACCHO Profile data, population metrics by year,[12,15,16] 2017 and 2021 Public Health Workforce Interests and Needs fielding data,[17,18] state-level governance structure data, and a member check on staffing reports in 2021 and 2022 from 18 State Associations of County and City Health Officials (e-mail communications, February–April 2024). We ran the multiple imputation algorithm in R version 4.3.3 (RStudio, Boston, MA). We pooled the resulting set of imputed data sets, averaged them to develop a single agency-level estimate, and then aggregated the estimates by state.

Differences in state governance structures necessitated tailored approaches to developing state-level employee estimates.[19] Once we developed statewide estimates, we sought to model potential uncertainty in data reporting or data collection. We chose an error allowance of 20%, the reported value for each of the potential data sources. We conducted a nonparametric resampling strategy,[20] taking 10 000 draws for each reported value, with the sample distribution being a standard normal distribution with a mean equal to the reported value and SD equal to 20% of the reported value. We matched and aggregated the 10 000 draws for each source by state (according to the state calculation) to develop a set of 10 000 state-level estimates, which we subsequently aggregated into regional and national estimates. The 95% credible interval for each estimate represents the 2.5th to 97.5th percentile range of this set.

We drew occupational profiles of prominent public health occupation groups from ASTHO and NACCHO profiles, but for 2019 to 2021, as the 2022 editions of each were not available at the occupation level of detail at the time of our analyses. We examined 16 occupation groups based on available data and definitions used among these sources. For the NACCHO Profile, which had a 59% response rate,[12,18] we used survey weights, accounting for nonresponse to create census-level estimates for each occupation category. ASTHO has a complete response rate from their state health agencies, although item-based nonresponse does occur.[10]

Public Health Nursing

PHNs are the largest occupational group in the public health workforce and are thought to be the most likely to be "countable" through alternative sources of data (e.g., licensure data sets, surveys).[21] We chose to examine this important component of the workforce for the sake of better characterizing PHNs themselves and as a means to consider alternative sources of workforce data that reflect the governmental public health workforce. We examined data obtained from the National Council of State Boards of Nursing (NCSBN) 2022 National Nursing Workforce Survey of Registered Nurses. These data reflected 2846 de-identified nurse respondents from 45 states and included information regarding their demographics, work setting, and primary specialty area of practice.

We used the literature[22,23] and expert review to identify the NCSBN items that would most closely define PHNs working in governmental public health settings. Our process resulted in a decision tree, using PHN "primary setting" and "primary specialty" variables that grouped respondents into a "broad government PHN" group and a "restricted government PHN" group, based on the setting and specialty they indicated. The broad government PHN group included all respondents indicating that their work setting was public health, school health, or correctional health, as we determined that these were likely government settings.

We combined these settings with respondents indicating their work was primarily in 1 of the 19 specialties we identified in the data set that could arguably include public health nursing work (e.g., family health, pediatrics, adult health). We devised the restricted government PHN group as a more narrowly defined set of specialties in the NCSBN data that consisted of public health, community health, maternal and child health, school health, and infectious diseases. Based on the literature[22,23] and expert review, we considered these to be the specialties most closely aligned with population-focused public health nursing practice. Applying the population weights provided in the data set, we calculated the total number of nurses in each of the setting and specialty combinations as well as the total count in each of the 2 groups.

RESULTS

State, local, and federal public health workforce estimates revealed notable trends in overall staffing levels and occupational composition.

Total Counts and Occupational Profiles

State and local public health agencies grew to approximately 239 000 staff in 2022, on par with total staffing in 2008. However, after we adjusted for population growth, state and local staffing totals decreased in the intervening period. Data indicated that local and regional employees made up slightly more than 70% of the total nonfederal workforce in 2022, with state central office employees constituting the remaining 30%.

Our analysis of federal staffing data showed that up to 74 federal entities (departments and their subunits) performed some public health activities. With respect to the federal workforce, approximately 14 000 staff were employed by the Centers for Disease Control and Prevention or the Health Resources and Services Administration, excluding contractors. There are many additional federal agencies and subunits that perform public health functions or services to varying degrees or that have public health responsibilities. Depending on the extent that these entities are included in federal counts, there are between 2 and 74 federal entities employing 14 000 (2 agencies) and 237 000 (74 agencies) staff, excluding contractors.

The distribution of state and local public health departments varies by state and region (Figure 1; Figures A and B, available as a supplement to the online version of this article at http://www.ajph.org). Staff size largely aligns by size of population served, with swaths of the coasts and population centers in Texas, Florida, New York, and California having the largest number of employees associated with those geographies. State central office estimates have somewhat more variability than local estimates, after accounting for the population size served. The number of public health workers varied regionally from 59 per 100 000 population to 97 per 100 000. Per 100 000 population, the median was 62 and the mean was 151. In absolute terms, the estimated median local health departments staff size was 20 (mean = 66) across the United States. A quarter of local health departments had an estimated 12 or

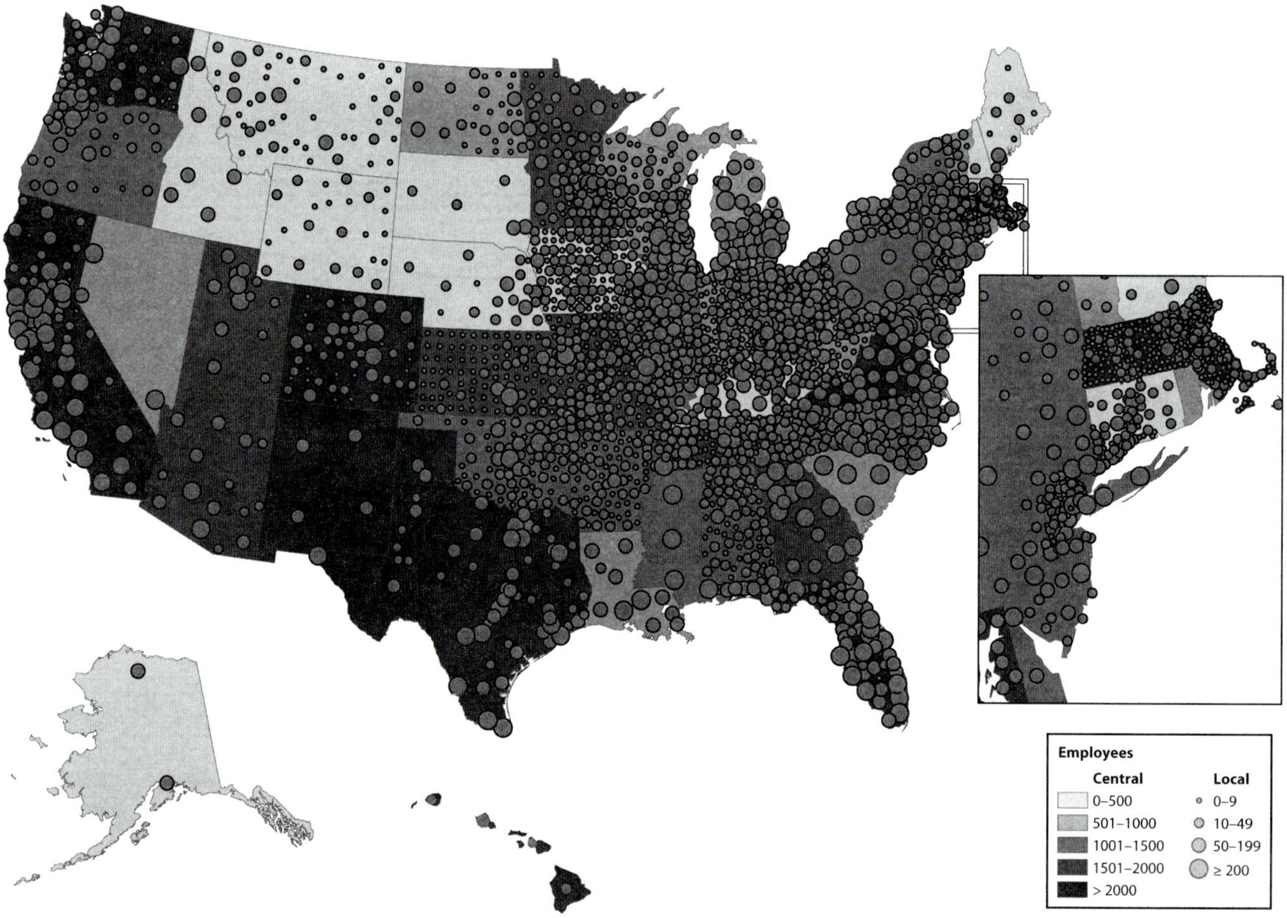

FIGURE 1— **Public Health Employees in State Central Offices Versus Local Offices: United States, 2022**

Note. Not pictured are US territories, freely associated states, and Tribal health organizations.

fewer staff and 11 or fewer FTEs. In absolute terms, the state health agency central office median was 1091, and the mean was 1328. A quarter of state health agency central offices had fewer than 470 staff, and a quarter had more than 1500.

Estimates of the state and local workforce in specific occupation groups can be found in Table 1. Among the occupation groups represented, the largest occupation groups included office and administrative support workers (37 576), public health or community health nurses (29 387), financial and operations business support workers (21 631), and environmental health workers (20 621). The smallest occupation groups were emergency preparedness and management workers (3468), information systems manager and information technology specialists (3009), oral health professionals (2551), public health physicians and other clinicians (2045), and public information specialists (616). Some occupations had larger total workforces at the state level (e.g., epidemiologists and statisticians, business support–financial and operations), whereas others had larger workforces at the local level (e.g., health educators, office and administrative support, environmental health workers).

Public Health Nursing

In our enumeration of the public health nursing workforce using NCSBN data and our 2 definitions of broad and restricted government PHNs, we found that 73 478 (1.8%) of the NCSBN's registered nurses fit our restricted government PHN definition out of the 4 047 872 registered nurses in NCSBN's weighted sample. Even when we expanded on this more narrowly defined set of restricted specialties most closely aligned with population-focused public health nursing practice and considered the broad government PHN definition, the broad government PHNs still made

TABLE 1— State and Local Full-Time Equivalent (FTE) Counts by Occupation Group: United States, 2022

Occupation Title	State FTEs (%)	Local FTEs (%)	Total FTEs
Office and administrative support	14 456 (38)	23 121 (62)	37 576
Public/community health nurse	8150 (28)	21 237 (72)	29 387
Business support—financial and operations	12 728 (59)	8 903 (41)	21 631
Environmental health worker	6 105 (30)	14 516 (70)	20 621
Behavioral health professional	9 033 (58)	6 669 (43)	15 702
Health educator	2 724 (27)	7 475 (73)	10 199
Agency leadership	1 668 (22)	5 792 (78)	7 460
Epidemiologists and statisticians	4 341 (60)	2 876 (40)	7 217
Nutritionist or dietitian	1 750 (25)	5 108 (75)	6 857
Laboratory workers	4 200 (67)	2 092 (33)	6 292
Community health worker	NA	5 564 (100)	5 564
Emergency preparedness/management worker	1 196 (34)	2 272 (66)	3 468
Information systems manager/information technology specialist	849 (28)	2 161 (72)	3 009
Oral health professional	347 (14)	2 203 (86)	2 551
Public health physicians and other clinicians	760 (37)	1 285 (63)	2 045
Public information specialist	NA	616 (100)	616

Note. NA = not available.

up only 147 957 (3.7%) of the total registered nurse workforce in this NCSBN data set. The preponderance of the PHNs in the restricted group indicated that they were working in a public health setting and described themselves as having a public health specialty (n = 35 678; 49%). The next largest segment of those in this restricted group were registered nurses who indicated that they worked in a school health setting and had a specialty in school health (n = 31 340; 43%).

Similar to the distributions we have described regarding our total counts and occupational profiles, our regional comparisons of PHNs using the NCSBN data demonstrated wide levels of variation by US Department of Health and Human Services region. This variation was especially apparent in the percentage of PHNs in the restricted government PHN group who indicated that they worked in public health settings and had a public health specialty versus those working in school health settings who had a school health specialty (Table 2).

TABLE 2— Percentage of Restricted Governmental Public Health Nurses by Health and Human Services Region, Overall and by Major Setting and Specialty: United States, 2022

US Department of Health and Human Services Region	% Restricted Governmental Public Health Nurses			
	Overall	Public Health Setting and Specialty	School Health Setting and Specialty	Other Settings and Specialties
1	1.6	0.7	0.7	0.2
2	2.6	0.6	1.9	0.1
3	1.7	0.8	0.6	0.3
4	1.5	0.7	0.6	0.1
5	1.6	0.9	0.6	0.1
6	1.7	0.5	1.0	0.2
7	1.9	0.9	0.8	0.3
8	2.1	1.2	0.6	0.3
9	2.2	1.7	0.5	0.1
10	1.6	1.0	0.4	0.2

DISCUSSION

Enumeration is essential if we are to gain an accurate understanding of the public health workforce. A count of public health workers facilitates knowledge of public health capacity and helps systems researchers understand trends and gaps in the workforce. This knowledge can then be translated into policy so that resources and funding can be triaged appropriately.

We estimated that there were approximately 239 000 state and local governmental public health workers as of 2022. In addition, approximately 14 000 individuals worked at the Centers for Disease Control and Prevention or the Health Resources and Services Administration. There are potentially hundreds of thousands more federal public health workers depending on which agencies are included in that count. The estimate of 239 000 is up from an estimated 206 500 in 2019. The 3-year increase amounted to 15.6%, placing staffing levels on par with pre-Great Recession numbers in 2008.[24]

Furthermore, the total count of 239 000 has increased since the 2012 enumeration,[5] but the increase is not enough to support the corresponding population increase during that time, let alone the rising needs of the population. The field is now approximately the same size it was before the onset of the Great Recession, which affected governmental workforces especially between 2010 and 2013.[24] Furthermore, our estimated total count is still less than half of the estimated 500 000 public health workers in 1980,[3] despite the vast increase in the US population in the past 40 years: in 1980, the US population was 226 545 805; in 2020, it had increased by 46% to 331 449 281.[25]

Although our estimates indicate that the public health field has gained workers in the past decade, a large proportion of workers are considering leaving the public health workforce in the near future, for retirement and other reasons.[26] Thus, attention to recruitment, onboarding, and retention must be ongoing, and generating related evidence regarding these practices should be a focus for public health systems researchers. More generally, it is worth noting that agencies were able to increase staffing before, during, and after the COVID-19 pandemic because of American Rescue Plan Act of 2021 funding (now expired) and the Public Health Infrastructure Grant program (a 1-time, 5-year award expiring in 2027); it is unclear whether monies from this program will be sustained.

It is important to note that this increase in staffing in state health agency central offices, alongside increases in staffing in local and regional health departments, was measured during the COVID-19 response and includes a substantial number of part-time or temporary workers. So although current staffing reflects an effort to fortify the nation's health defenses and amplify the public health system's capacity for service delivery and emergency readiness in the face of the COVID-19 pandemic, it is less clear whether these staffing levels will continue—and what the public health consequences of an again-reduced workforce might be.

The variation we identified in the distribution of the workforce suggests the need for a strategic and focused approach in policy development and resource allocation. As the population ages, changes, and migrates, the number of public health workers should be viewed not merely as a measure of potential capacity but also as a key performance indicator for future planning.

Our enumeration of occupation groups demonstrates the difference in size of each key public health occupation and the difference in their distribution between the state and local levels. In the PHN enumeration effort specifically, we found that PHNs made up less than 2% of the number of registered nurses in the country. Furthermore, about 90% of these PHNs work in either public health or school health.

It is worth highlighting the importance of a whole workforce enumeration when considering the needs of future governmental public health enterprises. The field is at an inflection point in a COVID-19 recovery environment: questions have shifted from how many staff do we have? to how many staff do we need? Before the COVID-19 pandemic, at least 80 000 additional staff were needed to ensure the delivery of the Foundational Public Health Services.[24] In a COVID-19 recovery environment, it is challenging to determine how many staff the field might need until we know how many we have.

In addition to the 14 000 federal and 240 000 state and local workforces, open questions remain about the Tribal and territorial workforces. These agencies often look different from state and local health departments, both in service mix and revenue streams. Available data suggest that at least 5600 staff work in territories and freely associated states as of 2022 (with missing data from 1 territory).[10] A Tribal workforce enumeration has not been conducted, but the most recently available information suggests that Tribes with Tribal Health Organizations have a median of 5 staff (mean = 13.4) working at agencies, with substantial variability in staffing totals.[27] To fully understand the US governmental public health workforce, robust data collection efforts should be supported across all settings—federal, state, local, Tribal, and territorial.

Limitations

Our enumeration is limited in certain aspects. The COVID-19 pandemic affected data collection, for example, response rates of the surveys used as our main data sources. The pandemic also resulted in fluctuating workforce numbers, as temporary workers were brought in to boost the response and then let go as funding streams ended.

We attempted to include contract workers in this enumeration, but we may have undercounted them if agencies underreported their contractual staff or, as in FEDSCOPE, contractors were excluded from available data. We also attempted to use licensure-related data from individual states to enumerate the number of PHNs, but we were able to obtain these data for only 4 states. Although we used FEDSCOPE data to count federal public health workers, there is no standardized definition of federal public health worker, so we created estimates of workers at various "tiers" of agencies ranked based on their relatedness to public health. Future enumeration work could more directly describe the US Public Health Service's workforce. These 6000 or more officers are represented in the federal analysis but could be described more precisely with other federal data.

Furthermore, the data we used were collected in 2021 and 2022; much has changed since they were collected. The occupation groups we identified were based on the definitions used by the available data sets. Occupation groups available in these data sets were not always defined in the same way, and occupations in public health are evolving, making estimates over time difficult to compare.

An additional major limitation of previous enumerations is that territorial and Tribal public health workers tend to not be counted.[9] This contributes to the "data genocide" and historical invisibility of Indigenous peoples.[28] There are 574 federally recognized Tribes in the United States, as well as many state-recognized Tribes in addition to unrecognized Tribal Nations. Furthermore, the public health work done in the US territories—American Samoa, Guam, the Commonwealth of the Northern Mariana Islands, Puerto Rico, and the US Virgin Islands—and freely associated states—the Federated States of Micronesia, the Republic of the Marshall Islands, and the Republic of Palau—is significant, and their workers need to be counted to give the discipline a more accurate understanding of the infrastructure in place.[4] Although we included estimates from the Tribes and territories from other sources, future enumerations would do well to more directly include these organizations in a common count.

Conclusions

This 2024 enumeration had the advantage of considering the recommendations of scholars who conducted previous enumerations,[4] and we continue to advocate similar recommendations. In particular, we call for more funding for reporting workforce numbers for public health agencies. Furthermore, we strongly advise that public health systems researchers adopt a standard taxonomy of public health workers, including a definition of what is considered public health work.

This enumeration serves as a baseline count of public health workers during the COVID-19 response. Part of this response involved focusing federal funding on public health infrastructure, including the workforce.[29] However, funding for these endeavors will expire in the near future, and there is no guarantee that additional funding will be authorized. Further enumeration in future years would enable comparisons to this baseline COVID-19 era estimate and facilitate the evaluation of whether recent funds allocated to the public health infrastructure contributed to stable or ongoing increases in public health staffing.

Evaluating the sufficiency of staffing and FTE growth is a separate matter from enumeration and requires consideration of the evolving and emerging demands on the public health system, the impact of domestic and global health challenges, and the specific needs of local and regional communities. Although the overall increase in workers is a positive step toward strengthening public health infrastructure, continuous assessment and strategic planning are essential with a goal to ensure that the public health system is resilient, responsive, and equipped to protect and promote the health of all communities against both current and future health threats.

Public Health Implications

As of 2022, the governmental public health workforce has returned to staffing levels last seen during the Great Recession. Approximately 240 000 staff are employed at the state and local levels—although a large proportion of new positions are temporary, term limited, or contractual. It is not clear whether increased staffing levels will remain as federal funds contract during COVID-19 recovery. AJPH

ABOUT THE AUTHORS

Jonathon P. Leider, Nicole M. Weiss, Abby Vogel, Sezen O. Onal, Xiao Zang, Harshada Karnik, Bibin Joseph, and Morgan Pak are with the Center for Public Health Systems, Division of Health Policy and Management, University of Minnesota School of Public Health, Minneapolis. Casey P. Balio and Nathan Dockery are with the Center for Rural Health Research, Department of Health Services Management and Policy, East Tennessee State University, Johnson City. Rachel Hogg-Graham is with the College of Public Health, University of Kentucky, Lexington. Paula Kett and Betty Bekemeier are with the Center for Health Workforce Studies, University of Washington, Seattle. Joyce Edmonds is with the Harvard T.H. Chan School of Public Health, Boston, MA. Amy Belflower Thomas is with the Public Health Accreditation Board, Alexandria, VA.

CORRESPONDENCE

Correspondence should be sent to Jonathon P. Leider, 420 Delaware St SE, Minneapolis, MN 55455 (e-mail: leider@umn.edu). Reprints can be ordered at https://www.ajph.org by clicking the "Reprints" link.

PUBLICATION INFORMATION

Full Citation: Leider JP, Balio CP, Hogg-Graham R, et al. Enumeration 2024: what we know and what we wish we knew about the governmental public health workforce in a COVID-19 recovery landscape. *Am J Public Health*. 2025;115(5):707–715.

Acceptance Date: November 21, 2024.

DOI: https://doi.org/10.2105/AJPH.2024.307960

ORCID iDs:

Jonathon P. Leider https://orcid.org/0000-0001-9905-476X

Casey P. Balio https://orcid.org/0000-0002-2987-4268

Rachel Hogg-Graham https://orcid.org/0000-0003-0555-4902

Nicole M. Weiss https://orcid.org/0000-0003-1704-3536

Abby Vogel https://orcid.org/0000-0001-5783-221X

Xiao Zang https://orcid.org/0000-0002-5722-8255

Paula Kett https://orcid.org/0000-0002-8524-6493

Harshada Karnik https://orcid.org/0000-0003-1687-8849

Nathan Dockery https://orcid.org/0009-0004-9398-9280

Bibin Joseph https://orcid.org/0009-0005-1506-8459

Morgan Pak https://orcid.org/0009-0004-0894-7503

Amy Belflower Thomas https://orcid.org/0009-0005-1871-9034

Betty Bekemeier https://orcid.org/0000-0002-9034-2746

CONTRIBUTORS

J. P. Leider, C. P. Balio, R. Hogg-Graham, N. M. Weiss, A. Vogel, P. Kett, N. Dockery, and B. Bekemeier analyzed the data and wrote the first draft of the article. S. O. Onal, X. Zang, J. Edmonds, H. Karnik, B. Joseph, M. Pak, and A. B. Thomas provided additional analytic support. All authors provided critical review.

ACKNOWLEDGMENTS

This work was supported by the Centers for Disease Control and Prevention (CDC), US Department of Health and Human Services (HHS), National Center for State, Tribal, Local, and Territorial Public Health Infrastructure and Workforce (grant OE22-2203: Strengthening US Public Health Infrastructure, Workforce, and Data Systems).

We obtained Public Health Workforce Interests and Needs data from the Public Health Workforce Interests and Needs Survey, a project supported through a collaboration of the ASTHO and the de Beaumont Foundation. Our use of the data does not imply ASTHO's or the de Beaumont Foundation's endorsement of the research, research methods, or conclusions contained in this article.

The authors thank the following data owners and contributors: the de Beaumont Foundation (Public Health Workforce Interests and Needs Survey), National Association of County and City Health Officials (NACCHO Profile), Association of State and Territorial Health Officials (ASTHO Profile), and the State Associations of County and City Health Officials and their members who participated in confirmation of their staffing levels. The authors also thank the Public Health Accreditation Board and the CDC for their partnership and the National Council of State Boards of Nursing for providing their data. The authors thank members of the Consortium for Workforce Research in Public Health for their feedback and guidance, including Heather Krasna, Beth Resnick, and Valerie Yeager.

Note. The contents of this article are those of the authors and do not necessarily represent the official views of, nor an endorsement by, the CDC, the HHS or the US government.

CONFLICTS OF INTEREST

The authors have no conflicts of interest to disclose.

HUMAN PARTICIPANT PROTECTION

No protocol approval was necessary because the project involved only a secondary data analysis of publicly available data.

REFERENCES

1. Merrill J, Btoush R, Gupta M, Gebbie K. A history of public health workforce enumeration. *J Public Health Manag Pract.* 2003;9(6):459–470. https://doi.org/10.1097/00124784-200311000-00005
2. Krasna H, Czabanowska K, Beck A, Cushman LF, Leider JP. Labour market competition for public health graduates in the United States: a comparison of workforce taxonomies with job postings before and during the COVID-19 pandemic. *Int J Health Plann Manage.* 2021;36(suppl 1):151–167. https://doi.org/10.1002/hpm.3128
3. US Department of Health, Education, and Welfare, Public Health Service. *A Report on Public and Community Health Personnel.* Washington, DC: Government Printing Office; 1980.
4. Gebbie KM. *The Public Health Workforce Enumeration 2000.* Washington, DC: US Department of Health and Human Services; 2000.
5. Beck AJ, Boulton ML, Coronado F. Enumeration of the governmental public health workforce, 2014. *Am J Prev Med.* 2014;47(5, suppl 3):S306–S313. https://doi.org/10.1016/j.amepre.2014.07.018
6. Tilson H, Gebbie KM. The public health workforce. *Annu Rev Public Health.* 2004;25:341–356. https://doi.org/10.1146/annurev.publhealth.25.102802.124357
7. Gebbie K, Merrill J, Sanders L, Gebbie EN, Chen DW. Public health workforce enumeration: beware the "quick fix." *J Public Health Manag Pract.* 2007;13(1):72–79. https://doi.org/10.1097/00124784-200701000-00012
8. Leider JP, Yeager VA, Kirkland C, Krasna H, Hare Bork R, Resnick B. The state of the US public health workforce: ongoing challenges and future directions. *Annu Rev Public Health.* 2023;44:323–341. https://doi.org/10.1146/annurev-publhealth-071421-032830
9. Leider JP, Balio CP, Hogg-Graham R, et al. *An Enumeration of the Public Health Workforce in 2024.* Available at: https://cworph.umn.edu/sites/cworph.umn.edu/files/2024-08/enumeration-2024.pdf. Accessed February 15, 2025.
10. Association of State and Territorial Health Officials. 2022 ASTHO profile dashboard. 2023. Available at: https://www.astho.shinyapps.io/profile. Accessed June 14, 2024.
11. US Office of Personnel Management. Federal workforce data. Available at: https://www.fedscope.opm.gov. Accessed June 25, 2024.
12. National Association of County and City Health Officials. National profile of local health departments. 2022. Available at: https://www.naccho.org/resources/lhd-research/national-profile-of-local-health-departments. Accessed February 15, 2025.
13. Rubin DB. Multiple imputation. In: van Buuren S. *Flexible Imputation of Missing Data.* 2nd ed. Boca Raton, FL: CRC Press; 2018. Available at: https://stefvanbuuren.name/fimd/ch-mi.html. Accessed February 17, 2025.
14. Azur MJ, Stuart EA, Frangakis C, Leaf PJ. Multiple imputation by chained equations: what is it and how does it work? *Int J Methods Psychiatr Res.* 2011;20(1):40–49. https://doi.org/10.1002/mpr.329
15. National Association of County and City Health Officials. *NACCHO National Profile of Local Health Departments.* 2019. Available at: https://www.naccho.org/uploads/downloadable-resources/Programs/Public-Health-Infrastructure/NACCHO_2019_Profile_final.pdf. Accessed February 15, 2025.

16. National Association of County and City Health Officials. *NACCHO National Profile of Local Health Departments*. 2016. Available at: https://www.naccho.org/uploads/downloadable-resources/ProfileReport_Aug2017_final.pdf. Accessed February 15, 2025.
17. de Beaumont Foundation. 2017 findings: key findings of PH WINS 2017. 2025. Available at: https://www.debeaumont.org/phwins/findings. Accessed February 15, 2025.
18. de Beaumont Foundation. 2021 Findings. 2025. Available at: https://www.debeaumont.org/phwins/2021-findings. Accessed February 15, 2025.
19. Vogel A, Onal SO, Zang X, et al. Enumerating the state and local public health workforce during the COVID-19 response. *Am J Public Health*. In press.
20. Hall P. Theoretical comparison of bootstrap confidence intervals. *Ann Stat*. 1988;16(3):927–953. https://doi.org/10.1214/aos/1176350933
21. Bekemeier B, Kett PM, Whitman G, Chadwick K, Edmonds JK. Distribution and Specialties of broadly versus narrowly defined public health nurses working in government settings in the United States, 2022. *Am J Public Health*. 2025; e1–e10. https://doi.org/10.2105/AJPH.2024.307950
22. Beck AJ, Coronado F, Boulton ML, Merrill JA. The public health workforce taxonomy: revisions and recommendations for implementation. *J Public Health Manag Pract*. 2018;24(5):E1–E11. https://doi.org/10.1097/PHH.0000000000000690
23. American Nurses Association. *Public Health Nursing: Scope and Standards of Practice*. 3rd ed. Silver Spring, MD: American Nurses Association; 2022.
24. Leider JP, McCullough JM, Singh SR, et al. Staffing up and sustaining the public health workforce. *J Public Health Manag Pract*. 2023;29(3):E100–E107. https://doi.org/10.1097/PHH.0000000000001614
25. US Census Bureau. Historical population change data (1910–2020). Available at: https://www.census.gov/data/tables/time-series/dec/popchange-data-text.html. Accessed May 30, 2024.
26. Weiss NM, Martin S, Onal SO, McDaniel N, Leider JP. Public health workforce survey data (2016–2021) related to employee turnover: proposed methods for harmonization and triangulation. *Front Public Health*. 2024;11:1306274. https://doi.org/10.3389/fpubh.2023.1306274
27. National Indian Health Board. Public Health Indian Country Capacity Survey (PHICCS) Project. Available at: https://www.nihb.org/public_health/proj_phiccs.php. Accessed July 22, 2024.
28. Urban Indian Health Institute. Data genocide of American Indians and Alaska Natives in COVID-19 data. Available at: https://www.uihi.org/projects/data-genocide-of-american-indians-and-alaska-natives-in-covid-19-data. Accessed May 28, 2024.
29. Centers for Disease Control and Prevention. Public health infrastructure grant. May 16, 2024. Available at: https://www.cdc.gov/infrastructure-phig/about/index.html. Accessed May 30, 2024.

Enumerating the State and Local Public Health Workforce During the COVID-19 Response

Abby Vogel, MS, Sezen O. Onal, PhD, Nicole M. Weiss, PhD, Xiao Zang, PhD, Morgan Pak, MPH, Bibin Joseph, MHA, MPH, and Jonathon P. Leider, PhD

See also Public Health Enumeration in 2024, pp. 698–715.

Objectives. To understand the landscape of the nonfederal governmental public health workforce and to identify replicable methods for future enumerations.

Methods. This enumeration of the state and local public health workforce was conducted from 2023 to 2024 and triangulated the National Association of County and City Health Officials (NACCHO) Profile 2022 and the Association of State and Territorial Health Officials (ASTHO) Profile 2022. We utilized Public Health Workforce Interests and Needs Survey (PH WINS) data from 2021 to assess demographic distributions across Department of Health and Human Services (HHS) regions in the United States.

Results. A total of 239 000 staff were employed in state and local health departments in 2022, a 2% increase since 2012. Sixteen states—including 6 in the Southeast—lost staff relative to population growth.

Conclusions. An uneven landscape of public health workforce density reflects chronic underinvestment in public health. The process of enumeration itself was also fraught with pitfalls and data limitations.

Public Health Implications. We recommend building on federal investments to develop dedicated funding streams for state and local public health. We also recommend amending federal efforts around enumeration to include governmental public health at all levels. (*Am J Public Health*. 2025;115(5): 716–725. https://doi.org/10.2105/AJPH.2024.307964)

AJPH May 2025, Vol. 115, No. 5

An accurate count of the public health workforce is essential for understanding the capacity of the governmental public health system, workforce trends, and policies needed to support public health infrastructure. However, governmental public health is not regularly enumerated by federal statistical agencies, with such cited reasons as lack of definition sets to capture all public health occupations and difficulty identifying public health agencies based on federal industry classifications.[1] Therefore, deriving total counts of employees is left to the field and occurs every 10 to 20 years. The infrequency of these cycles has proved challenging to a field facing transition and crises; in the decade after the Great Recession, state and local governmental public health is thought to have lost 15% to 20% of the workforce, which likely did not return by the onset of COVID-19.[2] During the COVID-19 pandemic, there was evidence of temporary increases in the workforce, though with substantial turnover.[3] Yet, without official estimates from the federal government or formal enumeration, this growth was not well-characterized.

Since 1964, the public health workforce has been counted via synthetic enumeration, which utilizes survey data of hundreds of agencies from multiple data sources to produce informed estimates.[4] Merrill et al. outlined the history of public health enumerations from 1923 through 2000, describing 19 unique enumerations during this period.[4] They described an approximately 10% reduction in the total governmental public health workforce (federal, state, and local) between 1980 and 2000,[4] from approximately 500 000[5] (representing 220 staff per

100 000 population) to roughly 448 254[6] (158 per 100 000), which, at the time, included many community health care workers in addition to other public health department employees. Merrill et al. discussed how the decrease might have been attributable to definitional changes in the public health worker taxonomy as well as actual decreases in the number of public health staff.[4]

In 2012, Beck et al. completed another synthetic enumeration of the public health workforce, which counted approximately 290 988 total public health workers (federal, state, and local), representing a further 35% reduction from 2000 levels.[7] Although changes in the definition of a public health worker partly explain this decrease, a real reduction in workforce numbers also contributed.[4,6] Beck et al. estimated the 2012 state and local workforce at 233 882 employees, or about 80% of the total workforce. They also emphasized several recommendations for future enumerations, such as adopting a "standardized methodology for continuously monitoring the size and composition of the public health workforce."[7(pS313)]

Other public health workforce researchers have provided recommendations to improve future enumerations. Tilson and Gebbie noted that defining the scope of work in public health was essential in conducting public health workforce research.[8] Gebbie et al. also cautioned against "quick fixes" to such research, which included relying on federal Bureau of Labor Statistics (BLS) data that are limited in their ability to properly characterize multidisciplinary fields like public health.[1] For example, historically, Standard Occupational Classification codes used by the BLS do not disaggregate the number of public health nurses from the group of registered nurses.[1] In 2023, Leider et al. called for an "overarching definition for workers across the collective public health workforce and a consensus-driven taxonomy of relevant occupations and disciplines."[3(p333)]

These recommendations provide a roadmap for navigating the challenges of public health enumeration. Building upon the foundations of prior enumerations, we updated the workforce enumeration ("Enumeration 2024") with a more comprehensive analysis of the number and distribution of public health workers a decade after the last enumeration of Beck et al.,[7] providing a methodology and baseline of comparison for future enumerations. This enumeration differs from previous workforce counts by including additional sources for triangulation, including Public Health Workforce Interests and Needs Survey (PH WINS) administrative fielding data and member reports from State Associations of County and City Health Officials (SACCHOs). We also used algorithmic missing data approaches to create more comprehensive estimates and credible intervals. In a parallel article in this issue (Leider et al., p. 707), we provide a full review of the enumeration of the public health workforce in 2022, including total counts, occupational profiles, and public health nursing workforce.[9] The current article outlines methods for and findings from the local and state total counts of Enumeration 2024.

METHODS

We estimated employee counts, including vacant positions, at the state and local levels using a synthetic enumeration approach. The synthetic enumeration of the state and local public health workforce was conducted by triangulating (cross-verifying data across disparate data sets[10]) two 2022 data sets: the National Association of County and City Health Officials (NACCHO) Profile 2022,[11] providing workforce information at the local agency level, and the Association of State and Territorial Health Officials (ASTHO) Profile 2022,[12] providing workforce information at the state agency level. Although every state provided employee estimates for state agencies via the ASTHO Profile, employee counts were only available for 37% of local agencies from the NACCHO Profile. To partially address the issue of missing data for the local public health workforce, we retrieved additional employee data for 2022 from 18 SACCHOs (e-mail communications, February–April 2024) and a small fielding of PH WINS[13] in 2022 that identified agency sizes. We interpolated these additional data with the NACCHO Profile 2022 responses, increasing the effective response rate for local agencies to 42%. For the remaining local agencies where employee and full-time equivalent (FTE) counts for 2022 were unavailable, we conducted multiple imputation by chained equations[14,15] using historical data as predictors, including the NACCHO Profile (employees and FTEs) in 2016 and 2019,[11,16,17] jurisdictional population within each local health agency in 2016, 2019, 2020, and 2022,[11,16,17] SACCHO reports (employees and FTEs) in 2021 (e-mail communications, February–April 2024), state-level governance information, and the PH WINS fielding data in 2017 and 2021.[13,18] We used predictive mean matching to impute all variables with missingness, and the algorithm conducted 20 imputations with 100 iterations for 2 imputation approaches representing 2 possible sequences for imputation.[9] We determined the number of imputations and iterations through a sensitivity analysis (see Methods Appendix, available as a supplement to the online version of this article at http://www.ajph.org), increasing these values until no significant improvement in convergence was observed. The resulting 40 sets of local workforce estimates (employee and FTE counts) were bootstrapped 1000 times, aggregated to the state sum, and averaged to serve as the "local imputed" estimate for each state.[19]

We then combined local imputed estimates for each state from the NACCHO Profile with state estimates from the ASTHO Profile. The ASTHO Profile had 3 data points of interest: state health agency central office counts, reported regional office counts, and reported local counts. To triangulate these data points into 1 state and local workforce estimate for each state, we analyzed each state's governance[20] and utilized 1 of 3 constructions to estimate total state and local staffing (see Methods Appendix for each state's construction). We aggregated state-level estimates into Department of Health and Human Services (HHS) region estimates where relevant. After developing state- and HHS region–wide estimates of total employee counts, we modeled 2 sources of uncertainty—that because of missingness and potential reporting error—and used them to develop reasonable 95% credible intervals (see Methods Appendix for more detail). For the following analysis, we allowed for a reporting error of up to 20%—the most conservative of our a priori identified reasonable error margins—as there were no empirical estimates of reporting uncertainty available. The sensitivity analysis in the Methods Appendix displays how different assumed uncertainty levels affected the 95% credible intervals.

To calculate the change in the public health workforce between 2019 and 2022, we used the same constructions of total state and local staffing using ASTHO Profile 2019 data and imputed local estimates for 2019 from the imputation process described in this section. We utilized PH WINS data from 2021[14] to estimate the distribution of demographic characteristics across HHS regions.

RESULTS

The total estimation of state and local governmental public health staff in 2022 was approximately 239 000 (95% credible interval = 227 963, 251 840), of which we estimated that 70% were embedded in local health departments. Staff were not evenly distributed across regions, as shown in Figure 1, which also shows that areas with fewer absolute staff tended to have more staff per capita. Regions 1, 7, 8, and 10 (which represent New England; IA, KS, MO, and NE; the Mountain West; and AK, ID, OR, and WA, respectively) had fewer than 15 000 total staff, but all had more than 84 staff per 100 000 population—that is, they had the smallest absolute workforces, but among the highest per capita workforces. This trend was observed in reverse as well: regions 4, 5, and 9, which comprise the Southeast (KY southeast to FL), the Midwest (MN east to OH), and the Southwest (CA, HI, NV, and AZ), all had large numbers of staff (especially region 4, which had almost 45 000 workers) but fewer than 72 workers per 100 000 population. However, region 6 (the South from LA to NM) had the fewest workers per 100 000: fewer than 60.

Sixty-two percent of states had a total workforce per 100 000 people served of between 50 and 100 (Figure 2). Although most states improved their staff-to-population ratio from 2019 to 2022, 16 states, mostly clustered in the South, lost staff relative to their population growth. Indiana and New Hampshire were unique in having lost staff relative to population between 2019 and 2022 and, in 2022, having fewer than 50 public health workers per 100 000, whereas Utah, Washington, and the District of Columbia all gained more than 25 staff per 100 000 in the prior 3 years and by 2022 had a density of more than 100 public health workers per 100 000.

The racial distribution of the workforce—broken out by HHS region in Table 1—was mostly consistent with each region's respective geography, with all regions except for regions 6 and 9 having majority-White workforces. Region 9, which comprised California, Hawaii, Nevada, and Arizona, had the largest proportions of Native Hawaiian/Other Pacific Islander, Asian, and Hispanic or Latino staff. Region 6 (the South from LA to NM) also had a large proportion of Hispanic or Latino staff. The largest proportion of Black or African American public health staff was in region 3 (the mid-Atlantic from WV to DE) and region 4 (the Southeast from KY to FL), consistent with the larger proportional population of Black or African American populations in the Mid-Atlantic and Southeast.[21] Regions 5, 7, and 8 (the Midwest, Plains States, and Mountain West) had the highest proportion of White staff. Region 5 also had the lowest proportion of Hispanic or Latino staff and region 8 (the Mountain West) had the fewest Black or African American staff.

Table 1 shows a minimal variation between HHS regions in the age distribution of the public health workforce. Of note is the fact that between 28.3%

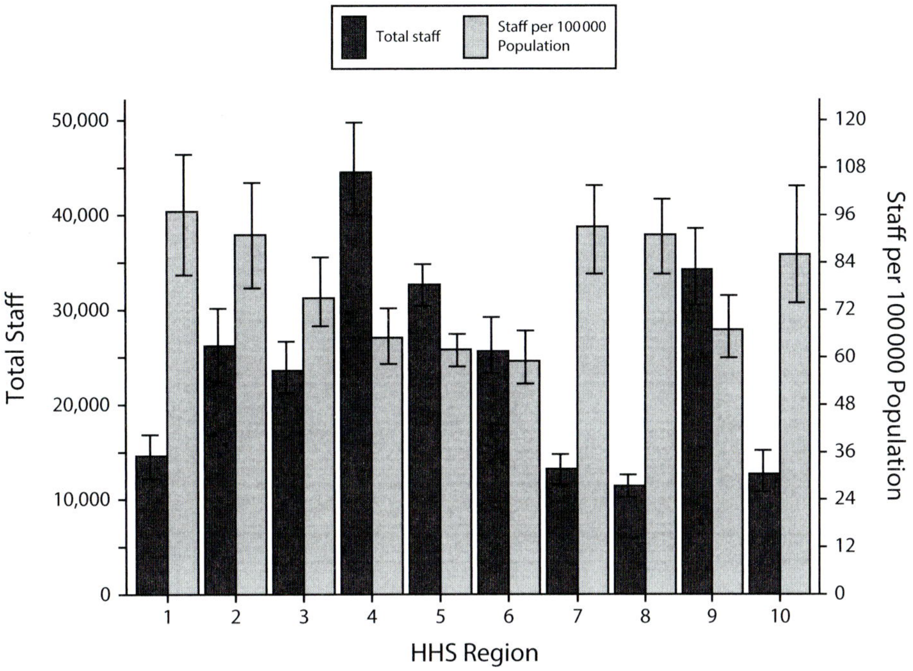

Region	Total Staff	Staff per 100000
1	14628	97
2	26228	91
3	23586	75
4	44521	65
5	32665	62
6	25648	59
7	13230	93
8	11444	91
9	34246	67
10	12698	86

FIGURE 1— Total State and Local Staff as Well as Staff per 100 000 Population by HHS Region: United States, 2022

Note. Only data from states and the District of Columbia are represented in the figure. Regions are defined by the Department of Health and Human Services (HHS).

(region 8) and 41.4% (region 3) of employees were older than 50 years.

The majority of the public health workforce across all 10 regions attained at least undergraduate degrees, as seen in Table 2. Undergraduate educational attainment (i.e., associate or bachelor's) ranged from 39.4% in region 1 to 53.2% in region 5. Between 26.4% (region 4) and 50.4% (region 1) held graduate degrees (i.e., master's or doctoral).

Public health job classifications are observed in Table 2 as well. The plurality of staff in all regions worked in public health sciences, although only a small proportion of staff were engaged in social services or other classifications. Compared with other measures, the distribution of job classifications had relatively little variation between regions.

Tables 1 and 2 are also displayed graphically in Figure A of the Appendix (available as a supplement to the online version of this article at http://www.ajph.org).

DISCUSSION

In conducting Enumeration 2024, the first look into the composition of a workforce responding to COVID-19 was made possible. Our estimates show a total of 239 000 public health employees at state and local agencies, a 15.7%

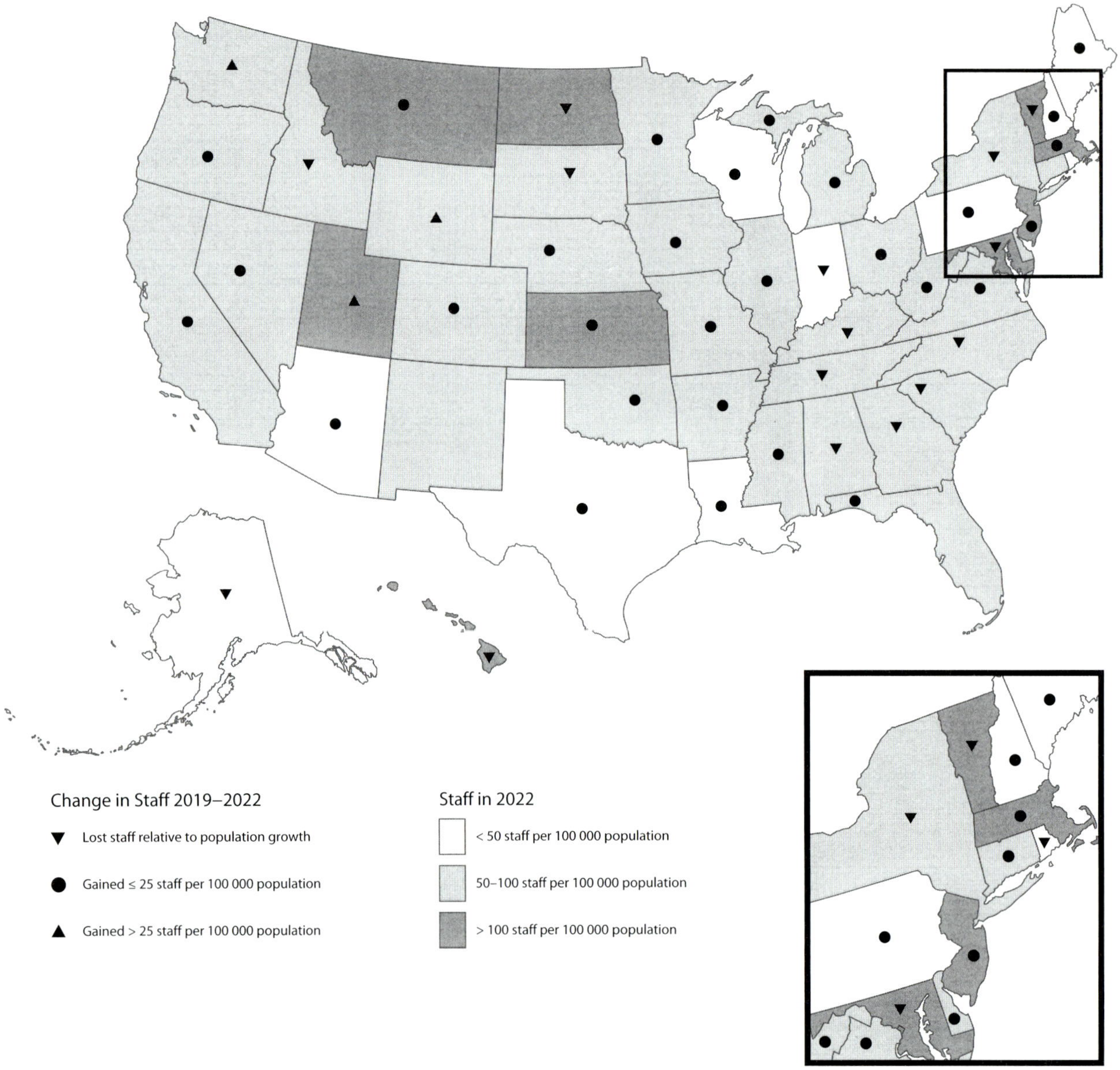

FIGURE 2— Public Health Workforce per 100 000 in 2022 and Change From 2019 Relative to Population Growth: United States

Note. No information regarding change in workforce since 2019 was available for New Mexico. Hawaii lost staff relative to population growth. The District of Columbia gained more than 25 per 100 000 population between 2019 and 2022 and had more than 100 staff per 100 000 population in 2022.

increase from 2019 (206 500).[3] Our estimates are comparable to those reported in the 2012 enumeration (roughly 234 000), although our approach and that undertaken in 2012 differed substantially, and the 2012 enumeration had not yet fully cataloged cuts associated with the Great Recession that saw the workforce fall to around 200 000.[7] However, although the growth over the past few years (from 2019 to 2022) is encouraging, overall this decade, the public health workforce increased by only about 2% despite the nation's population growing from about 309 million in 2010[22] to roughly 336 million in 2024 (an increase of almost 9%).[23] Thus, the public health workforce has failed to keep pace with the growth of the US population. This is particularly visible in the Southeast and Mountain West, where many states lost staff relative to population growth between 2019 and 2022.

Ratios of workers to population served varied across HHS regions, from 59 per 100 000 in region 6 to 97 per 100 000 in region 1, and 8 states had fewer than 50 workers per 100 000.

AJPH May 2025, Vol. 115, No. 5

TABLE 1— Distributions of Race/Ethnicity and Age of Public Health Workers by HHS Region: United States, 2021

	Region, %										
	1	2	3	4	5	6	7	8	9	10	National, %
Race/ethnicity											
American Indian or Alaska Native	0.7	0.9	0.9	0.7	0.6	1.9	1.4	1.1	0.8	1.2	0.9
Native Hawaiian or other Pacific Islander	0.2	0.1	0.4	0.2	0.1	0.2	0.2	0.4	1.2	0.4	7.4
Asian	4.8	11.3	5.6	2.4	3.4	4.0	2.5	2.9	20.2	6.8	15.3
Black or African American	17.3	20.0	25.8	23.3	11.1	18.2	6.2	2.0	7.5	4.6	18.0
Hispanic or Latino	14.4	12.9	10.2	17.1	7.2	30.0	11.0	12.0	33.7	13.6	0.4
White	59.5	50.2	53.1	51.5	74.9	41.2	75.2	78.1	31.0	69.6	53.7
≥ 2 races/ethnicities	3.1	4.7	4.0	4.8	2.8	4.4	3.5	3.6	5.5	3.9	4.3
Age, y											
< 31	16.2	10.7	13.6	12.8	15.3	12.0	14.8	14.9	12.3	14.3	13.3
31–40	23.1	24.8	22.4	19.5	25.3	24.3	24.4	29.3	26.2	27.6	24.0
41–50	25.6	24.9	22.5	24.4	24.9	25.6	23.7	27.6	26.9	25.7	25.1
51–60	23.1	27.2	25.6	28.5	22.6	25.5	23.9	19.9	24.1	21.5	25.0
≥ 61	12.0	12.4	15.8	14.8	11.9	12.6	13.2	8.4	10.5	10.9	12.6

Note. HHS = Department of Health and Human Services.
Source. Public Health Workforce Interests and Needs Survey (PH WINS) 2021.[13]

The geography of changes in the public health workforce merits further investigation, particularly as it relates to workforce and health policy differences between states. Public health worker demographics show that between 28.3% and 41.4% of employees were older than 50 years. This is notable because of the looming retirements of many in the Baby Boomer generation[24] as well as the low rates of recent public health graduates choosing to work in governmental public health agencies.[25] Individuals who identified as White constituted the majority of the workforce in all HHS regions except for regions 6 and 9, underscoring the necessity of efforts and funding dedicated to diversifying the workforce to reflect the changing racial makeup of the general population.[26,27] And regional educational attainment disparities may have impacts on the types of services that the public health workforce can provide.

This study affirms a major finding of past enumerations: incomplete data collected at different times by different organizations make it challenging and expensive to develop a clear picture of the workforce. Unlike staff in other fields, industries, and sectors, those in governmental public health are simply not counted by federal statistical agencies. Despite some work to modernize and include more public health occupation codes in federal lists, current federal occupation indices do not adequately capture the workforce[28]; that task falls to membership organizations, foundations, and academia, and thus is an imperfect solution to answering a critical, basic question: How many people work in public health? Only once we have answered this first question can the next question follow: How many more do we need?

TABLE 2— Distributions of Degree Attainment and Job Classification of Public Health Workers by HHS Region: United States, 2021

	Region, %										
	1	2	3	4	5	6	7	8	9	10	National, %
Highest degree											
No college degree	10.2	9.5	14.3	21.6	11.2	19.1	16.9	9.8	13.0	12.6	14.8
Associate	7.5	8.8	11.7	16.7	11.5	12.4	9.4	8.5	9.3	8.7	11.5
Bachelor's	32.0	34.3	36.7	35.3	41.7	35.6	41.4	41.2	38.2	37.2	37.2
Master's	43.3	38.1	30.4	22.6	32.0	27.8	28.5	35.7	31.4	34.8	30.6
Doctoral	7.0	9.3	6.9	3.8	3.7	5.1	3.8	4.8	8.1	6.7	5.9
Job classification											
Administrative	25.8	28.5	26.1	31.6	22.7	32.1	29.7	25.2	29.0	28.1	28.3
Clinical and lab	18.2	24.1	28.5	28.1	30.3	24.1	19.5	21.5	28.6	19.6	26.2
Public health sciences	54.5	45.2	44.3	36.7	44.4	40.3	44.6	52.6	40.2	51.3	42.9
Social services and all others	1.4	2.1	1.2	3.6	2.6	3.4	6.2	0.7	2.1	1.0	2.6

Note. HHS = Department of Health and Human Services.
Source. Public Health Workforce Interests and Needs Survey (PH WINS) 2021.[13]

Questions about how to grow the workforce sustainably are manifold in the field. A recent study from the Office of the Assistant Secretary for Planning and Evaluation (ASPE) and Mathematica finds similar challenges in scoping and scaling the workforce.[29] They offer a host of recommendations, including building pathways, leveraging nongovernmental partnerships, and explicitly planning surging strategies. Such surging strategies necessitate a larger initial base, or foundation, of the public health workforce in order to be able to surge when necessary.[3] One of the major challenges observed during COVID-19 was that response was performed sometimes to the exclusion of standard public health activities, even mandated ones.[30] This reality was born of an undersized workforce, though how undersized is difficult to know.[3]

We echo previous enumeration researchers who called for more funding and training on reporting public health agency workforce numbers. We also advocate for reaching a consensus as a field as to how to define a public health worker, including a potential tiered taxonomy of what is classified as such. This taxonomy must be adopted and utilized across the discipline. Furthermore, we recommend amending federal efforts around occupation- and industry-based enumeration to more explicitly include governmental public health at all levels. Mandating that enumerations be conducted by a federal agency should improve the consistency, coherence, and replicability of estimates over time, as well as provide more regular snapshots of the workforce.

Limitations

Although we were able to take many lessons from scholars who conducted prior enumerations, we were not able to incorporate all recommendations. For example, there remains debate on how to define public health workers, and lack of a universally accepted definition of a "public health worker" may have influenced who was reported, and thus counted, as working in public health. Furthermore, much of the data used in this work were collected during COVID-19. Because health agencies were triaging services at this time, it is possible that data are not as comprehensive or accurate as in other, nonpandemic years.

Our findings describe the public health workforce at the time the data were collected in 2022. This was at the beginning of the rollout for Centers for Disease Control and Prevention (CDC) funding for pandemic response. There is no guarantee that funding will be renewed by the government after it expires in some years. It is also unknown how the expiration of funding will affect workforce numbers into the future, and research endeavors over the next few years should explore this question.

There were a number of assumptions that had to be made to enable the development of the total counts estimates and the credible intervals, including decisions around the imputation algorithm, the triangulation of multiple data sources into statewide estimates, and the estimation of reporting error. Regarding multiple imputation, we must assume that data are missing at random—that is, that any patterns or underlying reasons for missing data are explained by other data elements present in the data set—which is an inherently unverifiable assumption.[31] To use predictive mean matching in our multiple imputation process, we must assume that the distribution of the missing data are the same as that of the observed data. Additionally, predictive mean matching cannot create estimates beyond the range of the observed data, which may cause bias.[32]

Lastly, public health staff serving in Tribes, Territories, and Freely Associated States were not included in this enumeration because of a lack of current and available data accessible to the Enumeration 2024 team. Future enumeration work should seek to incorporate data from these communities to more accurately reflect the state and local public health environment in every part of the United States. This article also did not include analysis of the federal public health workforce (e.g., the Commissioned Corps of the US Public Health Service, the CDC, and other related agencies), although they were counted as part of Enumeration 2024.[9]

Policy Implications

The state and local public health workforce, which provides the majority of public health services in the United States, increased only by about 2% in the last decade (from approximately 234 000[7] to approximately 239 000), despite the nation growing in population by nearly 9%. Sixteen states, including 6 in the Southeast, lost staff relative to their population growth between 2019 and 2022, and 8 states around the nation have fewer than 50 public health workers per 100 000 population.

This reality reflects the persistent environment of underinvestment and understaffing of state and local governmental public health. Although there have been substantive one-time investments in governmental public health by the federal government since the data collection for this enumeration,[33] we do not anticipate such efforts alone to be enough. Adding to the concern is the fact that the majority of public health workers in all regions are older than 40 years and that the workforce pipeline for governmental public health is inconsistent at best.[34] At this critical moment, when the COVID-19 pandemic is fresh in the minds of the citizenry and lawmakers, the nation, states, and localities should pursue dedicated funding streams to reinvest in governmental public health. Additionally, the federal government should invest in long-term efforts to develop a coherent and consistent method for enumerating the public health workforce at regular intervals. This has benefited other fields, and is of substantial importance to understanding the current state of governmental public health needs.[1]

This will likely prove to be challenging, however, as the current enumeration was funded by COVID-19 response allocations in the form of the Public Health Infrastructure Grant (PHIG). PHIG is unlikely to be renewed with the ending of the public health emergency.[33] Furthermore, even if funding were consistently allocated to public health enumeration efforts, systemic training in workforce data reporting would be needed across local health departments and state health agencies to ensure accurate counts and comparability of successive enumerations. Ideally, enumeration would be tasked to 1 federal agency—or potentially to the Public Health Accreditation Board as part of the accreditation process or as a component of evaluating agency performance—so that transfer of knowledge could be facilitated. Although challenging, these barriers must be addressed if future attempts at disinvestment of public health are to be anticipated and averted. AJPH

ABOUT THE AUTHORS

At the time of this study, all authors were with the Center for Public Health Systems, Division of Health Policy and Management, University of Minnesota School of Public Health, Minneapolis.

CORRESPONDENCE

Correspondence should be sent to Abby Vogel, D305 Mayo Bldg, 420 Delaware St SE, Minneapolis, MN 55455 (e-mail: abbymvogel97@gmail.com). Reprints can be ordered at https://www.ajph.org by clicking the "Reprints" link.

PUBLICATION INFORMATION

Full Citation: Vogel A, Onal SO, Weiss NM, et al. Enumerating the state and local public health workforce during the COVID-19 response. *Am J Public Health*. 2025;115(5):716–725.

Acceptance Date: November 26, 2024.

DOI: https://doi.org/10.2105/AJPH.2024.307964

ORCID iDs:

Abby Vogel https://orcid.org/0000-0001-5783-221X

Nicole M. Weiss https://orcid.org/0000-0003-1704-3536

Morgan Pak https://orcid.org/0009-0004-0894-7503

Bibin Joseph https://orcid.org/0009-0005-1506-8459

CONTRIBUTORS

A. Vogel, X. Zang, S. O. Onal, and J. P. Leider developed methods and analyzed data. N. M. Weiss, J. P. Leider, and A. Vogel completed first drafting. B. Joseph and M. Pak assisted with analytic development and visualization. All authors performed critical review.

ACKNOWLEDGMENTS

This work is supported by funds made available from the Centers for Disease Control and Prevention (CDC) of the US Dept of Health and Human Services (HHS), National Center for State, Tribal, Local, and Territorial Public Health Infrastructure and Workforce, through OE22-2203: Strengthening US Public Health Infrastructure, Workforce, and Data Systems grant.

PH WINS data from this study were obtained from the Public Health Workforce Interests and Needs Survey, a project supported through a collaboration of the Association of State and Territorial Health Officials (ASTHO) and the de Beaumont Foundation. The use of the data does not imply ASTHO's or the de Beaumont Foundation's endorsement of the research, research methods, or conclusions contained in this report.

We thank data owners and contributors: the de Beaumont Foundation (PH WINS), NACCHO (NACCHO Profile), ASTHO (ASTHO Profile), and especially the State Associations of County and City Health Officials and their members that participated in confirmation of their staffing levels. We thank the Public Health Accreditation Board and the CDC for their partnership. We also thank members of the Consortium for Workforce Research in Public Health for their feedback and guidance, including Heather Krasna, Beth Resnick, and Valerie Yeager.

Note. The contents are those of the authors and do not necessarily represent the official views of, nor an endorsement by, CDC/HHS, the US Government, or Public Health Accreditation Board.

CONFLICTS OF INTEREST

The authors have no conflicts of interest to disclose.

HUMAN PARTICIPANT PROTECTION

The project involved secondary data analysis of publicly available data.

REFERENCES

1. Gebbie K, Merrill J, Sanders L, Gebbie EN, Chen DW. Public health workforce enumeration: beware the "quick fix." *J Public Health Manag Pract.* 2007;13(1):72–79. https://doi.org/10.1097/00124784-200701000-00012
2. Leider JP, McCullough JM, Singh SR, et al. Staffing up and sustaining the public health workforce. *J Public Health Manag Pract.* 2023;29(3):E100–E107. https://doi.org/10.1097/PHH.0000000000001614
3. Leider JP, Yeager VA, Kirkland C, Krasna H, Bork RH, Resnick B. The state of the US public health workforce: ongoing challenges and future directions. *Annu Rev Public Health.* 2023;44:323–341. https://doi.org/10.1146/annurev-publhealth-071421-032830
4. Merrill J, Btoush R, Gupta M, Gebbie K. A history of public health workforce enumeration. *J Public Health Manag Pract.* 2003;9(6):459–470. https://doi.org/10.1097/00124784-200311000-00005
5. US Dept of Health, Education, and Welfare. A report on public and community health personnel. 1979. Available at: https://hdl.handle.net/2027/uc1.c3304068?urlappend=%3Bseq=3. Accessed October 29, 2024.
6. Gebbie KM. *The Public Health Work Force: Enumeration 2000.* Washington, DC: US Dept of Health and Human Services, Health Resources and Services Administration, Bureau of Health Professions, National Center for Health Workforce Information and Analysis; 2000.
7. Beck AJ, Boulton ML, Coronado F. Enumeration of the governmental public health workforce, 2014. *Am J Prev Med.* 2014;47(5):S306–S313. https://doi.org/10.1016/j.amepre.2014.07.018
8. Tilson H, Gebbie KM. The public health workforce. *Annu Rev Public Health.* 2004;25(1):341–356. https://doi.org/10.1146/annurev.publhealth.25.102802.124357
9. Leider JP, Balio CP, Hogg-Graham R, et al. An enumeration of the public health workforce in 2024. Consortium for Workforce Research in Public Health. 2024. Available at: https://cworph.umn.edu/sites/cworph.umn.edu/files/2024-08/enumeration-2024.pdf. Accessed October 29, 2024.
10. Weiss NM, Martin S, Onal SO, McDaniel N, Leider JP. Public health workforce survey data (2016–2021) related to employee turnover: proposed methods for harmonization and triangulation. *Front Public Health.* 2024;11:1306274. https://doi.org/10.3389/fpubh.2023.1306274
11. National Association of County & City Health Officials. 2022 National Profile of Local Health Departments. 2023. Available at: https://www.naccho.org/uploads/downloadable-resources/NACCHO_2022_Profile_Report.pdf. Accessed October 29, 2024.
12. Association of State and Territorial Health Officials. ASTHO Profile of State and Territorial Public Health, Volume 6. 2023. Available at: https://astho.shinyapps.io/profile. Accessed October 29, 2024.
13. de Beaumont Foundation. 2021 Public Health Workforce Interests and Needs Survey. 2021 findings. Available at: https://debeaumont.org/phwins/2021-findings. Accessed October 29, 2024.
14. Azur MJ, Stuart EA, Frangakis C, Leaf PJ. Multiple imputation by chained equations: what is it and how does it work? *Int J Methods Psychiatr Res.* 2011;20(1):40–49. https://doi.org/10.1002/mpr.329
15. Rubin D. Multiple Imputation. In: van Buuren S, ed. *Flexible Imputation of Missing Data.* 2nd ed. New York, NY: Chapman and Hall/CRC; 2018: 27–61.
16. National Association of County & City Health Officials. 2019 National Profile of Local Health Departments. 2020. Available at: https://www.naccho.org/uploads/downloadable-resources/Programs/Public-Health-Infrastructure/NACCHO_2019_Profile_final.pdf. Accessed January 16, 2024.
17. National Association of County & City Health Officials. 2016 NACCHO National Profile of Local Health Departments. 2017. Available at: https://www.naccho.org/uploads/downloadable-resources/ProfileReport_Aug2017_final.pdf. Accessed October 29, 2024.
18. de Beaumont Foundation. 2017 Public Health Workforce Interests and Needs Survey. 2017 key findings. Available at: https://debeaumont.org/phwins/findings. Accessed October 29, 2024.
19. Hall P. Theoretical comparison of bootstrap confidence intervals. *Ann Stat.* 1988;16(3):927–953. https://doi.org/10.1214/aos/1176350933
20. Meit M, Sellers K, Kronstadt J, et al. Governance typology: a consensus classification of state-local health department relationships. *J Public Health Manag Pract.* 2012;18(6):520–528. https://doi.org/10.1097/PHH.0b013e31825ce90b
21. US Census Bureau QuickFacts. United States. Available at: https://www.census.gov/quickfacts/geo/chart/US/RHI225223. Accessed October 29, 2024.
22. US Census Bureau. National population by characteristics: 2010–2019. Available at: https://www.census.gov/data/tables/time-series/demo/popest/2010s-national-detail.html. Accessed October 29, 2024.
23. US Census Bureau. US population on Jan. 1, 2024. Available at: https://www.census.gov/library/stories/2023/12/happy-new-year-2024.html. Accessed October 29, 2024.
24. Leider JP, Coronado F, Beck AJ, Harper E. Reconciling supply and demand for state and local

public health staff in an era of retiring baby boomers. *Am J Prev Med.* 2018;54(3):334–340. https://doi.org/10.1016/j.amepre.2017.10.026

25. Barna M. More public health grads being drawn to private sector jobs. *Nations Health.* 2019;49(6): 1–12.
26. Coronado F, Beck AJ, Shah G, Young JL, Sellers K, Leider JP. Understanding the dynamics of diversity in the public health workforce. *J Public Health Manag Pract.* 2020;26(4):389–392. https://doi.org/10.1097/PHH.0000000000001075
27. Bogaert K, Castrucci BC, Gould E, Sellers K, Leider JP. Changes in the state governmental public health workforce: demographics and perceptions, 2014–2017. *J Public Health Manag Pract.* 2019;25(suppl 2):S58–S66. https://doi.org/10.1097/PHH.0000000000000933
28. Krasna H, Czabanowska K, Beck A, Cushman LF, Leider JP. Labour market competition for public health graduates in the United States: a comparison of workforce taxonomies with job postings before and during the COVID-19 pandemic. *Int J Health Plann Manage.* 2021;36(suppl 1):151–167. https://doi.org/10.1002/hpm.3128
29. Lee KM, Bosold A, Alvarez C, Dada OO, Porterfield DS. Experiences and lessons learned from surging the governmental public health workforce during the COVID-19 pandemic. *J Public Health Manag Pract.* 2025;31(2):283–290. https://doi.org/10.1097/PHH.0000000000002051
30. Yeager VA, Madsen ER, Schaffer K. Qualitative insights from governmental public health employees about experiences serving during the COVID-19 pandemic, PH WINS 2021. *J Public Health Manag Pract.* 2023;29(suppl 1):S73–S86. https://doi.org/10.1097/PHH.0000000000001644
31. Donders ART, van der Heijden GJMG, Stijnen T, Moons KGM. Review: a gentle introduction to imputation of missing values. *J Clin Epidemiol.* 2006;59(10):1087–1091. https://doi.org/10.1016/j.jclinepi.2006.01.014
32. Kleinke K. Multiple imputation under violated distributional assumptions: a systematic evaluation of the assumed robustness of predictive mean matching. *J Educ Behav Stat.* 2017;42(4):371–404. https://doi.org/10.3102/1076998616687084
33. Centers for Disease Control and Prevention. Public Health Infrastructure Grant Program. December 15, 2023. Available at: https://www.cdc.gov/infrastructure/index.html. Accessed March 22, 2024.
34. Krasna H, Fried L. Generation public health: fixing the broken bridge between public health education and the governmental workforce. *Am J Public Health.* 2021;111(8):1413–1417. https://doi.org/10.2105/AJPH.2021.306317

Developing Indigenous-Centered Healing, Health, and Wellness Frameworks to Strengthen Indigenous Health Systems, Decolonize Public Health, and Achieve Health Equity

Christina E. Oré, DrPH, MPH, Em Loerzel, PhD, MSW, Erin Marziale, MPH, and Myra Parker, JD, PhD, MPH

See also Jernigan and Maudrie, p. 643.

AJPH May 2025, Vol. 115, No. 5

Over the past 20 years, national and global health initiatives have increasingly used resources, implemented tools, and proposed policies to change the social determinants of health contributing to health inequities. The World Health Organization and the US Centers for Disease Prevention and Control have applied their evidence-based frameworks to these efforts.

Yet, for tribal nations and Indigenous communities in the United States, these frameworks' relevance and applicability are limited. The disproportionate impact of the COVID-19 pandemic (e.g., incidence and mortality rates) highlighted Indigenous epistemologies and realities (e.g., tribal sovereignty, strained state–tribal health systems) that were either missing or did not conceptually fit in these social determinants of health frameworks.

We describe findings from the 2018 to 2024 Indigenous Social Determinants of Health Project completed by Seven Directions, an Indigenous public health institute. We propose constructs for Indigenous healing, health, and wellness frameworks developed by and for tribal nations and Indigenous communities. Practitioners and policymakers may use these tailored frameworks in collaboration across sectors (e.g., public health, social services, behavioral health) to align systems for transformational change, decolonize public health, and achieve health equity. (*Am J Public Health*. 2025;115(5):726–731. https://doi.org/10.2105/AJPH.2024.307958)

"As long as you remember what you have seen, then nothing is gone.

As long as you remember, it is part of this story we have together."

—Leslie Marmon Silko, Ceremony, 1978

Tribal nations and Indigenous communities (i.e., American Indian and Alaska Native [AIAN] peoples) in the United States have long viewed human existence and the environment as sharing essential connections with spiritual, physical, and mental wellness. In Indigenous peoples' epistemologies and sciences, humans and the physical world are one and the same; and wellness relies on the natural environment. This philosophy is passed from generation to generation.[1] Yet, AIAN peoples' epistemologies do not regularly inform US public health or equity research and policymaking,[2] although there were increasing acknowledgment and calls for inclusion under the Biden presidential administration (2021–2025).[3] This shortcoming is problematic, considering the persistence of health inequities associated with social determinants of health

(SDOH), which were exacerbated during the COVID-19 pandemic in tribal nations and Indigenous communities.[4]

Achieving AIAN health equity requires meaningful reflection and action from national, state, tribal, and urban public health rights holders, collaborators, and decision-makers.[2,5] We share findings from the Indigenous Social Determinants Project, which was completed by Seven Directions, an Indigenous public health institute at the University of Washington. Its aim was to propose shared constructs to develop Indigenous frameworks for healing, health, and wellness by and for tribal nations and Indigenous communities. Health practitioners and policymakers may use these tailored Indigenous frameworks across sectors to strengthen Indigenous health and health-related systems, decolonize public health, and achieve health equity.

The Indigenous Social Determinants of Health Project, funded by the National Network for Public Health Institutes through a US Centers for Disease Control and Prevention (CDC) cooperative agreement, was launched before the COVID-19 pandemic and has subsequently evolved. The Seven Directions approach to accomplishing the aims of the project was value based, iterative, and participatory. The aims were accomplished in 3 phases: (1) conducting a scoping review and critique of SDOH frameworks (2018–2021); (2) listening and learning at advisory board, community of practice, and community meetings (2021–2023); and (3) developing a 6-module training pilot to test and launch an Indigenous SDOH website (2023–2024). The findings we share in this essay reflect the scoping review findings, advisory board reflections, and peer–peer feedback given during 2 sessions (March 2022 and April 2023) of Gathering Grounds, an Indigenous public health community of practices hosted by Seven Directions.

FRAMEWORKS CRITIQUE

We describe and critique existing SDOH frameworks as they apply to describing health and equity in tribal nations and Indigenous communities. Health inequities stem from policies and systems (e.g., social structure, environment, economy, health) that do not fairly distribute or provide access to resources in support of individual- and population-level health and wellness.[5,6] They are perpetuated by power imbalances and seeming lack of political will to ensure systemic changes for equity.[5,7] There are 2 standard SDOH frameworks—those of the World Health Organization (WHO) and the US Centers for Disease Control and Prevention (CDC)—which were developed to understand the drivers of health inequities.[8,9]

The SDOH framework of the WHO identifies structural and intermediate determinants that create conditions for inequitable health outcomes, as shown in Figure 1.[8] This framework's conceptual foundation is that social circumstances (e.g., social status, cohesion) and context (e.g., governance, policies, culture, and societal values) determine the health outcomes of individuals.[8] The identified social determinants and their pathway have equal, if not greater, impact on individual and population health than do individual genetics, health behavior, and the health care delivery systems.[8]

The CDC provides a definition of SDOH as conditions in which individuals live, learn, work, and play that influence a wide range of health outcomes.[9] They propose that 5 domains contribute to creating the conditions that define SDOH:

1. economic stability,
2. education access and quality,
3. health care access and quality,
4. neighborhood and built environments, and
5. social and community contexts.[9]

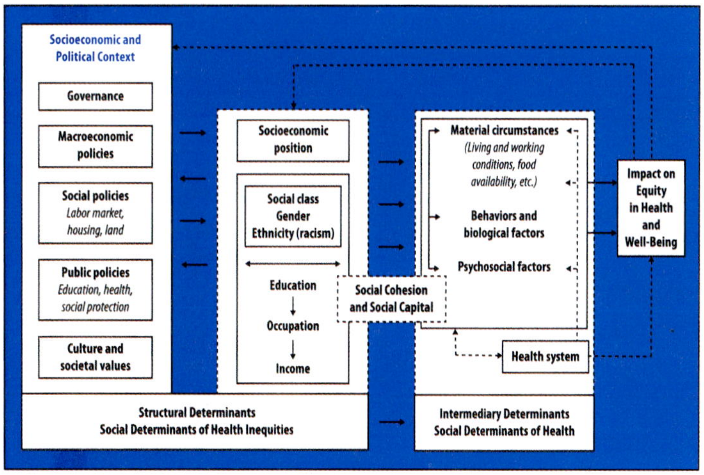

FIGURE 1— World Health Organization Commission on Social Determinants of Health Conceptual Framework for Social Determinants of Health; 2010

Source. Permission was granted to reproduce this diagram as it was originally published by the World Health Organization (WHO; 2010) on page 6 in A Conceptual Framework for Action on the Social Determinants of Health.

The conceptual foundation of this framework, based on the SDOH framework of the WHO, is that achieving improved health outcomes and equity is accomplished by using the evidence-based indicators in each domain.[9] It is an applied framework that uses Healthy People 2030 to fulfill the functions of public health: assessment, assurance, and program and policy development.[10,11] The SDOH frameworks of the WHO and the CDC contain broad social (e.g., systemic racism, housing policies) and intermediate (e.g., living and working conditions, access to quality care) determinants of health that affect tribal nations and Indigenous community health outcomes but are limited in their relevance and applicability.[8,9,12]

The disproportionate impact of the COVID-19 pandemic highlighted the need to address SDOH[4,13] and the limitations in the SDOH frameworks of the WHO and the United States. The frameworks do not consider cultural and contextual determinants such as health belief models, epistemologies, and ways of being and doing associated with healing, health, and wellness in and across tribal nations and Indigenous communities. The SDOH frameworks of the WHO and the CDC conceptually imply a linear, deterministic path to health that is individualistic rather than collective.

For more than 10 years, Indigenous scholars and global health entities have critiqued existing SDOH frameworks and raised awareness of the need to describe and map Indigenous determinants of health.[14,15] Commissioned reports described the SDOH framework of the WHO as prescriptive and unable to include the nuance and complexity of Indigenous social, political, and health realties.[15,16] There are 574 federally recognized tribal nations in the United States as well as many state and unrecognized tribes. Tribal nations and Indigenous communities have diverse histories, cultures, and traditions and unique political status and relationships with the federal government.[17] Standardizing an Indigenous SDOH (IsDOH) framework would reduce the complexity and diversity among tribal nations, and specificity ensures the relevance and applicability of the frameworks. With this confirmation, Seven Directions began to identify shared constructs that might guide tribal nations and Indigenous communities in developing their own frameworks.

ENSURING RELEVANCE

From a shared understanding of the limitations of the standard SDOH frameworks of the WHO and the CDC, the Seven Directions' team responded to calls by scholars and practitioners to go beyond social determinants and reclaim Indigenous health by identifying shared constructs of Indigenous healing, health, and wellness.[15,16]

Shared determinants of health that go beyond social determinants and toward reclamation of Indigenous health need to include (1) an understanding of the legacy of colonization, (2) the healing power of Indigenous knowledge and ways, and (3) the power of Indigenous voice and participation.[16] Although First Nations in Canada identified these, they are also shared among tribal nations and Indigenous communities in the United States.

In the United States, AIAN scholars of SDOH held roundtables with community members to describe IsDOH and identify areas of overlap. They created a figure that represented a typology of determinants of Indigenous healing, health, and wellness. The typology consists of broad Indigenous and non-Indigenous determinants as well as shared Indigenous and unique Indigenous determinants and health belief models.[15] These were later adapted and included in the 6-module training developed by Seven Directions.

The 4 IsDOH constructs described by Seven Directions are based on the need for specificity and 3 typologies (i.e., broad, shared, and unique) of determinants of Indigenous health.[15] They are illustrated in supplemental Figure A (available as a supplement to the online version of this article at http://www.ajph.org). The 4 constructs are (1) sovereignty and governance, (2) language and identity, (3) land and kinship, and (4) Indigenous knowledge and practices. All 4 constructs are understood to be relational and interconnected to create conditions for Indigenous community healing, health, and wellness.

Sovereignty and Governance

Tribal sovereignty predates European contact and has provided tribal nations the crucial status necessary to build and sustain systems that ensure the health, welfare, and safety of their communities.[17] Upon the formation of the United States, Congress and the federal courts recognized tribal sovereignty as inherent to tribal nations, noting that this political status exists above and beyond AIAN racial status.[17] The nature of tribal sovereignty sets Indigenous communities apart from other racial groups in the United States, both on and off the reservation.[17] Citizens of sovereign nations retain rights to specific services derived from the treaties and other formal legal processes that transferred land and resources from tribes to the federal government.[17]

Incorporating this political status into public health approaches can serve to improve SDOH in ways yet untapped. For example, AIAN nations, in the scope of inherent sovereignty, exercise public health authority to ensure the health, welfare, and safety of their citizens.[18] Tribal nations may express this authority through the adoption of tribal public health codes and cross-jurisdictional agreements that support data sharing and mutual aid with local non-AIAN jurisdictions.[18]

During the COVID-19 pandemic, tribal nations required masking on their lands and provided vaccines for everyone, which increased access for both enrolled members of the tribes and their neighboring communities. In some very rural areas, tribal health centers were the most accessible option for nonnatives.[19] Through public health governance, tribal nations develop and provide public health and health services with Indigenous worldviews and knowledge embedded in the care, programs, and policies,[18] furthering their goal of AIAN health equity.

Language and Identity

Tribal nations and Indigenous communities retain cultural and social systems, ways of being, and rich Indigenous knowledge systems that have sustained Indigenous peoples for generations.[1] However, with US colonization and assimilation policies (e.g., boarding schools, social welfare system), these systems were intentionally disrupted and, in many cases, purposefully destroyed. This resulted in a loss or dormancy of Indigenous knowledge (e.g., language, culture, practices) and identity, Indigenous health, and wellness approaches (e.g., medicines, ceremony) and the Indigenous knowledge systems or frameworks that served to connect knowledge and behaviors.[20] Indigenous knowledge–centered research is strengthening individual and community resilience for suicide prevention through positive coping mechanisms that come from intergenerational interactions, reconnection with culture and identity, and the resurgence and revitalization of Indigenous languages.[21]

Land and Kinship

For many tribal nations and Indigenous communities in the United States, wellness comes from maintaining geography and environmental relationships connected to collective health and healing practices.[1] The destruction and disruption of land-based wellness practices through land dispossession and removal and the destruction of sacred spiritual sites have been demonstrated to have negative health effects.[20] The desecration of lands contributes to a deep-seated sense of loss or grief that is felt in the collective soul of Indigenous individuals' communities.[22] In response, tribal nations and grassroots community organizations are partnering to engage youths, for example, in cultural practices that restore and maintain their ancestral connection to their lands. For example, the Healing of the Canoe study, a collaboration with Pacific Northwest Tribes, used the canoe journey as a metaphor and engaged youths in remembering and reengaging in the cultural practice for substance misuse and abuse prevention and promotion of tribal identity.[23]

Indigenous Knowledge and Practices

Indigenous epistemologies include the knowledge systems based in Indigenous cultural perceptions and understandings of the world, essential elements of wellness frameworks.[1] The ways tribal nations and Indigenous communities process, understand, and teach community members about wellness relies on language, story, and practices based on ancestral teachings maintained for generations.[21–23] History serves as a cornerstone of Indigenous epistemologies and theory, as the past affects the present and future generations of our communities.[22] Culturally based interventions not only add to the strength and resilience of a community but are also effective in improving population health outcomes.

The Healing of the Canoe study—an intervention aimed at reducing substance use in American Indian youths based on Salish cultural teachings and traditions—found that students exposed to their curriculum reported lower substance use rates.[23] Among AIAN epistemologies, physical and spiritual wellness are often intertwined, and one cannot exist without the other; ceremony and spiritual practices are essential to wellness.[1] Spirituality guides our understanding of this construct and conceptualization of frameworks for healing, health, and wellness and IsDOH with respect for the diversity of spiritual beliefs and practices of each Native nation and Indigenous community in the United States.[1,24]

For teams engaged in developing Indigenous frameworks, the 4 constructs are a starting point for story sharing and discussions. They prompt teams to reflect on their relationship to lands, kinship, language, identity, history, and sovereignty. For non-Indigenous team members or partners, they provide an opportunity to listen, learn, and advocate. Consequently, the discussions support identifying and mapping the typology of SDOH, shared and unique IsDOH, and broad SDOH.

RECOMMENDATIONS AND GUIDELINES

Tribal nations and Indigenous communities are continuously engaged with non-Indigenous private, nonprofit, and local, state, and federal government entities. They strengthen their cross-sector, long-term collaborations (e.g., health and human services, education, judicial, environmental) to address SDOH and improve health and wellness outcomes. The strengthening of tribal and Indigenous community systems ensures the safety, welfare, and health of their citizens and community members.

The following are actionable recommendations for developing Indigenous frameworks and establishing long term cross-sector collaborations among internal and external partners that serve tribal nations and Indigenous communities:

1. Establish and maintain long-term partnership built on trust, shared values, and purpose.
2. Develop an Indigenous framework for healing, health, and wellness for your tribal nations or Indigenous community based on meetings with community knowledge keepers, story work, and, if necessary, literature and environmental scans.
3. Host a community of practice or advisory board meetings to present the framework for feedback and revisions.
4. Work with partners to identify application of the framework. It may be applied in public health for screening and assessments, referrals and tracking, program development and evaluation, and policy development and funding allocations.
5. Apply and evaluate the framework.

These tailored frameworks are central to cross-sector alignment, decolonizing practices, and moving toward equity. Yet, they do not stand alone. Guidelines for integration with existing frameworks include the following:

1. describing health belief models,
2. identifying the typology of the determinants (i.e., broad, shared, or unique) and overlaps,
3. applying health belief models,
4. establishing criteria for use,
5. prioritizing IsDOH and SDOH, and
6. conducting an evaluation.

CONCLUSIONS

We have proposed the development of Indigenous frameworks of healing, health, and wellness (i.e., IsDOH frameworks) using constructs identified from scoping reviews and advisory board, peers, and community member feedback. The frameworks may be used in tandem with SDOH frameworks of the WHO and the CDC for the functions of public health (i.e., assessments, assurance, and program and policy development). The 4 constructs and subsequent IsDOH training developed by Seven Directions may be used in tribal nations, in Indigenous communities, and in partnership across sectors (e.g., public health, education, health, and social services) by practitioners and policymakers to strengthen Indigenous health and health-related systems, decolonize public health, and achieve health equity. AJPH

ABOUT THE AUTHORS

Christina E. Oré, Emily Loerzel, and Myra Parker are with Seven Direction, Center for the Study of Risk and Health Behavior, School of Medicine, University of Washington, Seattle. Erin Marziale is with the National Network for Public Health Institutes, New Orleans, LA.

CORRESPONDENCE

Correspondence should be sent to Christina E. Oré, 1959 NE Pacific St, Seattle, WA 98195-7238 (e-mail: core1@uw.edu). Reprints can be ordered at https://www.ajph.org by clicking the "Reprints" link.

PUBLICATION INFORMATION

Full Citation: Oré CE, Loerzel E, Marziale E, Parker M. Developing indigenous-centered healing, health, and wellness frameworks to strengthen indigenous health systems, decolonize public health, and achieve health equity. *Am J Public Health*. 2025;115(5):726–731.

Acceptance Date: November 20, 2024.

DOI: https://doi.org/10.2105/AJPH.2024.307958

ORCID iDs:
Christina E. Oré https://orcid.org/0000-0002-5511-4588

Erin Marziale https://orcid.org/0009-0004-2719-5319

Myra Parker https://orcid.org/0000-0003-4871-4304

CONTRIBUTORS

C. E. Oré updated the literature. C. E. Oré, E. Loerzel, and M. Parker conceptualized and wrote the original draft of the essay. C. E. Oré and E. Marziale edited the essay. All authors reviewed the final submission.

ACKNOWLEDGMENTS

This publication was supported by the Centers for Disease Control and Prevention (CDC), US Department of Health and Human Services (HHS) as part of a financial assistance award to the National Network of Public Health Institutes (NNPHI) totaling $300,000 with 100% funded by CDC, HHS (awards 1 NU38OT000303-01-00, 5 NU38OT000303-02-00, 5 NU38OT000303-03-00).

NNPHI collaborated on this effort with Seven Directions, University of Washington and the CDC's Office of Tribal Affairs and Strategic Alliances.

We would like to thank and acknowledge the contributions of Carmen Clelland, PharmD, MPA, MPH; Wendy Holmes, MS; Jessica Miller, MA; Lydia Mezenghie, MPH; and Joanne Odenkirchen, MPH, from the Office of Tribal Affairs and Strategic Alliances, Center for State, Tribal, Local, and Territorial Support, Centers for Disease Control and Prevention, Atlanta, GA.

Note. The contents of this essay are those of the authors and do not necessarily represent the official views of, nor an endorsement by, the CDC, the HHS, or the US government.

CONFLICTS OF INTEREST

The authors have no potential or actual conflicts of interest to declare from funding or affiliation-related activities.

HUMAN PARTICIPANT PROTECTION

No protocol approval was necessary because this essay was not a human participant research study; it was a public health resource development project.

REFERENCES

1. Cajete GA. Indigenous science, climate change, and indigenous community building: a framework of foundational perspectives for indigenous community resilience and revitalization. *Sustainability.* 2020;12(22):9569. https://doi.org/10.3390/su12229569
2. Trout L, Kramer C, Fischer L. Social medicine in practice: realizing the American Indian and Alaska Native right to health. *Health Hum Rights.* 2018;20(2):19–30.
3. White House. White House releases first-of-a-kind indigenous knowledge guidance for federal agencies. December 1, 2022. Available at: www.whitehouse.gov/ceq/news-updates/2022/12/01/white-house-releases-first-of-a-kind-indigenous-knowledge-guidance-for-federal-agencies. Accessed October 7, 2024.
4. Arias E, Tejada-Vera B, Kochanek KD, Ahmad FB. Provisional life expectancy estimates for 2021. *NCHS Vital Statistics Rapid Release Reports.* 2022; no 23. Available at: https://stacks.cdc.gov/view/cdc/118999. Accessed February 22, 2025. https://doi.org/10.15620/cdc:118999
5. Braveman P, Gottlieb L. The social determinants of health: it's time to consider the causes of the causes. *Public Health Rep.* 2014;129(suppl 2):19–31. https://doi.org/10.1177/00333549141291S206
6. Marmot M; Commission on Social Determinants of Health. Achieving health equity: from root causes to fair outcomes. *Lancet.* 2007;370(9593):1153–1163. https://doi.org/10.1016/S0140-6736(07)61385-3
7. Bowleg L. The White racial frame of public health discourses about racialized health differences and "disparities": what it reveals about power and how it thwarts health equity. *Front Public Health.* 2023;11:1187307. https://doi.org/10.3389/fpubh.2023.1187307
8. Solar O, Irwin A. *A Conceptual Framework for Action on the Social Determinants of Health.* Geneva, Switzerland: World Health Organization; 2010.
9. Centers for Disease Control and Prevention. Social determinants of health. January 17, 2024. Available at: http://www.cdc.gov/socialdeterminants/index.htm. Accessed August 3, 2023.
10. US Department of Health and Human Services. Healthy People 2030. Available at: https://www.healthypeople.gov. Accessed August 3, 2023.
11. Castrucci BC. The "10 essential public health services" is the common framework needed to communicate about public health. *Am J Public Health.* 2021;111(4):598–599. https://doi.org/10.2105/AJPH.2021.306189
12. Yearby R. Structural racism and health disparities: reconfiguring the social determinants of health framework to include the root cause. *J Law Med Ethics.* 2020;48(3):518–526. https://doi.org/10.1177/1073110520958876
13. Rodriguez-Lonebear D, Barceló NE, Akee R, Carroll SR. American Indian reservations and COVID-19: correlates of early infection rates in the pandemic. *J Public Health Manag Pract.* 2020;26(4):371–377. https://doi.org/10.1097/PHH.0000000000001206
14. US Commission on Civil Rights. *Broken Promises: Continuing Federal Funding Shortfall for Native Americans.* December 2018. Available at: https://www.usccr.gov/files/pubs/2018/12-20-Broken-Promises.pdf. Accessed February 22, 2025.
15. Carroll SR, Suina M, Jäger MB, et al. Reclaiming indigenous health in the US: moving beyond the social determinants of health. *Int J Environ Res Public Health.* 2022;19(12):7495. https://doi.org/10.3390/ijerph19127495
16. Greenwood M, De Leeuw S, Lindsay NM, eds. *Determinants of Indigenous Individuals' Health in Canada: Beyond the Social.* Toronto, ON: Canadian Scholars' Press; 2018.
17. Shelton BL. *Legal and Historical Roots of Health Care for American Indians and Alaska Natives in the United States.* Oakland, CA: Henry J. Kaiser Family Foundation; 2004.
18. Bryan RT, Schaefer RM, DeBruyn L, Stier DD. Public health legal preparedness in Indian country. *Am J Public Health.* 2009;99(4):607–614. https://doi.org/10.2105/AJPH.2008.146522
19. Healy J. Plenty of vaccines, not enough arms: a warning sign in Cherokee Nation. *New York Times.* March 16, 2021. Available at: www.nytimes.com/2021/03/16/us/vaccines-covid-cherokee-native-americans.html. Accessed October 7, 2024.
20. Walters KL, Beltran R, Huh D, Evans-Campbell T. Dis-placement and dis-ease: land, place, and health among American Indians and Alaska Natives. In: Burton EM, Matthews SA, Leung M, Kemp SP, Takeuchi DT, eds. *Communities, Neighborhoods, and Health: Expanding the Boundaries of Place.* New York, NY: Springer; 2011:163–199. https://doi.org/10.1007/978-1-4419-7482-2_10
21. Allen J, Wexler L, Rasmus S. Protective factors as a unifying framework for strength-based intervention and culturally responsive American Indian and Alaska Native suicide prevention. *Prev Sci.* 2022;23(1):59–72. https://doi.org/10.1007/s11121-021-01265-0
22. Hodge DR, Limb GE, Cross TL. Moving from colonization toward balance and harmony: a Native American perspective on wellness. *Soc Work.* 2009;54(3):211–219. https://doi.org/10.1093/sw/54.3.211
23. Donovan DM, Thomas LR, Sigo RLW, et al. Healing of the Canoe: preliminary results of a culturally tailored intervention to prevent substance abuse and promote tribal identity for Native youth in two Pacific Northwest tribes. *Am Indian Alaska Native Ment Health Res.* 2015;22(1):42–76. https://doi.org/10.5820/aian.2201.2015.42
24. Walters KL, Johnson-Jennings M, Stroud S, et al. Growing from our roots: strategies for developing culturally grounded health promotion interventions in American Indian, Alaska Native, and Native Hawaiian communities. *Prev Sci.* 2020;21(suppl 1):54–64. https://doi.org/10.1007/s11121-018-0952-z

Immigrant Inequities in Uninsurance and Postpartum Medicaid Extension: A Quasi-Experimental Study in New York City, 2016–2021

Teresa Janevic, PhD, MPH, Lauren Birnie, MPH, Kizzi Belfon, MPH, Lily Glenn, MPH, Sheela Maru, MD, MPH, Simone Reynolds, PhD, MPH, Folake Eniola, MPH, Heeun Kim, MPA, Frances M. Howell, MA, Ashley Fox, PhD, MPH, and Ellerie Weber, PhD, MBA

AJPH May 2025, Vol. 115, No. 5

Objectives. To determine if de facto postpartum Medicaid extension during the Families First Coronavirus Response Act (FFCRA) reduced immigrant versus US-born inequities in uninsurance.

Methods. We assessed self-reported uninsurance at 2 to 6 months postpartum among people with Medicaid-paid births using the New York City Pregnancy Risk Assessment Monitoring System (PRAMS), comparing immigrant and US-born people. We created a pre-FFCRA cohort of 2611 births from 2016 to 2019 and a post-FFCRA implementation cohort of 1197 births from 2020 to 2021. We calculated risk differences using log binomial regression.

Results. Self-reported postpartum uninsurance among immigrants decreased from 13.6% to 9.3% after FFCRA (adjusted risk difference = −4.9%; 95% confidence interval = −7.8%, −2.0%). Immigrant versus US-born inequities in postpartum uninsurance decreased except among Hispanic birthing people, among whom 1 in 6 reported they were uninsured during FFCRA, despite continued eligibility.

Conclusions. De facto postpartum Medicaid extension decreased immigrant inequities in insurance coverage, but Hispanic immigrants may have been unaware of continued coverage.

Public Health Implications. Postpartum Medicaid extension policies that are inclusive of all immigrants may decrease inequities, but community-integrated implementation is needed to raise awareness of coverage and advance postpartum maternal health equity. (*Am J Public Health*. 2025;115(5):732–735. https://doi.org/10.2105/AJPH.2024.307968)

In New York City (NYC), Hispanic and Black birthing people have 2 and 6 times the risk of pregnancy-related death as non-Hispanic White birthing people.[1] Inequities in maternal death extend into the postpartum period, and loss of Medicaid insurance after birth may contribute.[2] Lack of a federal requirement for Medicaid to insure undocumented and otherwise nonqualified immigrants means that immigrants are disproportionately uninsured in the postpartum period.[3] In New York State, before 2020, undocumented immigrants were eligible for pregnancy Medicaid, but coverage ended at 60 days after birth.[4] The Medicaid Maintenance of Eligibility in Families First Coronavirus Response Act (FFCRA) resulted in a de facto extension of Medicaid after birth.[5] In New York State, no Medicaid recipient was disenrolled after birth during FFCRA, regardless of immigration status. Our objective was to estimate if immigrant versus US-born inequities in postpartum uninsurance declined during FFCRA, overall and by race/ethnicity.

METHODS

We used 2016–2021 data from the NYC Pregnancy Risk Assessment Monitoring System (PRAMS), a population-based survey administered via mail and phone to individuals with a recent live birth, identified through a stratified, random sample of birth certificate records.[6] NYC PRAMS data are weighted to be representative of all live births to NYC residents. Over the study period (2016–2021), NYC PRAMS had an unweighted response rate of 61.7% and 8018 survey respondents. NYC PRAMS is unique to national PRAMS data because it links survey data to birth certificate details on birth country and years in the United States. We selected respondents with Medicaid-paid births, as ascertained by hospital staff (59.3%). We created a pre-FFCRA period of births (January 1, 2016–March 17, 2019; n = 2611) and a post-FFCRA implementation period of births (March 18, 2020–December 31, 2021; n = 1197). We considered March 18, 2019 to March 17, 2020 (n = 694) a "washout" period, so that our pre-FFCRA period included only those whose pregnancy-related Medicaid coverage would have expired prior to FFCRA implementation, whereas our post-FFCRA implementation period would include only those who gave birth during FFCRA and thus were "exposed" to continuous enrollment. We obtained self-reported race, ethnicity, country of birth, time in the United States, age, education, and parity from the birth certificate. We categorized self-reported postpartum insurance (none vs any) at survey response (2–6 months after birth) to ascertain "self-reported postpartum uninsurance" (henceforth "postpartum uninsurance"); we excluded from the analysis those with missing data on country of birth, race/ethnicity, or postpartum insurance status (3.2%). We created a 3-month time variable. Missingness was low for all variables, ranging from 0.0% (age) to 3.2% (postpartum insurance type).

We examined postpartum uninsurance graphically and sample characteristics by pre- and post-FFCRA implementation periods. We estimated marginal probabilities from logistic regression to calculate risk differences comparing the pre- and post-FFCRA implementation periods, adjusting for education, age, parity, and race/ethnicity. We used difference-in-difference (DID) parameterization to test immigrant versus US-born differences in postpartum uninsurance in the pre- and post-FFCRA implementation periods. We tested an interrupted time series approach; the time coefficient and post-FFCRA implementation period slopes were null, so we used DID models for simplicity. We used sampling weights and robust standard. We tested the parallel trends assumption visually, ran a placebo regression with a pre-FFCRA period of 2016 to 2017 and post-FFCRA implementation period of 2018 to 2019, and used alternate washout periods (October, 1 2019–March 17, 2020, March 18, 2019–January 16, 2020, and October 1, 2019–January 16, 2020).

RESULTS

Sociodemographic characteristics in the pre- and post-FFCRA implementation periods differed by years living in the United States (among immigrants), race/ethnicity, and education (Appendix Table A, available as a supplement to the online version of this article at http://www.ajph.org; $P < .05$ on χ^2 test). Appendix Figure A shows parallel trends between immigrants and US-born people in the pre-FFCRA period, followed by a decrease in postpartum uninsurance after FFCRA implementation.

Among immigrants, postpartum uninsurance decreased from 13.6% to 9.3% (adjusted risk difference [ARD] = −4.9%; 95% confidence interval [CI] = −7.8%, −2.0%), whereas among the US-born it changed from 1.2% to 0.7% (ARD = −0.5%, 95% CI = −5.6%, 4.6%; Table 1). Postpartum uninsurance decreased among all immigrant groups, but least among Hispanic immigrants, from 23.5% to 17.7% (ARD = −4.0%; 95% CI = −9.9%, 1.9; Table 1). Overall, the immigrant versus US-born disparity in postpartum uninsurance decreased 3.7 percentage points (adjusted DID = −4.0%; 95% CI = −7.1%, −0.9%). Disparity reductions of similar magnitude were present among Black and Hispanic subgroups. Results did not differ by years in the United States (Appendix Figure B).

The placebo analysis produced null results, as desired (Appendix Table B), and in sensitivity analyses, alternative washout periods produced similar results (Appendix Table C).

DISCUSSION

We found that continuous Medicaid enrollment during FFCRA was associated with a 4 percentage point decrease in postpartum uninsurance in NYC among immigrants, resulting in a reduction, but not elimination, of immigrant versus US-born inequities. However, 18% of Hispanic immigrants still reported they were uninsured.

Our equity impact analysis contributes to evidence that continuous Medicaid coverage during FFCRA decreased uninsurance. Medicaid-to-uninsured postpartum churn decreased nationally, from 10.3% in 2019 to 3.7% in 2021,[7] and Medicaid beneficiaries used more preventive services in the postpartum period.[8] We build on these findings by assessing the impact on equity on immigrants, the subpopulation most likely to lose coverage postpartum.

TABLE 1— Changes in Immigrant Versus US-Born Inequity in Self-Reported Postpartum Uninsurance Among Persons Insured by Medicaid at Birth Before and After Families First Coronavirus Response Act (FFCRA) Implementation: New York City, 2016–2021

	US-Born				Immigrant				Difference-in-Differences	
	Pre-FFCRA, % (95% CI)	Post-FFCRA, % (95% CI)	Risk Difference, % (95% CI)	Adjusted Risk Difference,[a] % (95% CI)	Pre-FFCRA, % (95% CI)	Post-FFCRA, % (95% CI)	Risk Difference % (95% CI)	Adjusted Risk Difference,[a] % (95% CI)	Difference-in-Difference, % (95% CI)	Adjusted Difference-in-Difference,[a] % (95% CI)
All race/ethnicities	1.2 (0.6, 2.3)	0.7 (0.2, 2.6)	−0.5 (−1.7, 0.007)	−0.5 (−5.6, 4.6)	13.6 (11.8, 15.6)	9.3 (7.1, 12.2)	−4.2 (−7.4, −1.0)	−4.9 (−7.8, −2.0)	−3.7 (−7.1, −0.3)	4.0 (7.1, 0.9)
Hispanic	1.9 (0.8, 4.4)	2.2 (0.6, 8.3)	0.3 (−3.1, 3.7)	−0.1 (−6.0, 5.8)	23.5 (20.0, 27.3)	17.7 (13.4, 22.9)	−5.8 (−11.8, 0.2)	−4.0 (−9.9, 1.9)	−6.1 (−13.0, 0.8)	−4.0 (−11.0, 3.0)
Non-Hispanic White[b]	0.4 (0.1, 2.8)	0.0	. . .	. . .	10.2 (6.3, 16.0)	0.4 (0.1, 2.6)	−9.8 (−14.6, −5.0)	−10.1 (−18.4, −1.8)	. . .	. . .
Non-Hispanic Black	1.5 (0.5, 4.2)	0.1 (0.0, 0.8)	−1.4 (−3.0, 0.2)	−1.3 (−21.6, 19.0)	5.7 (3.4, 9.5)	0.2 (0.0, 1.1)	−5.5 (−8.5, −2.5)	−5.4 (−8.5, −2.3)	−4.2 (7.5, −0.8)	−4.1 (−10.0, 1.8)
Non-Hispanic Asian or Pacific Islander[c]	. . .	. . .	. . .	. . .	5.8 (3.7, 9.0)	1.2 (0.3, 4.5)	−4.6 (−7.6, −1.6)	−4.7 (−9.0, −0.4)	. . .	. . .

Note. CI = confidence interval.
[a]Adjusted for education, age, parity, race/ethnicity, and nativity.
[b]Non-Hispanic White subgroup excluded from risk difference and difference-in-difference analyses because zero events of uninsurance were observed in the post-FFCRA implementation US-born subgroup, resulting in uninterpretable results.
[c]Non-Hispanic Asian or Pacific Islander US-born subgroup suppressed because of small sample size (< 30).

A strength of our study is the availability of birth country, years in the United States, and hospital-reported delivery payer. One limitation is that postpartum insurance was self-reported; however, this does yield the patient's perspective of coverage, which is vital to motivating patients to seek follow-up and preventive care. Another limitation is that we did not know the legal status of immigrants in our data, which would have allowed us to better understand the fraction of immigrants expected to gain coverage (Appendix Table D).

Public Health Implications

Many Hispanic immigrants reported no health insurance despite being eligible for continuous Medicaid coverage during FFCRA, suggesting a lack of awareness of their coverage. Other research has suggested that people enrolled in Medicaid during the pandemic thought they were uninsured.[9] One explanation for our findings is the fear and misunderstanding about Medicaid eligibility related to immigration status and public charge criteria among immigrants, which was thought to influence the uptake of Medicaid and Supplemental Nutrition Assistance Program (SNAP) at the onset of the pandemic.[10] Other explanations include poorer dissemination of information related to the continuous Medicaid provision in immigrant-serving health institutions or immigrant communities. The consequences of this Medicaid coverage knowledge gap could be profound: in 2020, postpartum maternal mortality increased 41% during the COVID-19 pandemic, with the largest increase for Hispanic people.[11] To combat this knowledge gap, agencies need targeted strategies to disseminate information on changes in postpartum Medicaid policy—for example, by working with community-based organizations and federally qualified health centers. However, these strategies will prove a challenge given the continued level of anti-immigrant sentiment in the United States and fear in some immigrant communities.[12]

Our findings have national implications. To date, of 47 states that implemented postpartum Medicaid extensions, New York and 11 other states include enrollees regardless of immigration status. As such, the gains in equity we identified in our natural experiment estimate what to expect in these states. However, states that exclude categories of immigrants may not see similar gains, thus reducing the effectiveness of the policy while leaving behind many immigrants.

Conclusion

Postpartum Medicaid extension policies have the potential to reduce inequities, but a targeted, community-integrated approach is needed to raise awareness of coverage and ensure optimal implementation to advance maternal health equity. AJPH

ABOUT THE AUTHORS

Teresa Janevic and Frances M. Howell are with the Department of Epidemiology, Columbia University Mailman School of Public Health, New York, NY. Lauren Birnie, Kizzi Belfon, Lily Glenn, and Folake Eniola are with the New York City Department of Health and Mental Hygiene, New York, NY. Sheela Maru is with the Department of Health System Design and Global Health, Icahn School of Medicine at Mount Sinai, New York, NY. Simone Reynolds is with the Department of Epidemiology and Biostatistics, SUNY Downstate Health Sciences University School of Public Health, New York, NY. Heeun Kim is with the Department of Population Health Sciences, Icahn School of Medicine at Mount Sinai, New York. Ashley Fox is with the Department of Public Administration and Policy, SUNY Albany Rockefeller College of Public Affairs and Policy, New York, NY. Ellerie Weber is with the Department of Population Health Science and Policy, Icahn School of Medicine at Mount Sinai, New York.

CORRESPONDENCE

Correspondence should be sent to Teresa Janevic, MPH, PhD, Columbia University Mailman School of Public Health, 722 W. 168th St, New York, NY 10032 (e-mail: Tmj2101@cumc.columbia.edu). Reprints can be ordered at https://www.ajph.org by clicking the "Reprints" link.

PUBLICATION INFORMATION

Full Citation: Janevic T, Birnie L, Belfon K, et al. Immigrant inequities in uninsurance and postpartum Medicaid extension: a quasi-experimental study in New York City, 2016–2021. *Am J Public Health*. 2025;115(5):732–735.

Acceptance Date: November 28, 2024.

DOI: https://doi.org/10.2105/AJPH.2024.307968

ORCID iDs:

Teresa Janevic https://orcid.org/0000-0002-9934-4406

Ashley Fox https://orcid.org/0000-0003-4106-7853

Ellerie Weber https://orcid.org/0000-0003-3179-7035

ACKNOWLEDGMENTS

This study was supported by the Robert Wood Johnson Foundation (grant #79625).

We thank the Health Data 4 New York City Project for initiating the initial collaborative working group contributing to this project.

CONFLICTS OF INTEREST

The authors have no conflicts of interest to report.

HUMAN PARTICIPANT PROTECTION

This study was approved by the institutional review board of the New York City Department of Health and Mental Hygiene.

REFERENCES

1. *Pregnancy-Associated Mortality in New York City, 2016–2020*. New York, NY: Maternal Mortality Review Committee, New York City Department of Health and Mental Hygiene; September 2024.
2. Society for Maternal-Fetal Medicine (SMFM). Electronic address: smfm@smfm.org; Stone J, Chandrasekaran S; SMFM Health Policy and Advocacy Committee. Society for Maternal-Fetal Medicine position statement: extending Medicaid coverage for 12 months postpartum. *Am J Obstet Gynecol*. 2024;231(1):B12–B14. https://doi.org/10.1016/j.ajog.2024.04.008
3. Maru S, Glenn L, Belfon K, et al. Utilization of maternal health care among immigrant mothers in New York City, 2016–2018. *J Urban Health*. 2021;98(6):711–726. https://doi.org/10.1007/s11524-021-00584-5
4. New York State Dept of Health. GIS 15 MA/022: continuous coverage for MAGI individuals. Available at: https://www.health.ny.gov/health_care/medicaid/publications/gis/15ma022.htm. Accessed December 5, 2024.
5. Ranji, U, Salganicoff A, Gomez I. Postpartum coverage extension in the American Rescue Plan Act of 2021. KFF. Available at: https://www.kff.org/policy-watch/postpartum-coverage-extension-in-the-american-rescue-plan-act-of-2021. Accessed December 5, 2024.
6. Shulman HB, D'Angelo DV, Harrison L, Smith RA, Warner L. The Pregnancy Risk Assessment Monitoring System (PRAMS): overview of design and methodology. *Am J Public Health*. 2018;108(10):1305–1313. https://doi.org/10.2105/AJPH.2018.304563
7. Eliason EL, Daw JR, Steenland MW. Changes in postpartum insurance coverage in the US during the COVID-19 pandemic. *JAMA Health Forum*. 2022;3(4):e220688. https://doi.org/10.1001/jamahealthforum.2022.0688
8. Wang X, Pengetnze YM, Eckert E, Keever G, Chowdhry V. Extending postpartum Medicaid beyond 60 days improves care access and uncovers unmet needs in a Texas Medicaid health maintenance organization. *Front Public Health*. 2022;10:841832. https://doi.org/10.3389/fpubh.2022.841832
9. Ding D, Sommers BD, Glied SA. Unwinding and the Medicaid undercount: millions enrolled in Medicaid during the pandemic thought they were uninsured. *Health Aff (Millwood)*. 2024;43(5):725–731. https://doi.org/10.1377/hlthaff.2023.01069
10. Touw S, McCormack G, Himmelstein DU, Woolhandler S, Zallman L. Immigrant essential workers likely avoided Medicaid and SNAP because of a change to the Public Charge Rule. *Health Aff (Millwood)*. 2021;40(7):1090–1098. https://doi.org/10.1377/hlthaff.2021.00059.
11. Thoma ME, Declercq ER. All-cause maternal mortality in the US before vs during the COVID-19 pandemic. *JAMA Netw Open*. 2022;5(6):e2219133. https://doi.org/10.1001/jamanetworkopen.2022.19133
12. Yang LH, Eger MA, Link BG. The human cost of politicizing immigration: migration stigma, US politics, and health. *JAMA*. 2024;332(8):619–620. https://doi.org/10.1001/jama.2024.11126

Occupational Determinants of Health and Well-Being for Indigenous Populations in the United States: Findings From the National Health Interview Survey, 2020–2022

Brett Shannon, MBBS, PhD, Courtney Ryder, PhD, Chibuzor Abasilim, PhD, Kirsten S. Almberg, PhD, Tessa Bonney, PhD, Linda Forst, MD, MPH, and Lee S. Friedman, PhD

See also Gunn et al. p. 634.

Objectives. To characterize occupational determinants of health and well-being for American Indian/Alaska Native (AIAN) populations in the United States using a nationally representative data set.

Methods. We conducted a descriptive analysis and multivariable logistic regression using National Health Interview Survey data (2020–2022) to compare demographic and work characteristics across 3 groups of AIAN individuals: non-Hispanic (n = 558), Hispanic (n = 304), and those with at least 1 other racial identity (n = 653). The total unweighted sample was 88 701.

Results. The 3 subgroups portrayed contrasting profiles by urbanicity, employment, region, and immigrant status. Specific groups had significantly lower odds of working and participating in the labor force and were more likely to have a family income below 200% of the poverty line, adjusting for age, education, and sex.

Conclusions. Differences among the groups highlight the need for future health research to account for cultural, social, spiritual, mental, and physical health factors across Indigenous nations. Expanding beyond broad AIAN classifications could improve the specificity of occupational health research.

Public Health Implications. The current definitions of Indigenous groups proposed by the US government directly impedes appropriate public health analysis to inform future work to address ongoing social, structural, and health disparities owing to colonization. (*Am J Public Health.* 2025;115(5):736–746. https://doi.org/10.2105/AJPH.2024.307959)

AJPH May 2025, Vol. 115, No. 5

The World Health Organization recognizes employment as an important social determinant of health.[1] Employment affects health and well-being and is an international policy area priority to reduce the gap in life expectancy for Indigenous people.[2] In 2023, the United States released its first ever American Indian/Alaska Native (AIAN) Worker Safety and Health Strategic Plan,[3] revealing the paucity of research, policy, and practice in Indigenous occupational health and safety and the links to underlying disparate health outcomes for Indigenous people.

In the United States, AIAN individuals have the highest unemployment rate (11.7% vs 7.3% for non-Hispanic White persons in 2020) and the lowest labor force participation rate (59.3%) and employment–population ratio (52.4%).[4] Despite this, there is a lack of information regarding employment barriers and employment characteristics for AIAN persons, in part because of the limitations of the existing race/ethnicity definitions and available data sources.[4] Data from the US Census Bureau's American Community Survey from 2009 to 2011 reveal that even when

Native Americans are similar to non-Hispanic White individuals in terms of age, sex, education level, marital status, and state of residence, their odds of being employed are 31% lower.[5]

Employment precarity in the United States is increasing, particularly for women, racial minorities, and those with less education.[6] Educational attainment is lower among AIAN populations than the dominant US population (80% vs 89% have a high school degree, respectively)[7]; this education disparity contributes to employment disparities[5] by restricting AIAN individuals' access to the workforce, narrowing the types of jobs available, increasing vulnerability to job termination, lowering the quality of working conditions, and reducing employment benefits. US unemployment rates increased markedly during the first months of the COVID-19 pandemic. The seasonally adjusted unemployment rate peaked at 14.7% in April 2020 and at 3.5% in February 2020 for US adults aged 16 years and older. In comparison, the AIAN unemployment rate was 7.5% in February 2020 and rose to 28.6% in April 2020, nearly double the rate of all US adults; however, this gap narrowed to 2.1% (AIAN unemployment = 13.1%; US adult unemployment = 11.0%) in June 2020.[8]

Stable employment is associated with better psychological and physical health as well as reduced mortality.[9,10] Researchers and policymakers are increasingly interested in identifying specific work characteristics that are indicators of employment quality,[11] particularly in a shifting labor market in which nonstandard work arrangements are on the rise. Researchers have considered various dimensions of employment quality, including wages, benefits, work hours, job security, contractual arrangements, job satisfaction, and promotional opportunities.[12] To date, population-based surveys regarding employment quality do not include Indigenous groups in race/ethnicity stratification,[13,14] limiting the current evidence on employment quality among US Indigenous workers.

Qualitative research among Australia's Indigenous communities that aimed to identify adults' priorities for well-being found that employment in a ranger program was associated with a number of well-being themes, including cultural education and training, meaningful work to reduce boredom and enhance self-respect, empowerment and strengthening Indigenous identity, women's empowerment enabling personal protection from violence, reduced substance abuse, increased physical activity, opportunities for formal qualifications, and a supportive environment for rehabilitation after release from prison.[15] To our knowledge, no national research has yet examined AIAN workers' access to employment and job quality, including labor force participation, industry- and occupation-specific employment patterns, and work limitations owing to mental and physical health. We aimed to characterize employment and employment quality for AIAN groups using secondary data from a US population-based survey.

METHODS

The National Health Interview Survey (NHIS) is a cross-sectional household survey with a multistage area probability design. We limited our analyses to adult files from the 3 most recent years of data: 2020 to 2022.[16] We first merged files by year, then appended the data sets for each year and divided the weight variable by 3 to adjust sampling weights for each survey cycle, consistent with recommended NHIS methodology when pooling multiple years of data. All participants in NHIS were asked all applicable survey questions, with skip patterns. We treated individual responses of "refuse to answer," "don't know," or "not ascertained" as missing data. Over the study period, the COVID-19 pandemic led to business closures and staff layoffs, which varied by region and state. It is impossible to determine the changes in employment over time during the pandemic from the NHIS data. However, the NHIS data provide the best picture currently available of the demographics, health, and employment distribution of the AIAN population at a time when employment was a key social determinant of health contributing to racial inequities.

Classification of Indigenous Populations

We divided participants into 3 mutually exclusive Indigenous subgroups based on their race and ethnicity survey responses: (1) non-Hispanic AIAN individuals ("AIAN-only"), (2) Hispanic AIAN individuals ("AIAN-Hispanic"), and (3) AIAN individuals with at least 1 other racial identity ("AIAN-other"). We used 2 comparison groups for descriptive statistics: (1) respondents who self-identified as non-Hispanic White and (2) those who identified as Hispanic, excluding those who also identified as AIAN to ensure an appropriate reference group for the AIAN-Hispanic population. Our methods statement on issues of Indigenous status collection in health data can be found in the "Indigenous Status Data Statement" section of the appendix (available as a supplement to the online version of this article at http://www.ajph.org).

In multivariable models, we compared the AIAN groups with all non-Indigenous participants. The total unweighted sample was 88 701; there was a 558 unweighted count of persons reporting AIAN-only (weighted count n = 1 870 867), 304 reporting AIAN-Hispanic (weighted count n = 1 026 383), and 653 reporting AIAN-other (weighted count n = 1 747 812).

Variables

We describe demographic and occupational characteristics across racial/ethnic categories, US regions, and remoteness. We separated the US regions into South, West, Midwest, and Northeast,[17] and we classified counties using the 2013 Urban–Rural Classification Scheme.[18] We captured employment status by whether participants worked during the previous week or were currently looking for work. Among those who were currently working, respondents reported whether they worked full time, whether they were self-employed, and whether their workplace offered health insurance or paid sick leave.

We measured all demographic and occupational characteristics, except industry and occupation, over the entire study period. Industry and occupation were available for only 2 years of data (2020, 2021) and were reported based on major codes of the 2007 North American Industry Classification System and the 2010 Standard Occupational Classification.[19,20] We used family income compared with the poverty threshold as an indicator for income, as respondents' wages were not available. Personal income and employment history were not available in the NHIS. Hours worked per week was a continuous variable in the data set that we changed to a binary variable of less than 35 hours versus 35 hours or more per week.

Statistical Analysis

We used SAS version 9.4 (SAS Institute Inc., Cary, NC) to conduct survey procedures accounting for the complex survey design of NHIS (strata, primary sampling units, and weights; PROC SURVEYFREQ, PROC SURVEYMEANS, and PROC SURVEYLOGISTIC). For categorical variables, we obtained the percentage (prevalence), and for continuous variables, we calculated the mean. For all descriptive statistics, we provide 95% confidence intervals (CIs) for the estimate. We measured the coefficient of variation (CV), the ratio of the SD to the mean, for all descriptive statistics to determine dispersion around the mean. We considered a CV between 0.3 and 0.5 acceptable but highlighted it in descriptive tables. We removed statistics with a CV of greater than 0.5.

We created 5 risk strata for industry and occupation for work-related injury or illness based on 2020 occupational and 2021 private and public industry Bureau of Labor Statistics rates of injury and illness cases.[21–23] Nonfatal work-related injury and illness rates by occupation ranged from 300.5 (health care support occupations) to 2.9 (legal occupations) per 10 000 full-time equivalent workers. We classified occupational risk strata from highest to lowest based on these rates as follows: first: 250 to 370, second: 140 to 250, third: 90 to 140, fourth: 30 to 90, fifth: 0 to 30. We used a similar method to define risk strata for industry groups by rate of work-related injuries and illnesses per 100 full-time equivalent workers as follows: first: 4 to 6, second: 3 to 4, third: 2 to 3, fourth: 1 to 2, fifth: 0 to 1. We did not include military-specific occupations in the risk stratification; however, persons employed by the military were kept in the denominator of total workers. We did not stratify military occupations into the 5 groups because they have a different level of risk, there were no Indigenous workers who identified as military workers, and less than 0.1% of Hispanic or non-Hispanic White workers reported military occupations.

We developed multivariable logistic models to examine employment and labor force participation, outcomes representing employment quality, and employment in high-risk professions by race/ethnicity, controlling for a priori confounders of age, education, and sex. The binary outcomes for the 5 models were labor force participation (based on employment status in past week), working full time, paid sick leave benefits at job in the previous week, health insurance offered at workplace for those who reported working the previous week, and income below 200% federal poverty level during the past year. We considered a 2-sided *P* value less than .05 statistically significant. We present odds ratios (ORs) from adjusted models, including the 95% CIs.

RESULTS

The 3 Indigenous subgroups portrayed contrasting population profiles based on urban–rural indices, US region where residing, and proportion born in the United States (Table 1). The AIAN-only subgroup was largely from the US Southern and Western regions, predominantly resided in nonmetropolitan areas, and was more likely to be born in the United States (95.6%; 95% CI = 92.6, 98.6) compared with other groups. The AIAN-Hispanic subgroup

TABLE 1— **Demographic Characteristics of Adults by Race/Ethnicity: National Health Interview Survey, United States, 2020–2022**

Characteristic	AIAN-Only (Unweighted n = 558), % (95% CI) or Mean (SE)	AIAN-Hispanic (Unweighted n = 304), % (95% CI) or Mean (SE)	AIAN-Other (Unweighted n = 653), % (95% CI) or Mean (SE)	Hispanic (Unweighted n = 11 553), % (95% CI) or Mean (SE)	Non-Hispanic White (Unweighted n = 59 990), % (95% CI) or Mean (SE)
Age, y					
18–29	27.2 (21.5, 32.8)	33.5 (25.7, 41.3)	20.6 (16.2, 25.1)	26.7 (25.6, 27.8)	17.4 (16.8, 18.0)
30–39	14.7 (11.7, 17.8)	17.2 (12.9, 21.4)	17.3 (13.5, 21.1)	20.9 (19.9, 21.8)	15.4 (15.0, 15.8)
40–49	17.0 (14.2, 19.9)	15.4 (10.9, 19.9)	16.2 (13.0, 19.4)	19.9 (18.9, 20.8)	14.7 (14.3, 15.0)
50–59	15.0 (9.2, 20.7)	13.6 (9.1, 18.1)	15.5 (12.4, 18.7)	15.0 (14.2, 15.7)	16.6 (16.3, 17.0)
60–69	14.5 (10.6, 18.4)	14.4 (9.1, 19.7)	16.2 (12.9, 19.6)	9.9 (9.2, 10.6)	17.6 (17.2, 17.9)
≥70	11.6 (8.8, 14.5)	5.9 (3.3, 8.6)	14.1 (11.2, 17.0)	7.6 (7.0, 8.3)	18.4 (17.9, 18.8)
Mean ±SE	45.3 ±42.9–47.7	41.3 ±38.6–44.1	47.6 ±45.7–49.4	42.6 ±42.2–43.1	50.5 ±50.2–50.8
Sex					
Male	45.8 (37.3, 54.3)	56.0 (48.7, 63.4)	46.3 (42.1, 50.6)	48.5 (47.4, 49.7)	49.1 (48.6, 49.6)
Female	54.2 (45.7, 62.7)	44.0 (36.6, 51.3)	53.7 (49.4, 57.9)	51.5 (50.3, 52.6)	50.9 (50.4, 51.4)
Education level					
< high school	19.9 (13.8, 25.9)	27.2 (19.8, 34.6)	8.6 (5.8, 11.5)	26.1 (24.8, 27.5)	6.1 (5.8, 6.5)
GED or high school	32.3 (28.1, 36.4)	28.2 (22.4, 34.1)	29.5 (25.4, 33.6)	30.7 (29.6, 31.9)	26.8 (26.1, 27.5)
Some college, associate's degree, or technical degree	35.0 (30.1, 39.8)	29.9 (23.4, 36.3)	41.8 (36.7, 46.9)	25.7 (24.7, 26.6)	29.8 (29.2, 30.4)
Bachelor's degree	8.0 (4.4, 11.5)	8.0 (4.5, 11.6)	12.9 (10.0, 15.9)	11.6 (10.8, 12.4)	22.9 (22.3, 23.5)
Graduate degree	4.0 (2.2, 5.9)	5.6 (3.2, 8.0)	6.4 (4.3, 8.4)	4.6 (4.2, 5.1)	14.0 (13.5, 14.4)
Missing	0.9 (0, 1.9)	1.0 (0.0, 2.5)	0.9 (0.0, 1.7)	1.2 (1.0, 1.5)	0.4 (0.4, 0.5)
Remoteness					
Large central metropolitan area	11.7 (4.6, 18.8)[a]	48.8 (39.8, 57.9)	19.6 (15.0, 24.1)	48.4 (43.6, 53.1)	22.8 (20.9, 24.6)
Large fringe metropolitan area	9.8 (3.1, 16.5)[a]	16.0 (9.8, 22.2)	20.2 (15.0, 25.3)	19.8 (17.1, 22.5)	26.4 (24.0, 28.8)
Medium and small metropolitan area	26.8 (10.7, 43)[a]	27.7 (18.8, 36.6)	36.4 (29.7, 43.0)	26.6 (21.3, 31.9)	33.2 (30.2, 36.3)
Nonmetropolitan area	51.7 (25.2, 78.2)	7.4 (3.5, 11.4)	23.9 (18.5, 29.3)	5.2 (2.7, 7.7)	17.6 (16.2, 19.1)
US region					
Northeast	4.3 (1.2, 7.4)[a]	12.5 (6.1, 18.9)	9.6 (6.3, 13.0)	13.3 (11.4, 15.3)	19.1 (17.6, 20.7)
Midwest	14.4 (4.9, 23.9)[a]	11.0 (6.7.0, 15.4)	23.2 (18.2, 28.2)	8.7 (6.9, 10.4)	26.2 (24.6, 27.9)
South	34.2 (13.4, 55)[a]	34.2 (26.6, 41.7)	44.3 (37.7, 50.9)	38.9 (34.4, 43.5)	34.7 (32.9, 36.5)
West	47.1 (18.4, 75.7)[a]	42.3 (34.2, 50.3)	22.8 (17.6, 27.9)	39.0 (34.9, 43.2)	20.0 (18.1, 21.8)
Marital status					
Married/living with partner	46.6 (40.2, 52.9)	45.6 (38.5, 52.7)	47.0 (42.5, 51.5)	56.9 (55.7, 58.1)	62.4 (61.9, 63.0)
Divorced or separated	12.0 (9.8, 14.3)	10.3 (7.0, 13.6)	15.6 (12.9, 18.4)	9.2 (8.6, 9.8)	9.6 (9.3, 9.9)
Single never married	30.0 (23.3, 36.8)	32.5 (25.6, 39.4)	25.4 (21.0, 29.8)	26.2 (25.2, 27.2)	18.5 (18.0, 19.0)
Widowed	6.5 (4.6, 8.3)	4.3 (0.9, 7.8)	7.4 (5.3, 9.4)	3.3 (2.9, 3.7)	6.4 (6.1, 6.6)
Missing	4.9 (2.7, 7.0)	7.3 (3.6, 10.9)	4.6 (2.6, 6.6)	4.4 (3.9, 4.9)	3.1 (2.9, 3.3)
Born in the US	95.6 (92.6, 98.6)	61.0 (53.0, 69.0)	94.1 (91.8, 96.3)	46.9 (45.2, 48.6)	92.2 (91.8, 92.6)

Note. AIAN = American Indian/Alaska Native; CI = confidence interval; GED = general equivalency diploma.
[a]Coefficient of variation = 0.3–0.5.

mirrored Hispanic individuals, with nearly half of participants located in central metropolitan areas and the majority residing in the Southern and Western parts of the United States; this subgroup had the lowest proportion of individuals born in the United States (61.0%; 95% CI = 53.0, 69.0) compared with other Indigenous subgroups. The AIAN-other group was more evenly distributed across urban regions and lived predominantly in areas across the Midwestern, Southern, and Western regions of the country (Table 1).

The AIAN-Hispanic and Hispanic groups had lower rates of high school completion or its equivalent, with more than one quarter of AIAN-Hispanic individuals (27.2%; 95% CI = 19.8, 34.6) not completing high school. Of the 3 Indigenous groups, AIAN-other had the highest level of having a bachelor's (12.9%; 95% CI = 10.0, 15.9) or postgraduate (6.4%; 95% CI = 4.3, 8.4) degree; however, these rates remained approximately 50% lower than the rate of non-Hispanic White participants with a bachelor's or graduate degree.

Labor Force Participation

Of those from the AIAN-only group, 45.9% (95% CI = 39.0, 52.9) were not working, and of those not working, only 12.6% (95% CI = 8.3, 16.8) were looking for work. These figures were comparable to the AIAN-other group, with 43.0% (95% CI = 37.8, 48.2) not working the previous week and only 7.1% (95% CI = 3.0, 11.2) of those not working looking for work. The AIAN-only and AIAN-other subgroups had the highest rates of participants unable to work for health reasons, with 25.2% (95% CI = 14.3, 36.1) and 30.6% (95% CI = 23.5, 37.7) of those not working, respectively. Particularly relative to non-Hispanic White individuals, the proportion of retired persons across all AIAN subgroups was substantially lower (Table 2). The Indigenous subgroups presented different employment patterns by industry and occupation (Table 3). Compared with all non-Indigenous participants, both the AIAN-only group and the AIAN-other group had significantly decreased odds of working during the previous week, after adjusting for age, education, and sex (Table 4).

The AIAN-only (54.5%; 95% CI = 48.9, 60.2) and AIAN-other (55.1%; 95% CI = 50.1, 60.1) subgroups had substantially lower labor force participation rates (i.e., currently working and looking for work combined). The labor force participation rate was highest in the Hispanic (68.0%; 95% CI = 66.8, 69.2) and AIAN-Hispanic (64.4%; 95% CI = 57.7, 71.2) subgroups. In addition, the differences in employment persisted when looking at employment during the year before the interview. Among AIAN-only persons, 59.5% (95% CI = 55.6, 63.5) reported doing any kind of work, as did 59.3% (95% CI = 54.4, 64.2) of AIAN-other persons. By contrast, the proportion was higher among AIAN-Hispanic (71.1%; 95% CI = 65.1, 77.1) and Hispanic (71.3%; 95% CI = 70.2, 72.5) persons, as well as non-Hispanic White persons (65.6%; 95% CI = 65.0, 66.3). Compared with all non-Indigenous participants, both AIAN-only and AIAN-other subgroups had significantly lower odds of participating in the labor force after adjusting for age, education, and sex (Table 4).

Compensation

Our analysis of income-level and income source indicators showed that the AIAN-only subgroup had the largest proportion (26.9%; 95% CI = 14.3, 39.5) with a family income below the federal poverty threshold (as determined by the National Center for Health Statistics in 2020–2022). Of current AIAN-only workers, more than one third (35.9%; 95% CI = 24.2, 47.6) had a family income below 200% the poverty threshold (Table 2). This figure was even higher in AIAN-Hispanic individuals, with 40.0% (95% CI = 30.0, 50.1) of current workers having a family income below the 200% poverty line. A large proportion of both the AIAN-only (25.8%; 95% CI = 13.3, 38.4) and the AIAN-other (17.3%; 95% CI = 13.8, 20.7) subgroups reported income from social security disability insurance.

In the adjusted model controlling for age, sex, and education, all 3 Indigenous groups had substantially higher odds of earning below 200% of the federal poverty level compared with all other races/ethnicities (Table 4).

Health Care Access and Employment Benefits

Employed Indigenous workers were less likely than were non-Indigenous workers to receive paid sick leave and health insurance from their workplace (Table 2). Of those who reported currently working, the Hispanic and AIAN-Hispanic groups had the lowest rates of employer-provided health insurance at 58.0% (95% CI = 49.0, 67.0), whereas the non-Hispanic White group had the highest rates of employer-provided health insurance (71.4%; 95% CI = 70.6, 72.1). AIAN-only workers (69.4%; 95% CI = 63.1, 75.7) and AIAN-other workers (66.6%; 95% CI = 60.0, 73.2) did not have a significantly lower proportion of health insurance than non-Hispanic White workers.

TABLE 2— Working Characteristics of Adults by Race/Ethnicity: National Health Interview Survey, United States, 2020–2022

Characteristic	AIAN-Only (Unweighted n = 558), % (95% CI)	AIAN-Hispanic (Unweighted n = 304), % (95% CI)	AIAN-Other (Unweighted n = 653), % (95% CI)	Hispanic (Unweighted n = 11 553), % (95% CI)	Non-Hispanic White (Unweighted n = 59 990), % (95% CI)
Worked last week					
Yes	48.7 (41.9, 55.6)	59.3 (52.2, 66.4)	52.1 (46.9, 57.2)	64.4 (63.2, 65.6)	59.4 (58.7, 60.1)
No	45.9 (39.0, 52.9)	34.4 (27.4, 41.5)	43.0 (37.8, 48.2)	31.2 (30.0, 32.4)	37.6 (36.9, 38.2)
Missing	5.3 (3.3, 7.3)	6.3 (2.8, 9.8)	4.9 (2.8, 7.0)	4.4 (3.9, 4.9)	3.0 (2.8, 3.3)
Labor force participation (worked last week or looking for work)	54.5 (48.9, 60.2)	64.4 (57.7, 71.2)	55.1 (50.1, 60.1)	68.0 (66.8, 69.2)	61.3 (60.6, 62.0)
Working or worked past 12 mo	59.5 (55.6, 63.5)	71.1 (65.1, 77.1)	59.3 (54.4, 64.2)	71.3 (70.2, 72.5)	65.6 (65.0, 66.3)
Main reason for not working					
Looking for work, laid off, unemployed	12.6 (8.3, 16.8)	15.0 (2.5, 27.5)[a]	7.1 (3.0, 11.2)	11.6 (10.2, 13.1)	5.2 (4.7, 5.6)
Retired	28.3 (22.0, 34.7)	21.4 (13.0, 29.9)	38.0 (31.9, 44.0)	29.2 (27.5, 30.9)	60.4 (59.4, 61.4)
Unable, health reasons	25.2 (14.3, 36.1)	15.7 (8.2, 23.1)	30.6 (23.5, 37.7)	15.9 (14.4, 17.4)	14.7 (14.0, 15.4)
Taking care of house or family	16.6 (7.6, 25.5)	24.9 (14.7, 35.1)	10.2 (6.3, 14.0)	25.7 (23.8, 27.6)	9.7 (9.2, 10.3)
Other	17.3 (10.4, 24.1)	20.8 (7.7, 34.0)[a]	14.2 (8.6, 19.8)	17.3 (15.5, 19.2)	10.0 (9.3, 10.6)
Missing		2.2 (0.0, 6.4)		0.2 (0.0, 0.4)	0.1 (0.0, 0.2)
Number of family members aged ≥ 18 y working last week					
0	28.9 (21.3, 36.5)	22.0 (16.1, 27.8)	29.2 (25.0, 33.4)	13.9 (13.1, 14.7)	25.4 (24.8, 26.0)
1	31.9 (26.9, 36.8)	31.9 (25.4, 38.5)	34.9 (30.3, 39.5)	31.0 (30.0, 32.1)	31.5 (31.0, 32.0)
≥ 2	36.9 (31.3, 42.4)	41.1 (33.9, 48.3)	34.1 (29.1, 39.1)	52.7 (51.3, 54.1)	41.6 (40.9, 42.2)
Of those who worked last week					
Usually work ≥ 35 h per week	79.1 (74.5, 83.7)	77.6 (69.2, 86.0)	83.3 (78.5, 88.1)	79.9 (78.7, 81.1)	81.2 (80.6, 81.8)
Paid sick leave	68.6 (63.0, 74.2)	51.9 (42.5, 61.2)	61.4 (54.7, 68.0)	60.5 (58.8, 62.2)	68.3 (67.5, 69.0)
Health insurance at job	69.4 (63.1, 75.7)	58.0 (49.0, 67.0)	66.6 (60.0, 73.2)	60.1 (58.6, 61.7)	71.4 (70.6, 72.1)
Family income < 200% poverty threshold[b]	35.9 (24.2, 47.6)	40.0 (30.0, 50.1)	32.1 (25.1, 39.1)	37.7 (36.0, 39.3)	13.0 (12.4, 13.6)

Note. AIAN = American Indian/Alaska Native; CI = confidence interval.
[a]Coefficient of variation = 0.3–0.5.
[b]As determined by National Center for Health Statistics in 2020–2022.

In the adjusted model controlling for age, sex, and education, the lower odds of workplace health insurance for the AIAN-Hispanic group was borderline nonsignificant compared with all other races/ethnicities (Table 4). Similarly, in the adjusted model controlling for age, sex, and education, the odds of having paid sick leave for those with an AIAN-Hispanic background was borderline nonsignificantly less than all other races/ethnicities (Table 4).

Industry and Occupation

Among participants who reported working during the past year, the most common industry for the AIAN-only subgroup was accommodation and food services (15.9%; 95% CI = 7.6, 24.2). The health care and social assistance industries were the most common industry in both the AIAN-Hispanic (12.3%; 95% CI = 5.4, 19.3) and AIAN-other (12.7%; 95% CI = 7.3, 18.2) subgroups. Results comparing industry and occupation data by race/ethnicity can be found in the "Industry and Occupation Results" section of the appendix (available as a supplement to the online version of this article at http://www.ajph.org).

DISCUSSION

The 3 Indigenous groups in the NHIS survey (i.e., AIAN-only, AIAN-Hispanic, AIAN-other) are very different population groups with respect to employment

TABLE 3— **Top 6 Industries and Occupations for Indigenous Workers by Indigenous Subgroup: National Health Interview Survey, United States, 2020–2021**

	Occupations		Industries	
Rank	**% (95% CI)**	**Occupation**	**% (95% CI)**	**Industry**
AIAN-only[a]				
1	13.5 (5.4, 21.5)	office and administrative support occupations[b]	15.9 (7.6, 24.2)	accommodation and food services industries
2	9.4 (5.8, 13.0)	building/grounds cleaning/maintenance occupations	13.8 (10.3, 17.4)	health care and social assistance industries
3	7.5 (3.8, 11.2)	management occupations	10.9 (6.3, 15.5)	public administration industries
4	7.3 (3.4, 11.2)	health care support occupations	9.8 (5.4, 14.1)	construction industries
5	6.9 (3.6, 10.1)	food preparation/serving related occupations	8.5 (1.0, 16.0)	retail trade industries[b]
6	5.2 (0.3, 10.1)	construction and extraction occupations[b]	7.0 (2.7, 11.3)	education services industries[b]
AIAN-Hispanic[c]				
1	13.8 (2.4, 25.1)	production occupations[b]	12.3 (5.4, 19.3)	health care and social assistance industries
2	11.1 (3.8, 18.4)	transportation/material moving occupations[b]	11.9 (1, 22.7)	administrative and support and waste management and remediation services industries[b]
3	8.7 (2.8, 14.6)	office and administrative support occupations[b]	9.9 (2.1, 17.6)	manufacturing industries[b]
4	8.5 (1.7, 15.4)	building/grounds cleaning/maintenance occupations[b]	9.1 (3.4, 14.7)	construction industries[b]
5	7.9 (2.4, 13.5)	management occupations[b]	8.4 (1.7, 15.2)	retail trade industries[b]
6	7.5 (2.2, 12.8)	construction and extraction occupations[b]	7.2 (3.1, 11.3)	education services industries
AIAN-other[d]				
1	16.4 (10.7, 22.2)	office and administrative support occupations	12.7 (7.3, 18.2)	health care and social assistance industries
2	11.0 (5.2, 16.8)	management occupations	11.2 (6.5, 15.8)	manufacturing industries
3	10.2 (5.6, 14.7)	transportation and material moving occupations	11.1 (5.8, 16.4)	accommodation and food services industries
4	9.1 (4.2, 14.1)	food preparation and serving related occupations	10 (5.5, 14.4)	retail trade industries
5	7.9 (4.4, 11.4)	sales and related occupations	8.7 (4.1, 13.2)	construction industries
6	6.1 (2.6, 9.6)	production occupations	7.1 (3.9, 10.3)	education services industries

Note. AIAN = American Indian/Alaska Native; CI = confidence interval.
[a]Unweighted n = 210.
[b]Coefficient of variation = 0.3–0.5.
[c]Unweighted n = 122.
[d]Unweighted n = 254.

quality. The AIAN-only group appears to be those born in US territories who are entitled to federal and state protections but have different employment needs and social determinants of health that may limit their access to resources such as health care and education.

The AIAN-Hispanic group was a unique group, with nearly one third of this national sample born outside the United States. Our analysis detailed a group with a high number of immigrants with less education, potentially including undocumented workers, who may be subject to prejudice as immigrants and be shunted into high-risk, low-wage jobs without benefits because of language and legal barriers.[24] This group potentially includes Indigenous groups from Latin America; further research is required to understand the makeup of this group. We identified the quality of employment, including access to regular full-time work and health benefits (e.g., paid sick leave, health insurance), as occupational inequities for this group, with worse

TABLE 4— Multivariable Model Evaluating Employment Characteristics Between Indigenous and Non-Indigenous Groups: National Health Interview Survey, United States, 2020–2022

	OR (95% CI)			
Multivariable Models[a]	Non-Indigenous (Ref)	AIAN-Only	AIAN-Hispanic	AIAN-Other
Model A: worked last week[b]	1	0.62 (0.45, 0.86)	0.96 (0.61, 1.52)	0.72 (0.57, 0.90)
Model B: labor force participation[c]	1	0.70 (0.53, 0.91)	0.95 (0.62, 1.45)	0.71 (0.57, 0.88)
Model C: family income below 200% poverty line[c]	1	2.36 (1.42, 3.91)	1.87 (1.36, 2.56)	2.06 (1.60, 2.65)
Model D: working with health insurance[d]	1	1.02 (0.73, 1.43)	0.74 (0.52, 1.06)	0.85 (0.64, 1.13)
Model E: working with sick leave[e]	1	1.08 (0.82, 1.43)	0.70 (0.48, 1.01)	0.85 (0.65, 1.10)
Model F: employment in high-risk occupation[f]	1	0.97 (0.70, 1.33)	0.98 (0.56, 1.72)	0.94 (0.64, 1.39)
Model G: employment in high-risk industry[f]	1	1.44 (0.97, 2.13)	1.07 (0.62, 1.84)	0.96 (0.67, 1.35)

Note. AIAN = American Indian/Alaska Native; CI = confidence interval; OR = odds ratio.
[a]Models adjusted for sex, age group, and education.
[b]Unweighted n = 85 162.
[c]Unweighted n = 88 244. Poverty line determined by the National Center for Health Statistics in 2020–2022.
[d]Unweighted n = 51 671.
[e]Unweighted n = 51 432.
[f]Unweighted n = 36 788, models F and G used only 2020 and 2021 National Health Interview Survey cycles.

employment conditions than those of the Hispanic comparison group.

The AIAN-other group resided in a more urban setting than did the AIAN-only group, more commonly resided in the US South or Midwest, and had attained a higher level of post–high school education. The ability to remain in the workforce appeared to be considerably affected by health issues in this group, and access to culturally appropriate health services may have been problematic.

Access to Employment

Using a nationally representative sample, we found that Indigenous groups were less likely to participate in the US labor force, with inequities in employment quality compared with other racial/ethnic groups. The disproportionate share of AIAN-only and AIAN-other subgroups who were not working specifically because of health reasons requires further examination. The role of excess morbidity and mortality, along with the specific physiological health parameters required for certain jobs, needs further investigation, particularly in relation to the number and quality of jobs available to Indigenous adults with underlying disabilities and chronic health conditions.

Characterizing the Workforce

In our analysis, the health care and social assistance industries ranked among the top 2 employment sectors for all 3 Indigenous subgroups, with each group having more than 12% of its workforce employed in these industries. In these industries, the AIAN-only subgroup was the only Indigenous group to record a health care occupation (i.e., health care support workers) in their top 6 occupation categories. Of note, for all races/ethnicities, health care support workers had the highest incidence of nonfatal occupational injuries and illnesses involving days away from work in 2020 of all occupation groups, at 360.1 per 10 000 full-time equivalent workers.[25] This period coincided with the first 12 months of the COVID-19 pandemic in the United States.

Having detailed occupational data on the AIAN groups would have aided policy and prevention efforts for Indigenous people in the early stages of the COVID-19 pandemic, when they had disproportionately high rates of COVID-19.[26] The health care industry will provide an important future area of occupational health research for Indigenous workers; however, this would need to include not only health professionals but also administration staff, maintenance workers, groundskeepers, and all other occupations in which Indigenous workers are likely disproportionately employed. Food preparation workers, servers, and maids were high-risk jobs for COVID-19 transmission during the pandemic, which would have disproportionality affected AIAN-only workers, who had increased workers in this industry.[27]

To our knowledge, there have been no studies conducted examining the occupational psychosocial or biological hazards for Indigenous workers in the health care industry in the United States or abroad.[28] The mining, construction, and transportation industries may allow specific partnerships with communities and other stakeholders in these employment groups to further explore Indigenous occupational health outcomes.

Quality of Work

The United States may be the only developed country to not have a national paid sick leave policy.[29] This is especially important for Indigenous workers, who experience disproportionately high rates of adverse health conditions compared with other racial/ethnic groups in the United States.[30] This makes AIAN individuals far more likely to require days off work, private physician consultations, and hospitalizations. The United States also lacks universal health care coverage, which disproportionally affects Indigenous people. In 2019, the percentage of those who identified as AIAN-only and reported no health insurance coverage was nearly 3-fold higher than that of non-Hispanic White individuals (14.90% vs 6.30%), and AIAN-only persons had lower rates of private health coverage than did non-Hispanic White persons (51.9% vs 74.7%).[31] With most US AIAN individuals today living in metropolitan areas, the location of most Indian Health Service sites has become a significant barrier to accessing health care.

Future Research

A review of the current definitions of race/ethnicity under the US directive on standards for the classification of federal data on race and ethnicity[32] is required given the limitations of their current format. As a next step, community-based participatory research approaches should be broadly introduced into Indigenous occupational health research to grow community skills in this area, empower community leaders, ensure veracity of results, and ultimately lead to improved occupational health policies and outcomes. Investment in training future Indigenous health researchers in this area would improve the quality of the research as well.

Limitations

This study has several limitations. First, NHIS estimates are based on self-reported employment status, and there are no comparison estimates from the Bureau of Labor Statistics for the Indigenous subgroups to validate our reported estimates. Second, there are numerous important factors not consistently identified in survey cycles—specifically, information on employment quality, including shift work, employment stability, current worker rights, cultural safety, and training and health promotion—which limits information on the current quality of self-reported employment.

Third we based our risk stratification of occupation and industry on national data that may not have been representative of the risk in Indigenous populations and across regions; however, studies have consistently demonstrated that high-risk industries and occupations have been shown to have increased injuries and illnesses among minority workers.[33] Fourth, the similarities between AIAN-Hispanic individuals and Hispanic individuals in terms of employment characteristics suggest that these 2 subgroups may represent a single group (i.e., Indigenous people who migrated from Latin America), rather than intermarried American Indians who originated in the United States. Immigration status is an important confounder for employment. Finally, national survey designs may be problematic for sampling small minority subpopulations, particularly AIAN adults, who are geographically clustered in some areas (e.g., rural Indian reservations) and dispersed and geographically invisible in other areas (e.g., urban centers).

Conclusions

Our findings demonstrate that there are 3 very different Indigenous worker populations that need to be addressed separately in future Indigenous occupational health research and strategic planning. The ability to report more detailed information on each of these 3 Indigenous groups would allow tailored research, policies, partnerships, and community-led occupational health and safety responses that align with the inaugural National Institute for Occupational Safety and Health's AIAN Worker Safety and Health Strategic Plan[3]; this needs to be carefully balanced with protecting privacy and confidentiality in future work. AJPH

ABOUT THE AUTHORS

Brett Shannon, Chibuzor Abasilim, Kirsten S. Almberg, Tessa Bonney, Linda Forst, and Lee S. Friedman are with the Division of Environmental and Occupational Health Sciences, School of Public Health, University of Illinois, Chicago. Courtney Ryder is with the College of Medicine and Public Health, Flinders University, Adelaide, Australia.

CORRESPONDENCE

Correspondence should be sent to Brett Shannon, Environmental and Occupational Health Sciences, School of Public Health, University of Illinois Chicago, 1603 W. Taylor St, Chicago, IL 60612 (e-mail: bshann3@uic.edu). Reprints can be ordered at https://www.ajph.org by clicking the "Reprints" link.

PUBLICATION INFORMATION

Full Citation: Shannon B, Ryder C, Abasilim C, et al. Occupational determinants of health and well-being for Indigenous populations in the United States—findings from the National Health Interview Survey, 2020–2022. *Am J Public Health*. 2025;115(5):736–746.

Acceptance Date: November 20, 2024.

DOI: https://doi.org/10.2105/AJPH.2024.307959

ORCID iDs:

Brett Shannon https://orcid.org/0000-0002-6257-5315

Chibuzor Abasilim https://orcid.org/0000-0002-8150-9970

Linda Forst https://orcid.org/0000-0003-4966-1929

Lee S. Friedman https://orcid.org/0000-0001-9312-6099

CONTRIBUTORS

B. Shannon and L. Friedman conceptualized and designed the study, conducted the analysis, reviewed the literature, and interpreted the data. B. Shannon, C. Ryder, C. Abasilim, K. S. Almberg, T. Bonney, and L. Forst, and L. Friedman drafted and revised the article. C. Ryder, C. Abasilim, K. S. Almberg, T. Bonney, and L. Forst contributed to the literature review. All authors approved the final version.

ACKNOWLEDGMENTS

B. Shannon is an Australian Aboriginal physician who received PhD funding from the John Monash Foundation, the American-Australian Association, and the Roberta Sykes Foundation.

Through this work, his aim is to support Indigenous and local community-led efforts in occupational health both in the United States and internationally.

CONFLICTS OF INTEREST

The authors have no conflicts of interest in regards to this study.

HUMAN PARTICIPANT PROTECTION

This study was considered nonhuman participants research, and the University of Illinois, Chicago institutional review board approved this work (no. 2023-0959).

REFERENCES

1. World Health Organization. A conceptual framework for action on the social determinants of health. 2010. Available at: https://iris.who.int/bitstream/handle/10665/44489/9789241500852_eng.pdf?sequence=1. Accessed February 15, 2024.
2. Australian Institute of Health and Welfare. Aboriginal and Torres Strait Islander health performance measures. 2020. Available at: https://www.indigenoushpf.gov.au/measures/2-07-employment. Accessed February 15, 2024.
3. Centers for Disease Control and Prevention. American Indian and Alaska Native Worker Safety and Health Strategic Plan. 2023. Available at: https://www.cdc.gov/niosh/docs/2023-123. Accessed February 15, 2024.
4. US Department of Labor, Bureau of Labor Statistics. Labor force characteristics by race and ethnicity, 2020. November 2021. Available at: https://www.bls.gov/opub/reports/race-and-ethnicity/2020/home.htm. Accessed February 16, 2024.
5. Austin A. Native Americans and jobs: the challenge and the promise. 2013. Available at: https://www.epi.org/publication/bp370-native-americans-jobs. Accessed February 16, 2024.
6. Oddo VM, Zhuang CC, Andrea SB, et al. Changes in precarious employment in the United States: a longitudinal analysis. *Scand J Work Environ Health*. 2021;47(3):171–180. https://doi.org/10.5271/sjweh.3939
7. US Census Bureau. American Community Survey 2017–2021 5-year data release. Available at: https://www.census.gov/newsroom/press-kits/2022/acs-5-year.html. Accessed February 16, 2024.
8. Bureau of Labor Statistics. Unemployment rate for American Indians and Alaska Natives at 7.9 percent in December 2021. January 26, 2022. Available at: https://www.bls.gov/opub/ted/2022/unemployment-rate-for-american-indians-and-alaska-natives-at-7-9-percent-in-december-2021.htm. Accessed September 12, 2024.
9. Henseke G. Good jobs, good pay, better health? The effects of job quality on health among older European workers. *Eur J Health Econ*. 2018;19(1):59–73. https://doi.org/10.1007/s10198-017-0867-9
10. Waddell G, Burton AK. *Is Work Good for Your Health and Well-Being?* 2006. Available at: https://cardinal-management.co.uk/wp-content/uploads/2016/04/Burton-Waddell-is-work-good-for-you.pdf. Accessed February 5, 2025.
11. Fujishiro K, Ahonen EQ, Winkler M. Investigating employment quality for population health and health equity: a perspective of power. *Int J Environ Res Public Health*. 2022;19(16):9991. https://doi.org/10.3390/ijerph19169991
12. Peckham T, Fujishiro K, Hajat A, Flaherty BP, Seixas N. Evaluating employment quality as a determinant of health in a changing labor market. *RSF*. 2019;5(4):258–281. https://doi.org/10.7758/RSF.2019.5.4.09
13. Bellisle D, Dickson A, Fugiel P, Golden L, Petrucci L, Bruno R. A good job, not just any job: defining and measuring employment quality in Illinois. September 1, 2022.Available at: https://lep.illinois.edu/wp-content/uploads/2022/09/A-Good-Job-Not-Just-Any-Job-9_1_22.pdf. Accessed February 15, 2024.
14. Gallup Inc. How COVID-19 affected the quality of work. Available at: https://www.gallup.com/education/267590/great-jobs-lumina-gates-omidyar-gallup-quality-report-2019.aspx. Accessed February 16, 2024.
15. Schultz R, Abbott T, Yamaguchi J, Cairney S. Injury prevention through employment as a priority for wellbeing among Aboriginal people in remote Australia. *Health Promot J Austr*. 2018;29(2):183–188. https://doi.org/10.1002/hpja.7
16. Centers for Disease Control and Prevention. National Health Interview Survey. Available at: https://www.cdc.gov/nchs/nhis/index.html. Accessed February 16, 2024.
17. Rose D. 2010 National Conference on Health Statistics: Exploring NHIS data by census division. Available at: https://www.cdc.gov/nchs/ppt/nchs2010/24_rose.pdf. Accessed February 16, 2024.
18. Centers for Disease Control and Prevention. NCHS urban–rural classification scheme for counties. Available at: https://www.cdc.gov/nchs/data-analysis-tools/urban-rural.html?CDC_AAref_Val=https://www.cdc.gov/nchs/data_access/urban_rural.htm. Accessed February 16, 2024.
19. US Census Bureau. North American industry classification system. Available at: https://www.census.gov/naics. Accessed February 5, 2025.
20. Bureau of Labor Statistics. Standard occupational classification. Available at: https://www.bls.gov/soc/2018/home.htm. Accessed February 16, 2024.
21. Bureau of Labor Statistics. Number and rate of nonfatal work injuries and illnesses in private industries. Available at: https://www.bls.gov/charts/injuries-and-illnesses/number-and-rate-of-nonfatal-work-injuries-and-illnesses-by-industry.htm. Accessed February 16, 2024.
22. Bureau of Labor Statistics. Injuries, illnesses, and fatalities. Available at: https://www.bls.gov/iif/nonfatal-injuries-and-illnesses-tables.htm. Accessed February 16, 2024.
23. Bureau of Labor Statistics. Table R98: Incidence rates for nonfatal occupational injuries and illnesses involving days away from work per 10, 000 full time workers by occupation and selected nature of injury or illness, private industry, 2020. Available at: https://www.bls.gov/web/osh/cd_r98.htm. Accessed February 16, 2024.
24. Pillai D, Artiga S. Employment among immigrants and implications for health and health care. June 12, 2023. Available at: www.kff.org/racial-equity-and-health-policy/issue-brief/employment-among-immigrants-and-implications-for-health-and-health-care. Accessed February 16, 2024.
25. Bureau of Labor Statistics. SNR05. Injury cases—rates, counts, and percent relative standard errors—detailed industry. Available at: https://www.bls.gov/iif/nonfatal-injuries-and-illnesses-tables.htm. Accessed February 16, 2024.
26. Centers for Disease Control and Prevention. COVID-19 among American Indian and Alaska Native persons—23 states, January 31–July 3, 2020. *MMWR Morb Mortal Wkly Rep*. 2020;69(34):1166–1169. https://doi.org/10.15585/mmwr.mm6934e1
27. Goldman N, Pebley AR, Lee K, Andrasfay T, Pratt B. Racial and ethnic differentials in COVID-19–related job exposures by occupational standing in the US. *medRxiv* [Preprint: 2021;2020.11.13.20231431; Update in: *PLoS One*. 2021;16(9):e0256085. https://doi.org/10.1371/journal.pone.0256085]. https://doi.org/10.1101/2020.11.13.20231431
28. Shannon B, Jennings W, Friedman L. Systematic scoping review of occupational health injuries

and illnesses among Indigenous workers. *Occup Environ Med* [Epub ahead of print: July 18, 2022]. https://doi.org/10.1136/oemed-2022-108264

29. US Department of Labor. Paid leave. Available at: https://www.dol.gov/agencies/wb/featured-paid-leave. Accessed February 16, 2024.
30. Indian Health Service. Disparities. October 2019. Available at: https://www.ihs.gov/newsroom/factsheets/disparities. Accessed February 5, 2025.
31. Office of Minority Health. American Indian/Alaska Native health. 2022. Available at: https://minorityhealth.hhs.gov/american-indianalaska-native-health. Accessed February 16, 2024.
32. Office of Management and Budget. Standards for maintaining, collecting, and presenting federal data on race and ethnicity. *Fed Regist.* 1997; 62(210):58788–58790. Available at: https://www.govinfo.gov/content/pkg/FR-1997-10-30/pdf/97-28653.pdf. Accessed February 16, 2024.
33. Seabury SA, Terp S, Boden LI. Racial and ethnic differences in the frequency of workplace injuries and prevalence of work-related disability. *Health Aff (Millwood)*. 2017;36(2):266–273. https://doi.org/10.1377/hlthaff.2016.1185

Polysubstance Use Profiles Among the General Adult Population, United States, 2022

Karilynn M. Rockhill, PhD, MPH, Joshua C. Black, PhD, Janetta Iwanicki, PhD, and Alison Abraham, PhD, MS, MHS

See also Xu et al., p. 646.

Objectives. To characterize present-day polysubstance use patterns in the general adult population.

Methods. From a 2022 nationally representative survey in the United States, we defined polysubstance use as last 12-month use of 2 or more drugs (n = 15 800). Latent class analyses included medical (as indicated) and nonmedical (not as directed) use of prescription opioids, stimulants, benzodiazepines, and antidepressants; recreational use of cannabis, psilocybin or mushrooms, other psychedelics, cocaine, methamphetamine, and illicit opioids; and concomitant use with alcohol, cannabis, prescriptions, or recreational drugs.

Results. The national prevalence of polysubstance use was 20.9% (95% confidence interval = 20.5%, 21.3%), broken down into the following 4 latent classes: (1) medically guided polysubstance use (11.5% prevalence, 6.1% substance use disorder [SUD]): prescribed drug use, some cannabis, and no concomitant use; (2) principal cannabis use variety (4.0% prevalence, 31.9% SUD): high probability of cannabis use with various drugs concomitantly used; (3) self-guided polysubstance use (3.4% prevalence, 14.5% SUD): nonmedical use of prescriptions and concomitant use; and (4) indiscriminate coexposures (2.1% prevalence, 58.9% SUD): concomitant drug use with indiscriminate drug preference.

Conclusions. Different polysubstance profiles show adults with untreated SUDs, and there are 2 previously unrecognized classes. Prevention and treatment strategies addressing polysubstance use should take a personalized perspective and tailor to individuals' use profile. (*Am J Public Health*. 2025; 115(5):747–757. https://doi.org/10.2105/AJPH.2024.307979)

AJPH May 2025, Vol. 115, No. 5

Polysubstance use of psychoactive drugs is a complex behavioral pattern described as use of multiple substances over one's lifetime or over the same timeframe, with inclusion of both prescription and recreational drugs.[1,2] Polysubstance use is a driver of morbidity and mortality in the United States. It is associated with increased risk of substance use disorders (SUDs).[3] In 2022, an estimated 40.3 million people experienced an SUD while only 6.5% received treatment.[4] Polysubstance use is also associated with unmet physical and mental health care needs,[5] poor SUD treatment retention or relapse,[2] increased risky behaviors (i.e., injection drug use or binge drinking[5]), and increased risk for overdose and death.[6] Opioid- and psychostimulant-related mortality has received the most attention given its contribution to the rise in overdose deaths.[7] However, an extensive review of US overdose death certificates indicated that an average of 2.4 drugs contributed to the cause of death, with many drugs involved (e.g., sedatives, antidepressants, antipsychotics).[8] Some research has signaled that the fourth wave of the overdose epidemic will be defined by death caused by co-involvement of multiple drugs.[9–11]

To better understand the complexity of polysubstance use, previous research has largely focused on either tabulations of common combinations[4] or latent class methods. Latent class methods are useful for identifying underlying subpopulations based on observed behaviors.[12] Two systematic reviews of polysubstance latent class profiles were conducted among adolescents in 2016[13] and among young adults in 2022.[14] These studies observed 2 common latent classes, a no use or single use of drugs or a predominately alcohol use with or without tobacco use.[13,14] Most studies included found only a low-prevalence polysubstance use class. de Jonge et al. concluded that discerning polysubstance use patterns was difficult when a study included highly prevalent behaviors like no use or single drug use groups, or alcohol or tobacco use; the authors recommended that future studies consider removing these behaviors to capture more nuanced polysubstance use behaviors.[14] Furthermore, few studies differentiated between prescription drug classes or nonmedical use (NMU) behaviors. This study directly addressed these previous limitations.

The objective of this study was to delineate polysubstance use patterns across psychoactive drugs and explore the associated risk profiles. No nationally representative study has looked at the general adult population to quantify and describe the totality of polysubstance use behaviors across multiple psychoactive drugs. The present-day patterns need to be more fully described to understand new populations that may be amenable to clinical or public health intervention if necessary. This research categorized polysubstance use behaviors by expanding the inclusion of drug types explored and differentiating prescription and recreational drug behaviors.[14] We also independently assessed profiles among those with and without likely SUDs.

METHODS

This research utilized a nationally representative survey of adults (aged ≥ 18 years) from the Survey of Non-Medical Use of Prescription Drugs (NMURx) Program, part of the Researched Abuse, Diversion and Addiction-Related Surveillance (RADARS) System. Details about this survey can be found elsewhere, including its reliability and concurrent validity of drug use estimates compared to multiple national surveys.[15] Briefly, NMURx is a semiannual, repeated, cross-sectional study consisting of a self-administered, confidential, online survey that measures drug use behaviors in all 50 states and Washington, DC. Importantly, it utilizes a calibration weighting scheme that corrects for any selection and nonresponse bias across both demographic and health measures to generate representative estimates. Data from 2022 (n = 59 041) collected across the 2 waves (April 15–June 3 and September 9–October 21) was used.

The survey collected behavioral information in the last 12 months across both prescription and recreational drugs. Respondents were asked about any use of 4 prescription drug classes (opioids, antidepressants, benzodiazepines, and stimulants) followed by NMU, defined as "use not directed by a health care professional." Other behavioral questions surrounding prescription drug use were concomitant (simultaneous) use with other drugs and drug sourcing (e.g., from own health care provider). The survey collected cannabis use, including use of marijuana, hashish, or any other preparation of the plant, but did not differentiate reason for use. Finally, questions on recreational or illicit drug use were asked as well as concomitant use with other drugs.

Measures and Definitions

We defined polysubstance use as any use of 2 or more of the following drugs in the last 12 months (n = 15 863): prescription opioids, prescription benzodiazepines, prescription stimulants, prescription antidepressants, cannabis, methamphetamine, cocaine powder, psilocybin or mushrooms, other psychedelics (including ketamine, lysergic acid diethylamide [LSD], 3,4-methylenedioxymethamphetamine [MDMA], mescaline, or phencyclidine [PCP]), or illicit opioids (including heroin, fentanyl, or fentanyl analogues). Prescription benzodiazepines and antidepressants were not commonly included in other studies, but drugs that affect the central nervous system can have abuse potential[16] and therefore we included them to be more comprehensive of dispensing in the general population. The recreational drugs included the most common used in the general population; inclusion of rarer drugs likely would not facilitate further delineation of behavioral profiles. We did not include alcohol and tobacco in the definition per previous research suggestions to understand more nuanced profiles.[14] We included concomitant drug use (simultaneous) as an additional behavior, defined by report of each drug listed here being used at the same time as alcohol, cannabis, recreational drugs, or other psychoactive prescriptions.

In addition, we collected information on demographics and other risk factors (e.g., drug treatment history, mental health diagnoses). The survey included the Drug Abuse Screening Test (DAST-10), a validated self-administered instrument measuring severity of problematic drug use found to discriminate well (scores ≥ 3) for patients with drug use disorders with or without diagnoses.[17,18] We used this measure as a proxy for likely SUD because the instrument has several beneficial characteristics: it can discriminate SUD without diagnoses, it is agnostic to which drugs are used, it can be used to compare people using different drugs,[19] and it intentionally excludes alcohol use disorder.

Statistical Analysis

We conducted a latent class analysis (LCA) of drug use behaviors exhibited in the last 12 months to identify subgroups among the population who reported polysubstance use. LCA takes a person-centered approach, examining patterns in the data and characterizing individuals into mutually exclusive groups.[12] The contribution to the models of both the drug used (individual drug indicators) and situational behaviors (medical use vs NMU, concomitant use) defined patterns of polysubstance use.

We classified the LCA model indicators as follows: (1) prescription drugs were treated as a 3-level categorical variable with NMU taking priority, then medical use, then no use; (2) cannabis and recreational drugs were treated as dichotomous use versus no use; and (3) concomitant use was summarized across any reported drug (if any drugs were used with alcohol then an indicator for concomitant alcohol use was included). Sample size considerations are evolving, but studies have posed that 300 or more observations per class is desirable.[20,21] Our sample size was therefore well powered to detect up to 5 latent classes.[22]

No a priori number of latent classes were assumed, and we determined model selection by evaluating model separation through goodness of fit tests using Bayesian Information Criterion in addition to qualitative model interpretability.[12,21] We reported other model fit and diagnostics based on best practices: Akaike Information Criterion, G^2 statistic, log-likelihood, smallest class size, entropy, and average posterior probabilities.[21] We incorporated the individual-level design weights from NMURx into the class estimation through the pseudo-maximum likelihood approach.[23] The chosen model was interpreted qualitatively based on the class probabilities and item-response probabilities.[12] We calculated posterior probabilities based on Bayes' Theorem and assigned individuals to the class with the highest probability.[24] We calculated proportions of demographics and other risk factors among the latent classes. Based on individual best class assignment, we used the weighted entire NMURx data to calculate prevalence of no drug use, single drug use, and each of the polysubstance use classes.

Finally, we were interested in a stratified analysis comparing LCA profiles among those with (n = 3473) and without (n = 12 390) likely SUD based on the DAST-10 (defined by scores ≥ 3 and < 3, respectively). We calculated measurement invariance across groups using a likelihood ratio test.[23] We estimated item-response probabilities independently within each SUD group. Given the cross-sectional nature of the survey, this approach was taken to generate independent latent profiles by SUD.

Given the online survey nature, respondents were required to answer all questions so that there were no item-level missing data. We conducted all analyses in SAS version 9.4 (Cary, NC).

RESULTS

Among adults in the United States in 2022, the prevalence of polysubstance use of 2 or more of the most common prescription and recreational drugs based on our definition was 20.9% (95% confidence interval [CI] = 20.5%, 21.3%), whereas the prevalence of use of only 1 drug was 26.5% (95% CI = 26.1%, 27.0%) and the prevalence of no drug use was 52.6% (95% CI = 52.1%, 53.1%). Compared to all adults, those using multiple drugs had higher proportions who self-reported being female, of White race, having annual household incomes of less than $50 000, and being current health care professionals or students (Table 1). Adults using multiple drugs also had higher proportions with a history of the mental health diagnoses, experience of acute or chronic pain, and use of alcohol or tobacco. Additionally, 17.6% of adults using multiple drugs had a likely SUD compared to 4.1% among those who used only a single drug.

Among the adults using multiple drugs, the most common behaviors included prescription opioid and antidepressant use (63.9% and 57.8%, respectively), followed by cannabis use (56.2%), then the remaining prescription drug classes (39.7% for benzodiazepines and 21.3% for stimulants), whereas all recreational drugs accounted for 8.7% or less (Table 1).

Latent Class Findings

The 4-latent-class model resulted in the best fit by Bayesian Information Criterion (Table A, which includes all diagnostics; available as a supplement to the online version of this article at http://www.ajph.org); models with more than 4 classes did not converge on a single solution. This 4-class model had an entropy of 0.83; entropy values of 0.8 or higher are acceptable, and it indicates how well the model defines the classes.[21] The average posterior class probability was 0.91, indicating that there was high certainty across individuals for class assignment, where 0.9 or higher is ideal.[21] After examination of the model inputs and the prevalence estimates, the following

TABLE 1— Weighted Characteristics of Total Adult Population vs Polysubstance Use Population: United States, 2022

Characteristics	Total Adult Population	Polysubstance Use
Unweighted no.	59 041	15 800
Estimated weighted no.	259 008 600	54 044 600
Age, y, mean (95% CI)	47.6 (47.4, 47.7)	44.3 (43.9, 44.6)
Male, % (95% CI)	51.2 (50.7, 51.7)	43.9 (42.9, 44.9)
Self-reported race,[a] % (95% CI)		
White	79.1 (78.6, 79.5)	83.3 (82.4, 84.1)
Black or African American	11.5 (11.1, 11.8)	9.9 (9.2, 10.5)
Any other race	12.6 (12.2, 12.9)	10.7 (10.0, 11.4)
Hispanic/Latino, % (95% CI)	11.5 (11.2, 11.9)	12.5 (11.8, 13.2)
Household annual income, $, % (95% CI)		
< 50 000	44.7 (44.2, 45.2)	48.6 (47.6, 49.7)
50 000 to < 75 000	35.2 (34.8, 35.7)	33.8 (32.8, 34.8)
≥ 75 000	20.1 (19.7, 20.5)	17.5 (16.7, 18.3)
Highest education, % (95% CI)		
High school or less	23.2 (22.8, 23.6)	23.8 (22.9, 24.7)
Some college or associate's degree	31.3 (30.9, 31.8)	35.9 (34.9, 36.9)
Bachelor's degree or trade school	30.5 (30.0, 31.0)	27.9 (26.9, 28.8)
Graduate degree	14.9 (14.6, 15.3)	12.5 (11.8, 13.1)
Current health care professional, % (95% CI)	5.4 (5.1, 5.6)	7.3 (6.7, 7.8)
Current student, % (95% CI)	7.2 (6.8, 7.5)	9.1 (8.4, 9.8)
History of mental health diagnoses, % (95% CI)		
Any anxiety disorder	23.5 (23.0, 23.9)	52.8 (51.7, 53.8)
Major depressive disorder	9.2 (8.9, 9.4)	23.9 (23.0, 24.8)
ADD/ADHD	6.9 (6.7, 7.2)	17.5 (16.7, 18.3)
PTSD	6.2 (6.0, 6.4)	16.3 (15.6, 17.0)
Any acute or chronic pain in last 12 mo, % (95% CI)	38.3 (37.8, 38.8)	59.1 (58.1, 60.2)
Likely SUD, DAST-10 Score 3–10, % (95% CI)	5.3 (5.1, 5.5)	17.6 (16.8, 18.4)
Drug use in last 12 mo, % (95% CI)		
Prescription opioids	21.4 (21.0, 21.8)	63.9 (62.9, 64.9)
Prescription antidepressants	18.1 (17.8, 18.5)	57.8 (56.8, 58.9)
Prescription benzodiazepines	10.1 (9.9, 10.4)	39.7 (38.7, 40.7)
Prescription stimulants	5.2 (5.0, 5.4)	21.3 (20.4, 22.1)
Cannabis	21.4 (21.0, 21.8)	56.2 (55.1, 57.2)
Other psychedelics[b]	1.9 (1.8, 2.1)	8.7 (8.1, 9.2)
Methamphetamine	1.8 (1.7, 1.9)	8.1 (7.6, 8.6)
Psilocybin or mushrooms	1.6 (1.5, 1.7)	7.5 (6.9, 8.1)
Cocaine powder	1.3 (1.2, 1.4)	6.0 (5.5, 6.5)
Illicit opioids	1.1 (1.0, 1.1)	4.8 (4.4, 5.2)
Alcohol	46.3 (45.8, 46.8)	52.7 (51.6, 53.7)
Tobacco smoker	12.0 (11.8, 12.2)	23.1 (22.5, 23.8)

Note. ADD/ADHD = attention deficit disorder/attention deficit hyperactivity disorder; CI = confidence interval; DAST-10 = drug abuse screening test; PTSD = posttraumatic stress disorder; SUD = substance use disorder. All estimates shown are weighted except the unweighted number to show sample size.
[a]Respondents may self-select multiple races, estimates may not sum to 100; any other race may include American Indian/Alaska Native, Asian, or Native Hawaiian/Pacific Islander.
[b]Other psychedelics included any use of: ketamine, LSD, MDMA, mescaline, or PCP.

4 classes were described and subjectively named (Figure 1, Table 2):

1. Medically guided polysubstance use (Figure 1a): national prevalence 11.5% (95% CI = 11.2%, 11.8%). This class was defined by the highest endorsement of medical use of multiple prescribed drugs classes (mean = 1.8 types) sourced from their own health care providers. There was 52.4% probability of cannabis use but negligible concomitant drug use. Among adults representing this class, in the last year 6.1% were estimated to have an SUD while 2.1% received substance use treatment.
2. Self-guided polysubstance use (Figure 1b): national prevalence 3.4% (95% CI = 3.2%, 3.5%). This class was defined primarily by NMU of multiple prescription drug classes (mean = 2.3 types) with some concomitant use with alcohol or other prescriptions. These prescriptions were likely to be sourced from providers, but approximately 25% sourced exclusively outside health care providers (data not shown). Among adults representing this class, in the last year 14.5% were estimated to have an SUD while 5.1% received substance use treatment.
3. Principal cannabis use variety (Figure 1c): national prevalence 4.0% (95% CI = 3.8%, 4.2%): This class was chiefly defined by high probability of cannabis use at 95.3% with smaller, but approximately equal, probabilities across NMU of prescriptions and recreational drugs. These drugs were used concomitantly with cannabis and alcohol. When we considered each drug type included in this analysis, there were on average 2.0 other drugs used besides cannabis. Among adults representing this class, in the last year 31.9% were estimated to have an SUD and only 8.1% received substance use treatment.
4. Indiscriminate coexposures (Figure 1d): national prevalence

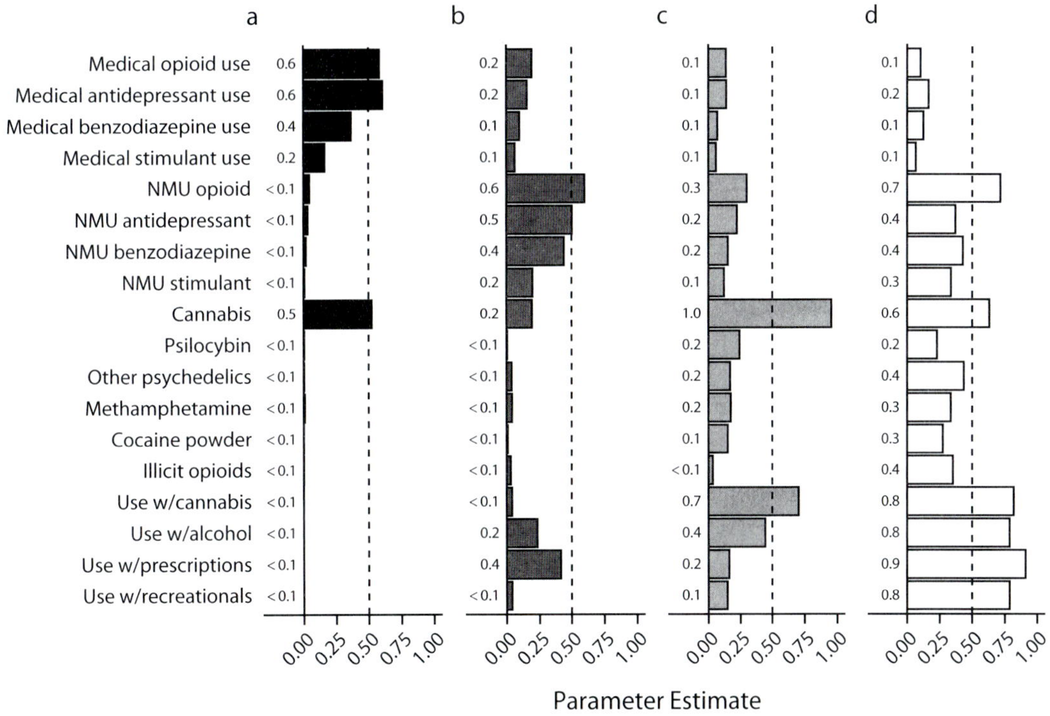

FIGURE 1— Model Parameters for 4 Polysubstance Use Latent Classes, (a) Medically Guided Polysubstance Use, (b) Self-Guided Polysubstance Use, (c) Principle Cannabis Use Variety, and (d) Indiscriminate Coexposures: United States, 2022

Note. NMU = nonmedical use. Four observed latent classes emerged among those who used 2 or more psychoactive drugs in the last 12 months in the United States in 2022 (standard errors of estimates in supplemental material). Medically guided polysubstance use (prevalence = 11.5%) and self-guided polysubstance use (3.4%) were primarily defined by medical or NMU of prescription drugs, respectively. Principal cannabis use variety (4.0%) had high probability of cannabis use with various prescription and recreational drugs concomitantly used. Indiscriminate coexposures (2.1%) indicated concomitant drug use with indiscriminate drug preference. The interpretation of the first bar would be that an individual belonging to the medically guided polysubstance use class had a 0.6 probability of using opioids medically in the last 12 months (standard errors shown in Table B, available as a supplement to the online version of this article at http://www.ajph.org).

TABLE 2— Weighted Characteristics Among 4 Polysubstance Use Latent Classes: United States, 2022

Measure	Medically Guided Polysubstance Use	Self-Guided Polysubstance Use	Principal Cannabis Use Variety	Indiscriminate Coexposures
Unweighted no.	7862	2719	3104	2115
Estimated weighted no.	29 718 900	8 696 200	10 268 000	5 361 500
Demographics and risk factors				
Age, y, mean (95% CI)	48.0 (47.4, 48.5)	44.3 (43.4, 45.1)	37.8 (37.1, 38.5)	36.2 (35.5, 37.0)
Male, % (95% CI)	36.2 (34.8, 37.6)	46.6 (44.1, 49.2)	52.8 (50.4, 55.3)	65.0 (62.2, 67.8)
Self-reported race,[a] % (95% CI)				
White	86.5 (85.4, 87.5)	82.9 (80.9, 85.0)	77.1 (74.9, 79.3)	78.1 (75.2, 81.1)
Black or African American	8.5 (7.7, 9.4)	8.7 (7.3, 10.1)	13.6 (11.8, 15.4)	11.9 (9.6, 14.1)
Any other race	9.1 (8.3, 10.0)	10.3 (8.6, 12.0)	14.3 (12.4, 16.2)	13.5 (11.0, 16.0)
Hispanic/Latino, % (95% CI)	9.2 (8.3, 10.0)	14.7 (12.8, 16.6)	16.2 (14.2, 18.1)	20.5 (17.9, 23.2)
Household annual income, $, % (95% CI)				
< 50 000	47.8 (46.3, 49.2)	45.5 (43.0, 48.0)	55.5 (53.0, 58.0)	45.6 (42.5, 48.7)
50 000 to < 75 000	34.3 (32.9, 35.6)	35.8 (33.3, 38.2)	29.7 (27.4, 32.0)	36.2 (33.3, 39.2)
≥ 75 000	18.0 (16.9, 19.1)	18.7 (16.7, 20.7)	14.8 (12.9, 16.6)	18.2 (16.0, 20.4)
Highest education, % (95% CI)				
High school or less	20.8 (19.6, 21.9)	23.7 (21.5, 25.9)	31.8 (29.5, 34.1)	25.2 (22.6, 27.8)
Some college or associate's degree	38.3 (36.9, 39.7)	30.3 (28.0, 32.6)	36.0 (33.7, 38.4)	31.3 (28.3, 34.2)
Bachelor's degree or trade school	28.1 (26.8, 29.4)	31.5 (29.1, 33.9)	23.9 (21.7, 26.0)	28.6 (25.8, 31.4)
Graduate degree	12.8 (11.9, 13.8)	14.5 (12.7, 16.2)	8.3 (7.0, 9.7)	15.0 (12.9, 17.0)
Current health care professional, % (95% CI)	6.4 (5.7, 7.1)	7.3 (6.0, 8.6)	6.0 (4.9, 7.2)	14.4 (12.1, 16.7)
Current student, % (95% CI)	7.7 (6.7, 8.6)	7.8 (6.2, 9.3)	9.8 (8.2, 11.5)	17.7 (15.2, 20.2)
History of mental health diagnosis, % (95% CI)				
Any anxiety disorder	55.8 (54.4, 57.2)	49.3 (46.8, 51.9)	49.7 (47.2, 52.2)	47.3 (44.2, 50.4)
Major depressive disorder	26.7 (25.4, 27.9)	21.1 (19.0, 23.1)	20.2 (18.3, 22.2)	19.7 (17.3, 22.1)
ADD/ADHD	17.3 (16.2, 18.4)	13.3 (11.5, 15.0)	19.2 (17.2, 21.2)	22.3 (19.8, 24.8)
PTSD	16.3 (15.3, 17.3)	13.3 (11.7, 14.9)	17.6 (15.8, 19.4)	18.3 (16.1, 20.5)
Any acute or chronic pain in last 12 mo, % (95% CI)	64.9 (63.5, 66.4)	51.2 (48.6, 53.7)	50.3 (47.8, 52.8)	56.7 (53.6, 59.8)
Substance use factors				
Likely SUD, DAST-10 Score 3-10, % (95% CI)	6.1 (5.4, 6.7)	14.5 (12.8, 16.2)	31.9 (29.6, 34.2)	58.9 (55.9, 62.0)
Received substance use treatment in last year, % (95% CI)	2.1 (1.7, 2.5)	5.1 (4.1, 6.1)	8.1 (6.8, 9.3)	23.2 (20.6, 25.8)
Concomitant use when using prescription drugs, % (95% CI)				
With alcohol	Rare[b]	23.8 (21.6, 26.0)	27.3 (25.0, 29.6)	65.4 (62.5, 68.2)
With cannabis	Rare	2.9 (2.1, 3.6)	47.8 (45.3, 50.3)	68.7 (65.9, 71.6)
With other prescription drugs	Rare	44.8 (42.3, 47.3)	12.2 (10.6, 13.8)	79.2 (76.7, 81.6)
With recreational drugs	Rare	3.7 (2.7, 4.6)	8.1 (6.8, 9.4)	66.7 (63.8, 69.6)
Concomitant use when using recreational drugs, % (95% CI)				
With alcohol	Rare	2.3 (1.6, 2.9)	24.4 (22.2, 26.5)	44.7 (41.7, 47.8)
With cannabis	Rare	Rare	34.9 (32.5, 37.2)	46.0 (42.9, 49.1)
With other prescription drugs	Rare	3.6 (2.6, 4.5)	3.5 (2.8, 4.3)	50.6 (47.5, 53.7)
With recreational drugs	Rare	0.3 (0.1, 0.5)	7.6 (6.3, 8.8)	39.8 (36.8, 42.8)

Continued

TABLE 2— Continued

Measure	Medically Guided Polysubstance Use	Self-Guided Polysubstance Use	Principal Cannabis Use Variety	Indiscriminate Coexposures
Prescription drug sourcing from own health care professional, % (95% CI)				
Among those using opioids	96.0 (95.3, 96.7)	74.1 (71.7, 76.5)	68.8 (65.5, 72.1)	59.8 (56.5, 63.1)
Among those using antidepressants	97.9 (97.4, 98.4)	78.0 (75.5, 80.5)	80.8 (77.5, 84.2)	62.8 (58.8, 66.9)
Among those using benzodiazepines	97.7 (97.1, 98.4)	70.6 (67.7, 73.6)	64.0 (59.3, 68.7)	53.1 (49.2, 57.1)
Among those using stimulants	98.3 (97.3, 99.3)	60.3 (55.4, 65.2)	58.2 (51.9, 64.5)	49.7 (44.7, 54.7)

Note. ADD/ADHD = attention deficit disorder/attention deficit hyperactivity disorder; CI = confidence interval; DAST-10 = drug abuse screening test; PTSD = posttraumatic stress disorder; SUD = substance use disorder. All estimates shown are weighted except the unweighted number to show sample size.
[a]Respondents may self-select multiple races, estimates may not sum to 100; any other race may include American Indian/Alaska Native, Asian, or Native Hawaiian/Pacific Islander.
[b]Sparse data cells (< 5 respondents) were suppressed.

2.1% (95% CI = 1.9%, 2.2%). This class was defined by concomitant use of cannabis, alcohol, prescriptions, and recreational drugs with patterns indicating indiscriminate drug preferences. When we considered each drug included in this analysis, there were on average 4.6 drugs used in the last 12 months. When prescription drugs were used, they were commonly sourced outside of health care providers. Among adults representing this class, in the last year 58.9% were estimated to have an SUD and only 23.2% received substance use treatment.

Table 2 shows the demographic characteristics and other risk factors for members of the 4 classes. Those belonging to the medically guided polysubstance use and self-guided polysubstance use classes generally were older and there were slightly more females than males. The principal cannabis use variety and indiscriminate coexposures classes had the highest proportions of self-reported minority groups compared to other classes without noticeable differences in income or education.

Sensitivity Analysis by Substance Use Disorder

The measurement invariance likelihood ratio test indicated that there were differences in the measurement model across the SUD groups ($P < .001$). When modeled independently, 4 analogous latent classes were observed among those with and without likely SUD by subjective interpretation, albeit in different proportions (Figure 2). The difference in class membership probabilities was likely driving the measurement invariance findings more than item-response probabilities. The group without a likely SUD comprised 82.4% of the sample, so latent class proportions were similar to the proportions of each class in the overall analysis. The medically guided polysubstance use class was 6% larger proportionally compared to the overall findings, the self-guided polysubstance use class was similar in size, while the other 2 classes were smaller. The indiscriminate coexposures class in this group was indicated with an asterisk because the item-response probabilities for recreational drugs were slightly lower than the overall findings with high probabilities for NMU of prescription drugs (online Figure A). The group with likely SUD constituted 17.6% of the sample and had almost equal proportions of the 4 latent classes, with principal cannabis use variety being largest at 34.5% (Figure 2). The self-guided polysubstance use class was also indicated with an asterisk because the item-response probabilities for recreational drugs and concomitant use were slightly higher than the main findings (Figure A).

DISCUSSION

This study, which utilized a general population survey among adults in the United States, found that 21% used 2 or more psychoactive drugs in 2022. This research elucidated the landscape of polysubstance use by using methods to reduce the dimensionality of this multifaceted behavior. Four unique behavioral classes were found that crossed multiple drug classes and drug types (prescription or recreational), and they were partially defined by patterns of concomitant drug use.

The most prevalent profile contained individuals with fewer markers of SUD and was categorized primarily by prescription drugs used as intended, sourced by their own providers. Although

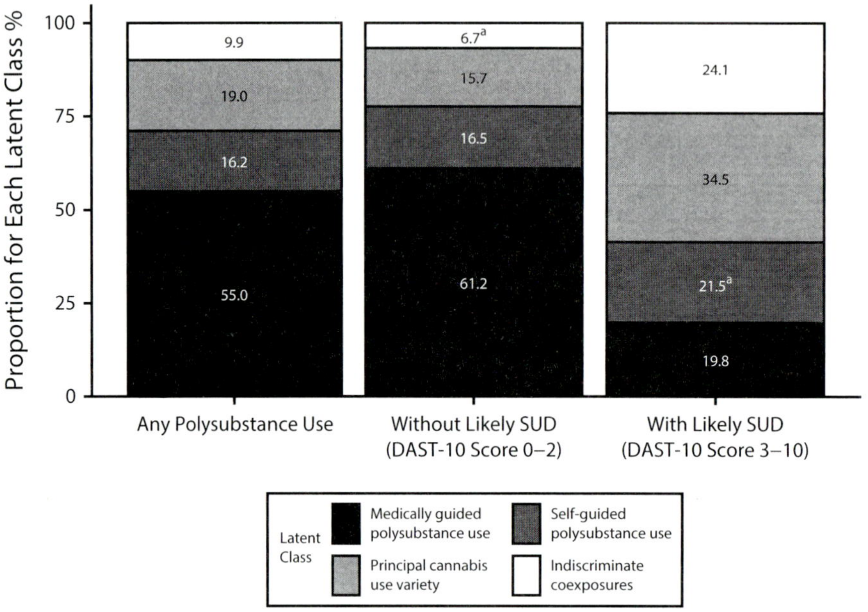

FIGURE 2— Proportion of 4 Polysubstance Use Latent Classes Comparing Those With or Without Substance Use Disorders: United States, 2022

Note. DAST-10 = drug abuse screen test; SUD = substance use disorder. Those adults without likely SUD constituted 82.4% of the polysubstance sample, while those with likely SUD were 17.6% of sample. An analogous 4 latent classes were observed in both SUD groups as observed in the main analysis, albeit in different proportions, indicating that SUD could arise in someone belonging to any of these classes.

[a]Indicates analogous classes upon interpretation but different contributions in latent class item-response probabilities (provided in Table B and Figure A, available as a supplement to the online version of this article at http://www.ajph.org).

this group is unsurprising in the context of common behaviors, it is not commonly discussed in the context of polysubstance use. This group equates to about 11.5% of all adults, and it had other health concerns such as pain history and high proportion of comorbidities. Additionally, about half of this group reported also using cannabis throughout a similar timeframe. This medically guided polysubstance use group is a new contribution to the polysubstance use literature, although it is consistent with prior studies linking cannabis use with increased use of psychoactive prescriptions.[25] More research examining this association and the interplay of mental health disorders is warranted, because these use patterns of multiple drugs, even under the direction of a health care provider, could represent individuals attempting to treat complex comorbidities. This group reports interactions with health care providers, where identification, education, or prevention strategies could be helpful to address underlying mental health concerns or prevent potential prescription drug interactions.

The second largest latent class found, the principal cannabis use variety, constitutes 4.0% of all adults. Cannabis was the primary drug, but there are about equal proportions of people using other prescription drugs nonmedically, recreational drugs, or both. Of note, while there is variety in the other drugs of choice, these other drugs in the profile are commonly used concomitantly with cannabis or alcohol. Approximately one third of this group has a likely SUD, but with the variety in the other contributing drug, education tactics or prevention strategies would need to be more customized to the individual. With this being the second largest profile and as more states continue to legalize cannabis, there might be opportunities to explore intervention points through other environments outside health care providers. This group reported only modest interaction with health care, so new places to add "connect to care" opportunities may be required, such as dispensaries or cannabis retail outlets.

The smallest 2 latent classes found are the ones that are already discussed in the literature but are often grouped into a single, low-prevalence class that combines both recreational drug use with NMU of prescription drugs, often called "the polysubstance use class."[14,26] This work separates it into 2 distinct profiles. First, the self-guided polysubstance use class (3.4%) consists of those primarily nonmedically using prescription medications and mixing with other prescriptions or alcohol. This group has also been identified in other studies, particularly around prescription opioid or stimulants use[27,28] and around use of alcohol with sedatives.[29] Although this class still has an opportunity for health care provider intervention, it could be a group that would benefit from different screening and early referral; 14.5% had markers for a SUD. Many in the class could benefit from prevention of potential drug interactions or education around advancement to SUDs.

Finally, the indiscriminate coexposures class is consistent with other studies and is the most often cited polysubstance group, despite it having the lowest prevalence (2.1%). It is typically associated with high risk for acute advanced health outcomes like overdose and has major clinical and public health implications. We observed a large discrepancy between those with a likely SUD (58.9%) and those reporting getting treatment (23.2%) who could benefit from psychosocial or pharmacological treatment.[30] A better understanding of treatment access or barriers to access among this group would be beneficial. Pharmacological treatments typically address single substances, and new treatments that address psychostimulant use or concomitant use should be explored given that there are currently none approved by the Food and Drug Administration.[31] There is likely a subset of this group who do not believe they are at risk for acute health events, despite commonly sourcing their drugs from illicit sources and mixing drugs concomitantly.[32]

After stratifying the analysis by those with likely SUD, 4 similar classes appeared with differing prevalence, demonstrating that SUD is not a defining feature of the classes. This is a shift in perspective that is necessary. Most literature describes those with SUDs as being more aligned with specific high-risk profiles, which was shown here, but this work shows that an SUD could arise in someone belonging to any of these classes. Therefore, there is a need to take a more personalized approach where identification into an individual's total drug use behaviors is quantified and their health care approaches them more holistically. "Polysubstance use" lacks diagnostic specificity, and these individuals can be clinically complex cases with ranging profiles of drug use histories and high rates of comorbidities or mental health disorders.[26,33,34] Approaches to identifying these individuals should be expanded to capture a wide range of drugs and use behaviors. Given that an SUD can cause a spectrum of difficulties in an individual's life, an SUD may manifest differently across these profiles, which would be important to explore in the future.

Strengths and Limitations

One strength of this large population study was the person-centric analysis approach, which helps elucidate behavior profiles not described in the context of polysubstance use. Within our classes, we found parallels to polysubstance use features seen in other studies, giving strength to the novel findings of this study. The weighted analysis accounts for both health and demographic metrics to make more generalized drug use prevalence estimates. Limitations to this study include possible drug recall bias within the last year. Online formats have been shown to be less prone to social desirability bias, which is important for accuracy of self-report.[35] Also, the latent class approach can be sensitive to inclusion criteria, although we found that profiles were defined across drug classes and behaviors; it did not appear to be sensitive to inclusion of any 1 drug. Additionally, class interpretation can be subject to the naming fallacy based on qualitative interpretation of the probabilistic assignment. It is important to note that the landscape of drug use is rapidly evolving in the United States. These observed profiles could change over time, such as with the introduction of new substances or changes in use patterns (e.g., use of xylazine, changes in prescribing guidelines or decriminalization of substances).

Public Health Implications

About 1 in 5 US adults have used multiple psychoactive drugs in the last year across 4 distinct profiles. Current diagnostic criteria for identifying polysubstance use lack the ability to identify the extensive combinations of drug use patterns.[26,33] No one-size-fits-all prevention approach is likely to succeed given the clear existence of subpopulations with very different behaviors and histories.

Both clinical practice and public health should adapt the current approaches. First, for more effective clinical care, the education of providers around these profiles and correlated behaviors would be beneficial. Knowledge of use behaviors obtained from current screening tools could prompt future questioning into correlated harmful behaviors in a nonaccusatory manner. Second, improved screening tools could help determine appropriate clinical risk stratification, which dictates education, future screening, or next steps to reduce adverse health effects. Third, an SUD can manifest in different ways, and understanding which behaviors are leading to problematic areas of a patient's life would improve overall patient care, both physical and mental. Not everyone in these profiles interacts regularly with health care providers, so public health professionals should consider alternative access points to interact with individuals in their own communities to educate about risks, encourage safe use patterns, or implement programs to eliminate use patterns, depending on individuals' goals and health risks. AJPH

ABOUT THE AUTHORS

Karilynn M. Rockhill and Alison Abraham are with the Department of Epidemiology, University of Colorado Anschutz Medical Campus, Aurora, CO. Karilynn M. Rockhill, Joshua C. Black, and Janetta Iwanicki are with Rocky Mountain Poison & Drug Safety, Denver Health & Hospital Authority, Denver, CO.

CORRESPONDENCE

Correspondence should be sent to Karilynn Rockhill, 1391 N. Speer Blvd, Suite 600, Denver, CO 80204 (e-mail: Karilynn.rockhill@rmpds.org). Reprints can be ordered at https://www.ajph.org by clicking the "Reprints" link.

PUBLICATION INFORMATION

Full Citation: Rockhill KM, Black JC, Iwanicki J, Abraham A. Polysubstance use profiles among the general adult population, United States, 2022. *Am J Public Health*. 2025;115(5):747–757.

Acceptance Date: December 8, 2024.

DOI: https://doi.org/10.2105/AJPH.2024.307979

ORCID iDs:

Karilynn M. Rockhill https://orcid.org/0000-0003-2831-4055

Joshua C. Black https://orcid.org/0000-0002-7329-2740

Janetta Iwanicki https://orcid.org/0000-0001-9608-391X

Alison Abraham https://orcid.org/0000-0002-6863-0565

CONTRIBUTORS

K. M. Rockhill and A. Abraham conceptualized the study question. K. M. Rockhill and J. C. Black conceptualized the statistical approach. J. Iwanicki contributed to obtaining the data set. K. M. Rockhill conducted all analyses and drafted the manuscript. All authors participated in interpreting results and editing the manuscript and approved it for publication.

ACKNOWLEDGEMENTS

Research reported in this publication was supported by the National Institute on Drug Abuse of the National Institutes of Health (award no. R36DA057413).

This work was presented at the 2023 annual meeting of the American Public Health Association.

Note. The contents are solely the responsibility of the authors and do not necessarily represent the official views of the National Institutes of Health.

CONFLICTS OF INTEREST

The authors have no conflicts of interest to report.

HUMAN PARTICIPANT PROTECTION

Secondary data research application for this analysis was approved by the Colorado Multiple Institutional Review Board (COMIRB) on March 7, 2023 (#23-0373). The NMURx Program study was given a certificate of exemption by COMIRB on July 5, 2016 (#16-0922).

REFERENCES

1. Connor JP, Gullo MJ, White A, Kelly AB. Polysubstance use: diagnostic challenges, patterns of use and health. *Curr Opin Psychiatry*. 2014;27(4):269–275. https://doi.org10.1097/YCO.0000000000000069
2. Crummy EA, O'Neal TJ, Baskin BM, Ferguson SM. One is not enough: understanding and modeling polysubstance use. *Front Neurosci*. 2020;14:569. https://doi.org/10.3389/fnins.2020.00569
3. Salom CL, Betts KS, Williams GM, Najman JM, Alati R. Predictors of comorbid polysubstance use and mental health disorders in young adults—a latent class analysis. *Addiction*. 2016;111(1):156–164. https://doi.org/10.1111/add.13058
4. *Key Substance Use and Mental Health Indicators in the United States: Results From the 2020 National Survey on Drug Use and Health*. Rockville, MD: Substance Abuse and Mental Health Services Administration; 2021. HHS Publication No. PEP21-07-01-003, NSDUH Series H-56. https://www.samhsa.gov/data/sites/default/files/reports/rpt35325/NSDUHFFRPDFWHTMLFiles2020/2020NSDUHFFR1PDFW102121.pdf
5. Lorvick J, Browne EN, Lambdin BH, Comfort M. Polydrug use patterns, risk behavior and unmet healthcare need in a community-based sample of women who use cocaine, heroin or methamphetamine. *Addict Behav*. 2018;85:94–99. https://doi.org/10.1016/j.addbeh.2018.05.013
6. Gilmore D, Zorland J, Akin J, Johnson JA, Emshoff JG, Kuperminc GP. Mortality risk in a sample of emergency department patients who use cocaine with alcohol and/or cannabis. *Subst Abus*. 2018;39(3):266–270. https://doi.org/10.1080/08897077.2017.1389799
7. Mattson CL, Tanz LJ, Quinn K, Kariisa M, Patel P, Davis NL. Trends and geographic patterns in drug and synthetic opioid overdose deaths—United States, 2013–2019. *MMWR Morb Mortal Wkly Rep*. 2021;70(6):202–207. https://doi.org/10.15585/mmwr.mm7006a4
8. Black JC, Rockhill KM, Dart RC, Iwanicki J. Clustering patterns in polysubstance mortality in the United States in 2017: a multiple correspondence analysis of death certificate data. *Ann Epidemiol*. 2023;77:119–126. https://doi.org/10.1016/j.annepidem.2022.03.011
9. Ciccarone D. The rise of illicit fentanyls, stimulants and the fourth wave of the opioid overdose crisis. *Curr Opin Psychiatry*. 2021;34(4):344–350. https://doi.org/10.1097/YCO.0000000000000717
10. Jenkins RA. The fourth wave of the US opioid epidemic and its implications for the rural US: a federal perspective. *Prev Med*. 2021;152(pt 2):106541. https://doi.org/10.1016/j.ypmed.2021.106541
11. Townsend T, Kline D, Rivera-Aguirre A, et al. Racial/ethnic and geographic trends in combined stimulant/opioid overdoses, 2007–2019. *Am J Epidemiol*. 2022;191(4):599–612. https://doi.org/10.1093/aje/kwab290
12. Collins LM, Lanza ST. *Latent Class and Latent Transition Analysis: With Applications in the Social, Behavioral, and Health Sciences*. Hoboken, NJ: John Wiley and Sons Inc; 2010.
13. Tomczyk S, Isensee B, Hanewinkel R. Latent classes of polysubstance use among adolescents—a systematic review. *Drug Alcohol Depend*. 2016;160:12–29. https://doi.org/10.1016/j.drugalcdep.2015.11.035
14. de Jonge MC, Bukman AJ, van Leeuwen L, Onrust SA, Kleinjan M. Latent classes of substance use in young adults—a systematic review. *Subst Use Misuse*. 2022;57(5):769–785. https://doi.org/10.1080/10826084.2022.2040029
15. Black JC, Rockhill K, Forber A, et al An online survey for pharmacoepidemiological investigation (Survey of Non-Medical Use of Prescription Drugs Program): validation study. *J Med Internet Res*. 2019;21(10):e15830. https://doi.org/10.2196/15830
16. Dart RC. Monitoring risk: post marketing surveillance and signal detection. *Drug Alcohol Depend*. 2009;105(suppl 1):S26–S32. https://doi.org/10.1016/j.drugalcdep.2009.08.011
17. Skinner HA. The drug abuse screening test. *Addict Behav*. 1982;7(4):363–371. https://doi.org/10.1016/0306-4603(82)90005-3
18. Bohn M, Babor T, Kranzler H. Validity of the Drug Abuse Screening Test (DAST-10) in inpatient substance abusers. *Probl Drug Depend*. 1991;119:233–235.
19. Janulis P, Luo J, Tang X, Schalet BD. Can severity of substance use be measured across drug classes? Estimating differential item functioning by drug class in two general measures of substance use severity. *Drug Alcohol Depend*. 2023;250:110877. https://doi.org/10.1016/j.drugalcdep.2023.110877
20. Nylund-Gibson K, Choi AY. Ten frequently asked questions about latent class analysis. *Transl Issues Psychol Sci*. 2018;4(4):440–461. https://doi.org/10.1037/met0000486
21. Weller BE, Bowen NK, Faubert SJ. Latent class analysis: a guide to best practice. *J Black Psychol*. 2020;46(4):287–311. https://doi.org/10.1177/0095798420930932
22. Dziak JJ, Lanza ST, Tan X. Effect size, statistical power and sample size requirements for the bootstrap likelihood ratio test in latent class analysis. *Struct Equ Modeling*. 2014;21(4):534–552. https://doi.org/10.1080/10705511.2014.919819
23. Lanza ST, Collins LM, Lemmon DR, Schafer JL. PROC LCA: a SAS procedure for latent class analysis. *Struct Equ Modeling*. 2007;14(4):671–694. https://doi.org/10.1080/10705510701575602
24. Bakk Z, Kuha J. Relating latent class membership to external variables: an overview. *Br J Math Stat Psychol*. 2021;74(2):340–362. https://doi.org/10.1111/bmsp.12227

25. Rognli EB, Bramness JG, von Soest T. Cannabis use in early adulthood is prospectively associated with prescriptions of antipsychotics, mood stabilizers, and antidepressants. *Acta Psychiatr Scand.* 2020;141(2):149–156. https://doi.org/10.1111/acps.13104
26. Connor JP, Leung J, Chan GCK, Stjepanović D. Seeking order in patterns of polysubstance use. *Curr Opin Psychiatry.* 2023;36(4):263–268. https://doi.org/10.1097/YCO.0000000000000881
27. Chan GCK, Butterworth P, Becker D, et al. Longitudinal patterns of amphetamine use from adolescence to adulthood: a latent class analysis of a 20-year prospective study of Australians. *Drug Alcohol Depend.* 2019;194:121–127. https://doi.org/10.1016/j.drugalcdep.2018.08.042
28. Rockhill KM, Olson R, Dart RC, Iwanicki JL, Black JC. Differing behaviors around adult nonmedical use of prescription stimulants and opioids: latent class analysis. *J Med Internet Res.* 2023;25:e46742. https://doi.org10.2196/46742
29. Quek LH, Chan GC, White A, et al. Concurrent and simultaneous polydrug use: latent class analysis of an Australian nationally representative sample of young adults. *Front Public Health.* 2013;1:61. https://doi.org/10.3389/fpubh.2013.00061
30. Ray LA, Meredith LR, Kiluk BD, Walthers J, Carroll KM, Magill M. Combined pharmacotherapy and cognitive behavioral therapy for adults with alcohol or substance use disorders: a systematic review and meta-analysis. *JAMA Netw Open.* 2020;3(6):e208279. https://doi.org/10.1001/jamanetworkopen.2020.8279
31. Lee JC, Janda KD. Development of effective therapeutics for polysubstance use disorders. *Curr Opin Chem Biol.* 2022;66:102105. https://doi.org/10.1016/j.cbpa.2021.102105
32. Carroll JJ, Marshall BDL, Rich JD, Green TC. Exposure to fentanyl-contaminated heroin and overdose risk among illicit opioid users in Rhode Island: a mixed methods study. *Int J Drug Policy.* 2017;46:136–145. https://doi.org/10.1016/j.drugpo.2017.05.023
33. Shearer RD, Bart G, Reznikoff C. Rethinking the use of "polysubstance" to describe complex substance use patterns. *J Gen Intern Med.* 2022;37(12):3174–3175. https://doi.org/10.1007/s11606-022-07424-5
34. Ellis JD, Rabinowitz JA, Ware OD, Wells J, Dunn KE, Huhn AS. Patterns of polysubstance use and clinical comorbidity among persons seeking substance use treatment: an observational study. *J Subst Use Addict Treat.* 2023;146:208932. https://doi.org/10.1016/j.josat.2022.208932
35. van Gelder MM, Bretveld RW, Roeleveld N. Web-based questionnaires: the future in epidemiology? *Am J Epidemiol.* 2010;172(11):1292–1298. https://doi.org/10.1093/aje/kwq291

Behavioral Interventions for Increasing Seat Belt Use and Decreasing Distracted Driving Using Telematics: A National Randomized Trial

Jeffrey P. Ebert, PhD, Ruiqi Yan, MS, Sadie Friday, BA, Dylan Small, PhD, Catherine C. McDonald, RN, PhD, Kelsey Bartolozzi, BA, and M. Kit Delgado, MD, MS

Objectives. To test low-cost, scalable interventions designed to encourage seat belt use (primary outcome) and discourage handheld phone use while driving.

Methods. A randomized controlled trial assigned 1139 consenting General Motors–connected vehicle customers in the United States to 1 of 4 groups for a 10-week intervention: (1) control, (2) behavioral engagement, (3) behavioral engagement plus raffle, and (4) behavioral engagement plus shared pot. Behavioral engagement involved education, personalized tips, a "wish outcome obstacle plan" exercise, and weekly feedback about buckling and handheld-free streaks. Participants in the behavioral engagement plus raffle group also earned a chance at a $125 prize each week they had a buckling or handheld-free streak. Those in the behavioral engagement plus shared pot group earned an equal share of this prize for each streak. The intervention was delivered virtually in spring 2023.

Results. Participants in the behavioral engagement plus shared pot group had a higher buckling rate (91.3%) than those in the behavioral engagement plus raffle (89.5%), behavioral engagement (89.4%), or control (88.3%) groups—differences that remained significant at follow-up. Handheld phone use did not differ significantly.

Conclusions. A behavioral intervention with a shared pot incentive could be delivered at scale to reduce injuries and deaths associated with vehicular crashes.

Trial Registration. ClinicalTrials.gov identifier: NCT05469477. (*Am J Public Health*. 2025;115(5):758–768. https://doi.org/10.2105/AJPH.2024.307980)

AJPH May 2025, Vol. 115, No. 5

Worldwide, 1.2 million people die and 50 million suffer nonfatal injuries annually because of road traffic crashes.[1] Wearing a seat belt in the front seat of a car decreases the risk of serious injury by 50% and death by 45%,[2] but, globally, fewer than half of drivers and front-seat passengers report regular seat belt use.[3] In high-income countries, front-seat buckling rates are 90% or greater,[4,5] partly because of primary enforcement laws and campaigns.[6] Still, individuals at highest risk for crash are least likely to wear a seat belt, and the rate of crash fatalities involving unrestrained occupants in the United States has risen to 50%.[7]

A significant contributor to crash risk is distracted driving, which is responsible for about 1 million crashes per year in the United States alone.[8] Handheld phone use while driving increases the odds of crash by 2 to 12 times.[9,10] Telematics data from mobile applications have revealed that 1 in 3 drivers was distracted by their phone before a crash and that distracted drivers take longer to brake, increasing crash severity.[11] Despite these risks and laws banning certain kinds of handheld use,[12–14] 5% of US drivers are visibly engaged in handheld use at any given time.[15]

Innovations in telematics and automobile insurance enable an individualized approach to encourage safer driving.[16] Vehicle and mobile telematics measure hard braking, speeding, and other risky driving behaviors. Vehicle telematics also measure seat belt use, and mobile telematics measure phone use. Usage-based insurance programs use these data to calculate drivers' risk of crash and price policies.[17,18] As these programs become more popular,[19] so does the opportunity to measure, encourage, and incentivize safer driving. Previous research with usage-based insurance customers has found that structuring incentives according to behavioral economics principles, providing motivating feedback, and allowing adequate time to form new habits can lead to sustained reductions in distracted driving.[20,21] Similar interventions have increased self-reported buckling behavior,[22,23] but their impact on telematics-measured buckling has not been tested.[23]

We conducted a preregistered, randomized controlled trial testing low-cost, scalable interventions designed to simultaneously increase seat belt use and decrease handheld phone use, both measured by telematics. Consenting drivers of General Motors (GM)–connected vehicles were randomly assigned to control or 1 of 3 treatment arms for a 10-week intervention period. Behavioral engagement participants were given (1) safety and other reasons to buckle up and avoid handheld phone use, (2) a goal visualization and planning exercise, (3) weekly personalized safety tips, and (4) weekly feedback about whether they achieved perfect buckling and "phone-free" streaks. Behavioral engagement plus raffle participants received behavioral engagement and were entered into a $125 raffle for each weekly streak attained. Behavioral engagement plus shared pot participants received behavioral engagement and an equal share of $125 for each weekly streak. The primary outcome was seat belt use; the secondary outcome was handheld phone use. We predicted that, relative to control, all 3 treatment arms would show more seat belt use and less handheld use, with the shared pot arm changing the most.

METHODS

GM determined customer eligibility on August 15, 2022, based on a preceding 5-week period. The research team intended for customers to be eligible for invitation if they were aged 18 years or older, had at least 5 weeks of baseline data averaging at least 8 trips per week, and had baseline seat belt use of 75% or less for short trips (<2 miles) and 90% or less for longer trips (≥ 2 miles). During analysis, it was discovered that customers were invited if they had at least 8 trips over the entire 5-week baseline period, and it appears that no buckling-related exclusions were applied (Appendix Figure A, available as a supplement to the online version of this article at https://ajph.org).

Between January 30 and March 2, 2023, GM sent e-mails inviting customers to participate. Participants could earn, via ClinCard virtual debit card, $20 for completing a survey and $50 for installing the Way to Drive app. The e-mail listed the customer's vehicle year, make, and model and stated the invitation was solely for them. The e-mail linked to a consent form in Qualtrics; the link included a random ID used to associate GM trip data with the participant. Those who consented provided their name, e-mail address, phone number, and date of birth, then advanced to an intake survey that collected sociodemographic information.

Survey completers were randomized to a study arm by Qualtrics. Control participants were simply thanked and encouraged to buckle up and avoid handheld phone use for the next 15 weeks. Treatment arm participants proceeded to the initial parts of behavioral engagement. First, they received education about the safety, legal, financial, and social benefits of putting their phone down and buckling up when driving (Appendix Figure B). Next, they were asked what would encourage them to engage in these behaviors and selected from a menu of options derived from previous research.[24,25] Based on their selections, participants received personalized tips via text message throughout the intervention (Appendix Figure C). Last, they completed a wish outcome obstacle plan (WOOP) exercise (Appendix Figure D) that has been shown to increase goal attainment.[26,27]

Afterward, participants in the behavioral engagement group were told to expect text messages with safe driving tips and feedback on whether they had perfect buckling and phone-free driving streaks, which they could opt out of by texting "bye." Streak feedback increases engagement and motivation[28] and has been effective in abstinence-based addiction treatment.[29,30] Positive, gain-framed language was used to keep acceptability high and because buckling and avoiding handheld use while driving are prevention behaviors, which respond well to such framing.[31–33]

Participants in the behavioral engagement plus raffle group were additionally told that, for each weekly streak they had, they would be entered into a $125 raffle. Raffles and lotteries are widely used as an affordable, scalable incentive to encourage healthy behaviors of large groups. Their motivational power draws on people's tendency to inflate the value of low-probability large rewards and on variable reinforcement.[34] Despite their widespread use in public health contexts, lotteries have a mixed record of success.[34–37]

Participants in the behavioral engagement plus shared pot group were instead told they would split a $125 pot with others who had a perfect streak.[21] In a repeated context, this may be more motivating than a raffle incentive, where the typical experience of someone who earns raffle chances is that they win nothing.[38] A shared pot may also be more motivating than a small guaranteed prize of similar value because it advertises a much larger total purse, has an element of unpredictability given that the take-home reward amount is not prospectively known,[39] and communicates a social norm that others are engaging in the desired behavior.[40]

On March 8, 2023, participants were enrolled into the Way to Health platform, which processed incoming trip data and delivered messages. Participants were notified that the study was about to start and asked to install the Way to Drive app. Those who texted "bye" in response were unenrolled before the intervention period. The 10-week intervention period began March 12 and ended May 20. A 5-week follow-up period began immediately afterward. GM data on seat belt use were securely transferred to Way to Health early each morning; Way to Drive data on phone use were transferred continuously. Participants who withdrew from the study after the intervention period began were retained in the analysis until the point of withdrawal.

For each GM trip, seat belt use was a binary variable indicating whether the driver's seat belt was latched at any point. GM estimates it has accurate latch data for 98% of connected vehicles. To achieve a perfect buckling streak, participants needed to wear their seat belt on every trip during the week. Trips of less than 0.1 miles were excluded. For each Way to Drive trip, handheld phone use as a proportion of drive time was measured. The Way to Drive app uses information about a phone's motion and handsfree audio connectivity to distinguish between handheld and handsfree use with 82% accuracy.[21]. The app has an algorithm that classifies trips as driver or nondriver with 97% accuracy[41]; nondriver trips were excluded. To achieve a perfect phone-free streak, participants needed to engage in handheld phone use less than 1/60 (1.7%) of their drive time on every trip during the week.

Each Sunday of the intervention, treatment participants received a text encouraging them to buckle up and avoid handheld use every time they drove. Beginning the second Sunday, the text informed them which, if any, perfect streaks they had achieved the previous week (Appendix Figure E). Those with a perfect streak were shown how many weeks in a row they had achieved this streak. Raffle participants were also told they had been entered into a $125 raffle for their streak, along with how many others were entered (Appendix Figure F); shared pot participants were told how many others would share the $125 prize (Appendix Figure G). All incentive arm participants were reminded they could get a prize for each perfect streak. In addition, each Wednesday, those on track for 1 or both perfect streaks were sent an encouraging text.

Each Tuesday, treatment participants received a personalized safety tip via text, based on their intake survey responses. The first reminded them of their WOOP responses. On even-numbered weeks, they got a personalized tip related to seat belt use; on odd-numbered weeks, they got a tip about avoiding handheld phone use. The final text asked how they would make sure to buckle up and stay off their phone in the future.

Analysis Plan

We determined that 211 participants per arm would be needed to achieve 80% power to detect a 7.5-percentage-point difference in seat belt use between an intervention arm and control. This assumed use of Bonferroni–Holm adjustment to maintain a family-wise type I error rate of 0.05 for the 3 comparisons of active intervention arms to control. To account for potential attrition, we planned to recruit at least 250 participants per arm.

The primary outcome was proportion of intervention period trips during which participants used their seat belt. We used fractional regression with a logit link function in our unweighted primary analytic model, applying heteroskedasticity-consistent covariance matrix estimation to compare each of the 3 active intervention arms to control.[42] Holm-adjusted P values are reported for these 3 comparisons; adjusted P values may be evaluated against an α threshold of 0.05.[43] Exploratory analyses compared each of the active intervention arms against each other. The secondary outcome was proportion of drive time engaged in handheld phone use (e.g., calls, texting, swiping, and typing). Way to Drive trips were included if they were (1) classified as driver by the app and not reclassified by the participant or (2) reclassified as driver by the participant. Analytic models included the prespecified covariates in Table 1. Participants missing covariate data were excluded from the complete case analyses. We report outcomes after adjusting for model covariates. For both outcomes, analyses were repeated for the postintervention period to test whether any behavior change was sustained.

We tested for moderators of any significant intervention period treatment effects by sequentially adding to the model each covariate's dummy-coded covariate by treatment arm interaction terms, conducting a Wald test for each covariate and applying Bonferroni–Holm to the resulting 12 *P* values. We also explored whether treatment arms' rates of perfect weekly streaks differed from control, using logistic generalized estimating equations with the same covariates as the primary and secondary models.

RESULTS

A total of 1139 individuals from 49 US states and the District of Columbia participated, with 280 assigned to control, 285 to behavioral engagement, 287 to behavioral engagement plus raffle, and 287 to behavioral engagement plus shared pot (Appendix Figure H, CONSORT diagram). Mean participant age was 51 (SD = 14) years; nearly 60% were male and 81% were White (Table 1). Mean buckling rate at baseline was 83% (SD = 20%). After excluding participants who withdrew or were missing prespecified variables, 1001 remained for the primary analysis of seat belt use. Only 60% of participants installed and enabled the Way to Drive app to collect trip data during the intervention period, which resulted in a smaller sample of 682 for the secondary analysis of phone use.

Seat Belt Use

Weekly buckling trends across the 3 study periods are shown in Figure 1. In the primary model, intervention period buckling among those in the behavioral engagement plus shared pot group (adjusted mean = 91.3%) was greater than control (adjusted mean = 88.3%; adjusted *P* = .002). Participants in the behavioral engagement plus raffle group (adjusted mean = 89.5%) and the behavioral engagement group (adjusted mean = 89.4%) did not differ from control (adjusted *P*s = 0.37). Exploratory analyses found that the buckling rate in the behavioral engagement plus shared pot group was greater than in both the behavioral engagement plus raffle group (*P* = .015) and the behavioral engagement group (*P* = .037). Figure 2 shows these results in terms of unbuckled rate, where lower is better; Appendix Figure I provides unadjusted results. At follow-up, the buckling rate of behavioral engagement plus shared pot participants (adjusted mean = 92.0%) remained greater than control (adjusted mean = 88.1%; adjusted *P* < .001). The behavioral engagement plus raffle group (adjusted mean = 89.6%) did not differ from control (adjusted *P* = .12), but the behavioral engagement group did (adjusted mean = 90.2%; adjusted *P* = .041). Exploratory analyses again found that the buckling rate in the behavioral engagement plus shared pot group was greater than in both the behavioral engagement plus raffle group (*P* = .005) and the behavioral engagement group (*P* = .026).

Handheld Phone Use

During the intervention, handheld phone use among behavioral engagement plus shared pot (adjusted mean = 139 seconds per hour [s/h]), behavioral engagement plus raffle (adjusted mean = 149 s/h), and behavioral engagement (adjusted mean = 189 s/h) participants did not differ from control (adjusted mean = 170 s/h; adjusted *P*s > .46; Figure 3). This remained true at follow-up: participants in the behavioral engagement plus shared pot group (adjusted mean = 147 s/h), behavioral engagement plus raffle group (adjusted mean = 176 s/h), and behavioral engagement group (adjusted mean = 179 s/h) did not differ from control (adjusted mean = 174 s/h; adjusted *P*s > .65). See Appendix Figure J for weekly trends and Appendix Figure K for unadjusted model results.

Effect Moderators

There was no evidence that the effectiveness of the behavioral engagement plus shared pot intervention on buckling depended on participants' age, race, ethnicity, education, rurality, residence in a state with a primary or secondary enforcement law, proportion of short trips, number of reported crashes, or baseline seat belt use (adjusted *P*s > .99); number of reported tickets (adjusted *P* = .50); or income (adjusted *P* = .39). The participant sex by behavioral engagement plus shared pot interaction was not significant (adjusted *P* = .053) but warranted further inspection; the intervention was relatively ineffective among participants who did not disclose sex (*P* < .001), but there was no difference between females and males (*P* = .41).

TABLE 1— Participant Sociodemographic Characteristics and Seat Belt Use at Baseline: United States, July 10–August 14, 2022, and March 12–May 20, 2023

	Overall, No. (%) or Mean ±SD	Control, No. (%) or Mean ±SD	Behavioral Engagement, No. (%) or Mean ±SD	Behavioral Engagement Plus Raffle, No. (%) or Mean ±SD	Behavioral Engagement Plus Shared Pot, No. (%) or Mean ±SD
No.	1139	280	285	287	287
Age, y	51.3 ±14.4	50.6 ±15.4	52.2 ±14.6	50.9 ±13.7	51.3 ±13.9
Sex					
Female	454 (39.9)	106 (37.9)	107 (37.5)	116 (40.4)	125 (43.6)
Male	679 (59.6)	171 (61.1)	177 (62.1)	170 (59.2)	161 (56.1)
Intersex	1 (0.1)	1 (0.4)	0 (0.0)	0 (0.0)	0 (0.0)
Undisclosed	5 (0.4)	2 (0.7)	1 (0.4)	1 (0.3)	1 (0.3)
Race					
White or Caucasian	926 (81.3)	221 (78.9)	230 (80.7)	230 (80.1)	245 (85.4)
Black or African American	102 (9.0)	27 (9.6)	30 (10.5)	22 (7.7)	23 (8.0)
Other	67 (5.9)	20 (7.1)	13 (4.6)	23 (8.0)	11 (3.8)
Undisclosed	44 (3.9)	12 (4.3)	12 (4.2)	12 (4.2)	8 (2.8)
Ethnicity					
Hispanic	116 (10.2)	31 (11.1)	28 (9.8)	27 (9.4)	30 (10.5)
Non-Hispanic	1003 (88.1)	242 (86.4)	253 (88.8)	255 (88.9)	253 (88.2)
Undisclosed	20 (1.8)	7 (2.5)	4 (1.4)	5 (1.7)	4 (1.4)
State seatbelt enforcement[a]					
None	6 (0.5)	1 (0.4)	1 (0.4)	1 (0.3)	3 (1.0)
Primary	866 (76.4)	212 (76.3)	209 (74.4)	232 (80.8)	213 (74.2)
Secondary	261 (23.0)	65 (23.4)	71 (25.3)	54 (18.8)	71 (24.7)
Missing, no.	6	2	4	0	0
Residence rurality[a]					
Rural	141 (12.4)	29 (10.4)	34 (12.1)	34 (11.8)	44 (15.3)
Suburban	214 (18.9)	54 (19.4)	54 (19.2)	46 (16.0)	60 (20.9)
Urban	778 (68.7)	195 (70.1)	193 (68.7)	207 (72.1)	183 (63.8)
Missing, no.	6	2	4	0	0
Education level					
High school or less	149 (13.1)	48 (17.1)	32 (11.2)	33 (11.5)	36 (12.5)
Some college or college degree	710 (62.3)	164 (58.6)	179 (62.8)	183 (63.8)	184 (64.1)
Above college	271 (23.8)	67 (23.9)	69 (24.2)	70 (24.4)	65 (22.6)
Undisclosed	9 (0.8)	1 (0.4)	5 (1.8)	1 (0.3)	2 (0.7)
Annual Income, $					
< 50 000	155 (13.6)	35 (12.5)	48 (16.8)	37 (12.9)	35 (12.2)
50 000–100 000	348 (30.6)	98 (35.0)	71 (24.9)	82 (28.6)	97 (33.8)
> 100 000	543 (47.7)	131 (46.8)	137 (48.1)	143 (49.8)	132 (46.0)
Undisclosed	93 (8.2)	16 (5.7)	29 (10.2)	25 (8.7)	23 (8.0)
Traffic violations in previous 5 y					
0	872 (76.6)	219 (78.2)	206 (72.3)	225 (78.4)	222 (77.4)
1	216 (19.0)	53 (18.9)	59 (20.7)	47 (16.4)	57 (19.9)
2	41 (3.6)	8 (2.9)	14 (4.9)	12 (4.2)	7 (2.4)
≥ 3	10 (0.9)	0 (0.0)	6 (2.1)	3 (1.0)	1 (0.3)

Continued

TABLE 1— Continued

	Overall, No. (%) or Mean ±SD	Control, No. (%) or Mean ±SD	Behavioral Engagement, No. (%) or Mean ±SD	Behavioral Engagement Plus Raffle, No. (%) or Mean ±SD	Behavioral Engagement Plus Shared Pot, No. (%) or Mean ±SD
Car crashes in previous 5 y					
0	879 (77.2)	224 (80.0)	214 (75.1)	217 (75.6)	224 (78.0)
1	214 (18.8)	47 (16.8)	55 (19.3)	60 (20.9)	52 (18.1)
2	35 (3.1)	4 (1.4)	12 (4.2)	8 (2.8)	11 (3.8)
≥3	11 (1.0)	5 (1.8)	4 (1.4)	2 (0.7)	0 (0.0)
State seatbelt enforcement[a]					
None	6 (0.5)	1 (0.4)	1 (0.4)	1 (0.3)	3 (1.0)
Primary	866 (76.4)	212 (76.3)	209 (74.4)	232 (80.8)	213 (74.2)
Secondary	261 (23.0)	65 (23.4)	71 (25.3)	54 (18.8)	71 (24.7)
Missing, no.	6	2	4	0	0
Baseline seat belt use proportion[b]	0.83 ±0.20	0.83 ±0.20	0.83 ±0.20	0.82 ±0.20	0.83 ±0.18
Missing, no.	62	18	14	15	15
Intervention short trip proportion[c]	0.28 ±0.14	0.28 ±0.15	0.28 ±0.15	0.28 ±0.14	0.28 ±0.13
Missing, no.	75	18	17	17	23

Note. All variables were included as covariates in the primary analytic model. For the secondary outcome, the last 3 were not included as covariates because they were hypothesized only to predict seat belt use. In addition, the secondary model included "valid usage time," defined as the proportion of drive time during which the Way to Drive app was able to detect distraction events and the vehicle was traveling at least 9 miles per hour. For the follow-up period, the primary and secondary models included, respectively, postintervention short trip proportion and postintervention valid usage time as covariates.

[a]Derived from zip code.[44,45]

[b]Proportion of General Motors (GM) trips during the baseline period on which the driver buckled.

[c]Proportion of GM trips during the intervention period less than 2 miles long; drivers are less likely to buckle on short trips.

Exploratory Analysis of Perfect Streaks

During the intervention, the rate of perfect weekly buckling streaks was higher in the behavioral engagement plus shared pot (31.9%; adjusted $P = .003$) and behavioral engagement plus raffle (30.6%; adjusted $P = .004$) groups relative to control (22.9%; Appendix Figure L). At follow-up, the behavioral engagement plus shared pot (36.1%; adjusted $P < .001$) and behavioral engagement plus raffle (29.4%; adjusted $P = .032$) groups remained above control (22.8%). Similarly, during the intervention, the rate of perfect weekly phone-free streaks was higher in the behavioral engagement plus shared pot (21.7%; adjusted $P = .003$) and behavioral engagement plus raffle (18.4%; adjusted $P = .039$) groups relative to control (12.7%; Appendix Figure M). At follow-up, the behavioral engagement plus shared pot group (17.5%; adjusted $P = .002$) remained significantly above control (8.7%), but the behavioral engagement plus raffle group (13.3%; adjusted $P = .072$), did not.

DISCUSSION

In this national randomized trial of scalable interventions designed to increase objectively measured seat belt use, we report 3 key findings. First, a behavioral intervention with modest financial incentives led to a sustained increase in seat belt use. Second, structuring incentives as a shared pot was more effective than a raffle of similar expected value. Third, none of the interventions significantly reduced handheld phone use while driving, a major source of distraction.

Specifically, we found that an intervention involving education, personalized tips, a goal planning exercise, weekly streak feedback, and a shared pot incentive reduced unbuckled drives by 26% relative to control. The absolute 3-percentage-point effect is comparable to the difference between US states that do and do not have primary enforcement seat belt laws.[46] At follow-up, the reduction was even greater—33% in relative terms, 4% in absolute—suggesting drivers built lasting habits that no longer required feedback or incentives.[21] Although our sample was

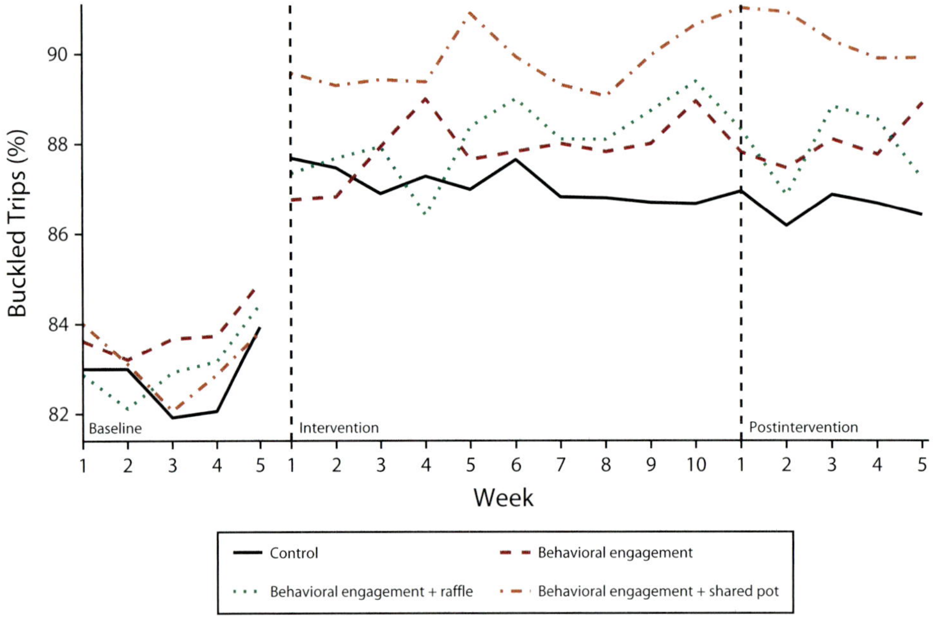

FIGURE 1— **Mean Weekly Buckling Rates Across Baseline, Intervention, and Postintervention Periods: United States, July 10–August 14, 2022, and March 12–June 24, 2023**

Note. The break depicted between the baseline and intervention periods represents the nearly 7-month delay between these 2 periods.

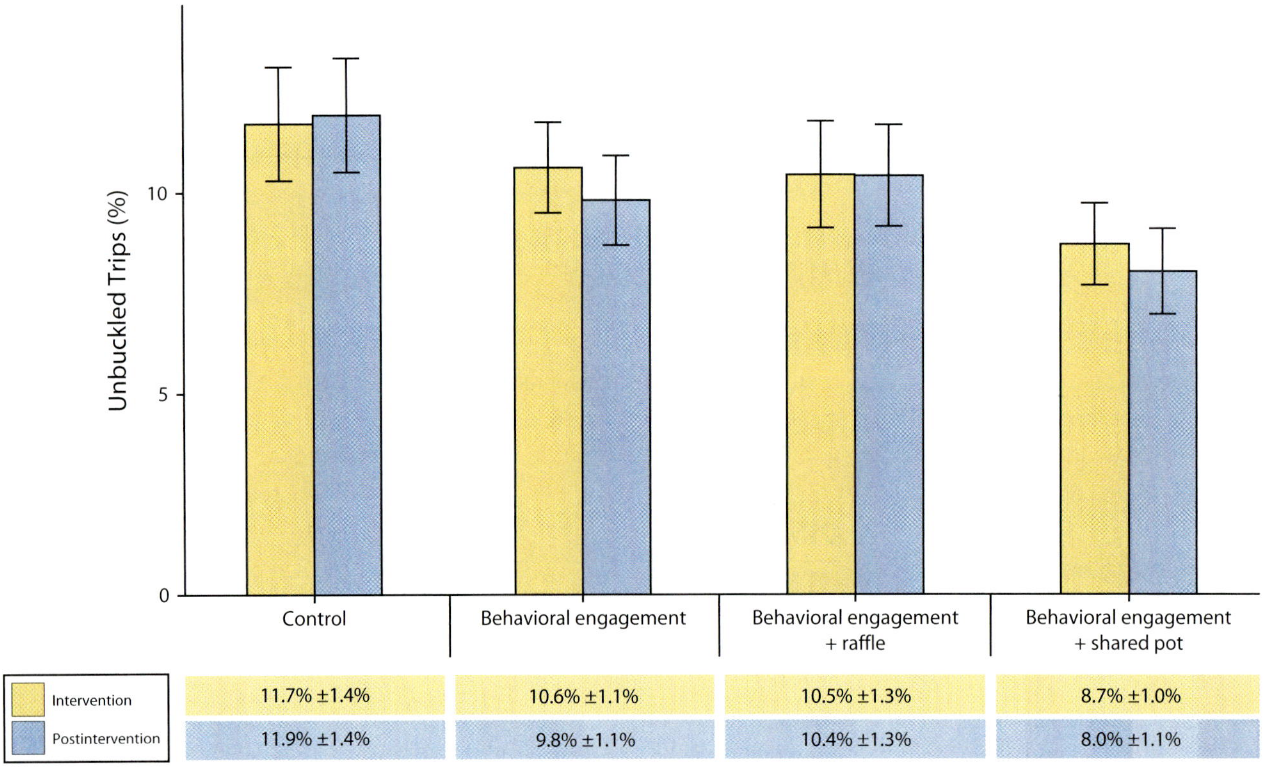

FIGURE 2— **Adjusted Mean Percentage of Trips When Driver Was Unbuckled: United States, March 12–June 24, 2023**

Note. Error bars represent 95% confidence intervals.

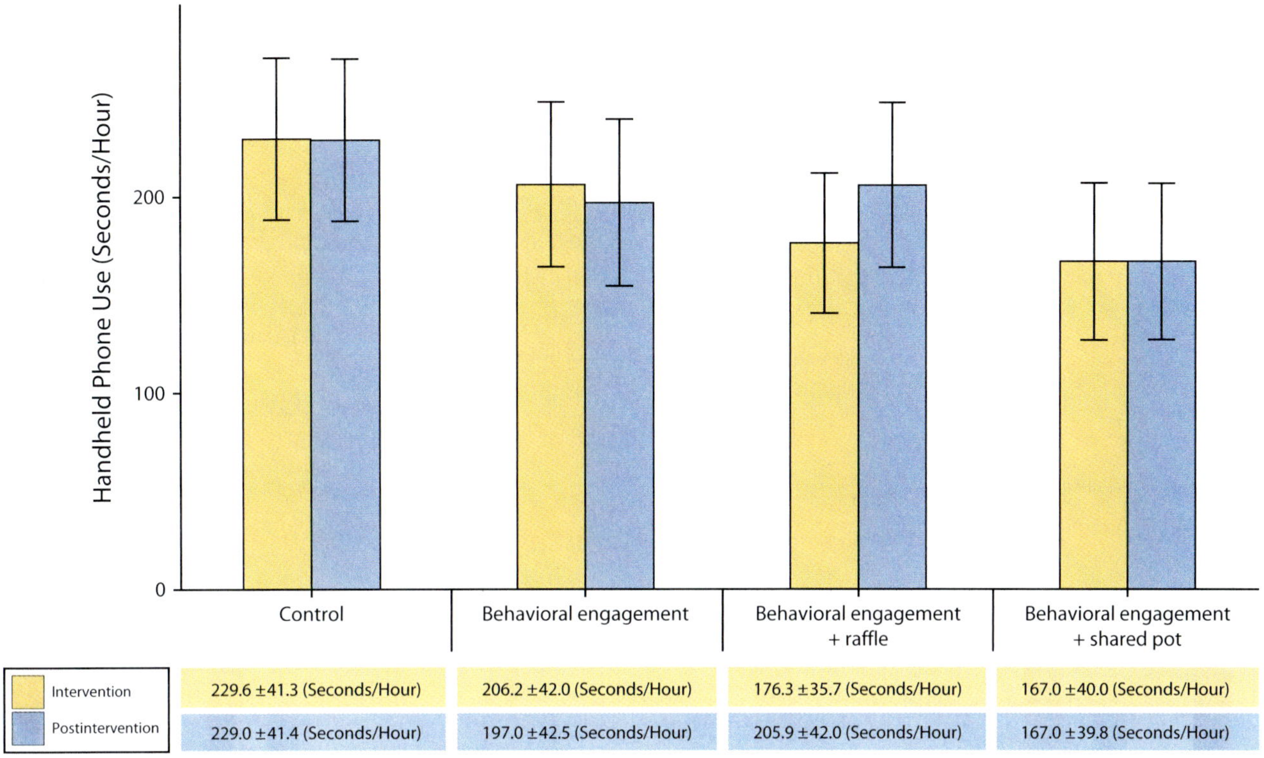

FIGURE 3— Adjusted Mean Handheld Phone Use While Driving: United States, March 12–June 24, 2023

Note. For each participant and study period, seconds of handheld phone use per hour of drive time was calculated. Error bars represent 95% confidence intervals.

more likely to be older, White, and male than the US population, the intervention was similarly effective across demographic groups, suggesting results would generalize to more diverse samples. However, only 17 (1.5%) participants were in the 18- to 24-year age range; more research is needed to determine intervention effectiveness with young adult and adolescent drivers, who are at greatest risk of unrestrained crash.[7] The intervention was equally effective in states with and without primary or secondary enforcement laws, suggesting that the benefits of the intervention and seat belt laws are additive. Incentive costs were $0.44 per driver-week.

Incentive structure mattered for behavior change. The shared pot incentive was superior to a raffle of approximately equal expected value, suggesting that, in a repeated game, a guaranteed 1/Nth share of a prize is more motivating than a 1-in-N chance at the full prize. This novel behavioral economics finding warrants replication in other contexts, as it could enhance the effectiveness of public health interventions that have relied on lottery incentives.[34–37] Because it equally rewards everyone who engages in the desired behavior, the shared pot structure may be especially attractive in highly regulated industries like insurance. Future research should investigate potential mechanisms underlying the shared pot's superiority over a raffle, such as its guarantee of a reward, uncertainty about the reward's amount, or the prosocial norm it communicates.

Previous research has found positive effects of behavioral or educational interventions on seat belt use, regardless of whether financial incentives were also offered,[23] whereas the present trial found that behavioral engagement alone was insufficient. A key difference is that nearly all previous trials have used self-reported buckling as the outcome, whereas the present trial used telematics-measured buckling. It is unknown whether previous behavioral or educational interventions would, by themselves, increase telematics-measured buckling. Regardless, the present research suggests that their effectiveness could be enhanced by incorporating modest, time-limited financial incentives tied to objectively measured performance.

None of the interventions significantly reduced the overall proportion of drive time engaged in handheld phone use, the secondary outcome.

However, exploratory analyses found that raffle participants had 45% more and shared pot participants 71% more phone-free streaks than control participants. Together, these results suggest that incentivizing perfect streaks may have been effective among those who already had low handheld phone use but ineffective for heavier users who account for most handheld phone use. Incentivizing attainable goals tailored to each driver may be a more effective approach.[20,21,47,48]

This study had limitations. First, its opt-in nature means we cannot gauge the acceptability and effectiveness of interventions if scaled to all customers. We note that the study's inadvertent inclusion of customers across the full distribution of buckling behavior likely increases its external validity and usefulness to insurers and other entities seeking to scale interventions to drivers regardless of their baseline buckling behavior. Second, we did not know whether a seat belt was worn properly for the duration of a trip. Third, we did not know if the participant was the driver of their GM vehicle on any given trip (drives by nonparticipants would have diluted the measured impact of interventions). Fourth, 40% of enrollees did not install Way to Drive; the resulting smaller sample for the secondary outcome means that strong conclusions cannot be drawn about the efficacy of interventions for curbing handheld use. The low installation rate also opens the possibility of self-selection bias; however, there was no evidence of differential installation across study arms (Appendix Figure H), and the adjusted model controlled for potential confounders (see Appendix Figure K for a discussion). Fifth, we do not know how long heightened levels of buckling were sustained beyond the 5-week follow-up period.

Delivered at scale, the best-performing intervention could substantially reduce deaths and costs associated with vehicular crashes. An estimated 2677 lives could be saved annually in the United States if all motor vehicle passengers wore a seat belt.[2] A 26% reduction in the unbuckled rate would translate to about 700 lives saved each year. At a total economic cost per crash fatality of $1 778 000,[49] this would mean $1.2 billion in annual savings. A promising channel for scaling incentivized behavioral interventions to promote seat belt use is usage-based insurance programs, which make up 17% of the US auto insurance market.[50] These programs already provide drivers feedback on risky driving behaviors and pay out $5 billion in safe driving discounts annually.[51,52] As these programs grow in popularity and more vehicles are equipped with telematics measuring seat belt use, so, too, does the opportunity to leverage behavioral science to have a meaningful impact on safe driving. We recommend that policymakers clear remaining regulatory hurdles to offering discounts and incentives to drivers for engaging in safe behavior[53] while taking steps to ensure the privacy of customers' telematics data. AJPH

ABOUT THE AUTHORS

Jeffrey P. Ebert, Ruiqi Yan, Sadie Friday, Dylan Small, and M. Kit Delgado are with the Perelman School of Medicine, University of Pennsylvania, Philadelphia. Catherine C. McDonald is with the Perelman School of Medicine and the School of Nursing, University of Pennsylvania, Philadelphia. Kelsey Bartolozzi is with General Motors Financial, Fort Worth, TX.

CORRESPONDENCE

Correspondence should be sent to Jeffrey P. Ebert, University of Pennsylvania, 3535 Market St, Suite 1500, Philadelphia, PA 19104 (e-mail: jeffrey.ebert@pennmedicine.upenn.edu). Reprints can be ordered at https://www.ajph.org by clicking the "Reprints" link.

PUBLICATION INFORMATION

Full Citation: Ebert JP, Yan R, Friday S, et al. Behavioral interventions for increasing seat belt use and decreasing distracted driving using telematics: a national randomized trial. *Am J Public Health*. 2025;115(5):758–768.

Acceptance Date: December 8, 2024.

DOI: https://doi.org/10.2105/AJPH.2024.307980

ORCID iDs:

Jeffrey P. Ebert https://orcid.org/0009-0004-4044-0972

Sadie Friday https://orcid.org/0009-0006-1482-6593

Dylan Small https://orcid.org/0000-0003-4928-2646

Catherine C. McDonald https://orcid.org/0000-0003-3856-8542

M. Kit Delgado https://orcid.org/0000-0002-2248-8401

CONTRIBUTORS

J. P. Ebert conceptualized and designed the study, interpreted data, and drafted and revised the article. R. Yan analyzed and interpreted data. S. Friday designed the study and acquired data. D. Small conceptualized and designed the study and analyzed and interpreted data. C. C. McDonald acquired data and revised the article. K. Bartolozzi conceptualized and designed the study, acquired data, and revised the article. M. K. Delgado conceptualized and designed the study, acquired and interpreted data, and revised the article. All authors approved the final article.

ACKNOWLEDGMENTS

This research was supported by funding from the Abramson Family Foundation (M. K. Delgado) and General Motors, as well as by Centers for Disease Control and Prevention (CDC) grant R49CEE003083 (C. C. McDonald).

The authors wish to thank Skip Coon and Michael Kopinsky of the Penn Medicine Way to Health team, Amy Brassell of General Motors, Katie DeGraaf of General Motors Financial, and Dina Abdel-Rahman, Neda Khan, Maya Nelson, Arjun Patel, and Ruiying (Aria) Xiong of the Penn Medicine Nudge Unit.

Note. The content is solely the responsibility of the authors and does not necessarily represent the official views of the funders. The Abramson Family Foundation and the CDC had no role in the study design or in the collection, analysis, and interpretation of data.

CONFLICTS OF INTEREST

The authors declare that they have no competing interests.

HUMAN PARTICIPANT PROTECTION

The study protocol was approved by the institutional review board of the University of Pennsylvania.

Participants consented and were compensated for their time.

REFERENCES

1. World Health Organization. Road traffic injuries. Available at: https://www.who.int/news-room/fact-sheets/detail/road-traffic-injuries. Accessed December 20, 2024.
2. National Center for Statistics and Analysis. Lives saved in 2017 by restraint use and minimum-drinking-age laws. *Traffic Safety Facts.* National Highway Traffic Safety Administration. March 2019. Available at: https://crashstats.nhtsa.dot.gov/Api/Public/Publication/812683. Accessed February 27, 2025.
3. Kargar S, Ansari-Moghaddam A, Ansari H. The prevalence of seat belt use among drivers and passengers: a systematic review and meta-analysis. *J Egypt Public Health Assoc.* 2023;98(1):14. https://doi.org/10.1186/s42506-023-00139-3
4. World Health Organization. Seat-belt wearing rate data by country. Available at: https://apps.who.int/gho/data/view.main.51416. Accessed May 31, 2024.
5. National Center for Statistics and Analysis. Seat belt use in 2023 – overall results. *Traffic Safety Facts.* DOT HS 813 543. National Highway Traffic Safety Administration. February 2024. Available at: https://crashstats.nhtsa.dot.gov/Api/Public/Publication/813543. Accessed February 27, 2025.
6. Richard CM, Magee K, Bacon-Abdelmoteleb P, Brown JL. *Countermeasures That Work: A Highway Safety Countermeasure Guide for State Highway Safety Offices, Ninth Edition.* DOT HS 812 478. National Highway Traffic Safety Administration. 2018. Available at: https://www.nhtsa.gov/sites/nhtsa.gov/files/documents/812478_countermeasures-that-work-a-highway-safety-countermeasures-guide-9thedition-2017v2_0.pdf. Accessed February 27, 2025.
7. National Center for Statistics and Analysis. Occupant protection in passenger vehicles: 2021 data. 2023. *Traffic Safety Facts.* DOT HS 813 449. National Highway Traffic Safety Administration. May 2023. Available at: https://crashstats.nhtsa.dot.gov/Api/Public/ViewPublication/813449. Accessed February 27, 2025.
8. National Center for Statistics and Analysis. Distracted driving 2019. Traffic Safety Facts. DOT HS 813 111. National Highway Traffic Safety Administration. April 2021. Available at: https://crashstats.nhtsa.dot.gov/Api/Public/Publication/813111. Accessed February 27, 2025.
9. Dingus TA, Guo F, Lee S, et al. Driver crash risk factors and prevalence evaluation using naturalistic driving data. *Proc Natl Acad Sci U S A.* 2016;113(10):2636–2641. https://doi.org/10.1073/pnas.1513271113
10. Dingus TA, Owens JM, Guo F, et al. The prevalence of and crash risk associated with primarily cognitive secondary tasks. *Saf Sci.* 2019;119:98–105. https://doi.org/10.1016/j.ssci.2019.01.005
11. *The State of US Road Risk in 2024.* Cambridge, MA: Cambridge Mobile Telematics; 2024.
12. Cheng C. Do cell phone bans change driver behavior? *Econ Inq.* 2015;53(3):1420–1436. https://doi.org/10.1111/ecin.12166
13. Oviedo-Trespalacios O. Getting away with texting: behavioural adaptation of drivers engaging in visual-manual tasks while driving. *Transp Res Part A Policy Pract.* 2018;116:112–121. https://doi.org/10.1016/j.tra.2018.05.006
14. Rudisill TM, Baus AD, Jarrett T. Challenges of enforcing cell phone use while driving laws among police: a qualitative study. *Inj Prev.* 2019;25(6):494–500. https://doi.org/10.1136/injuryprev-2018-042931
15. National Center for Statistics and Analysis. Driver electronic device use in 2022. *Traffic Safety Facts.* DOT HS 813 531. National Highway Traffic Safety Administration. January 2024. Available at: https://crashstats.nhtsa.dot.gov/Api/Public/ViewPublication/813531.pdf. Accessed February 27, 2025.
16. Stevenson M, Harris A, Wijnands JS, Mortimer D. The effect of telematic based feedback and financial incentives on driving behaviour: a randomised trial. *Accident Anal Prev.* 2021;159:106278. https://doi.org/10.1016/j.aap.2021.106278
17. Arumugam S, Bhargavi R. A survey on driving behavior analysis in usage based insurance using big data. *J Big Data.* 2019;6(1):86. https://doi.org/10.1186/s40537-019-0249-5
18. Tselentis DI, Yannis G, Vlahogianni EI. Innovative motor insurance schemes: a review of current practices and emerging challenges. *Accid Anal Prev.* 2017;98:139–148. https://doi.org/10.1016/j.aap.2016.10.006
19. Fortune Business Insights. Automotive usage based insurance market size, share & COVID-19 impact analysis, 2023–2030. Available at: https://www.fortunebusinessinsights.com/automotive-usage-based-insurance-market-104103. Accessed June 1, 2024.
20. Delgado MK, Ebert JP, Xiong RA, et al. Feedback and financial incentives for reducing cell phone use while driving: a randomized clinical trial. *JAMA Netw Open.* 2024;7(7):e2420218. https://doi.org/10.1001/jamanetworkopen.2024.20218
21. Ebert JP, Xiong RA, Khan N, et al. A randomized trial of behavioral interventions yielding sustained reductions in distracted driving. *Proc Natl Acad Sci U S A.* 2024;121(32):e2320603121. https://doi.org/10.1073/pnas.2320603121
22. Suffoletto B, Pacella-LaBarbara ML, Huber J, Delgado MK, McDonald C. Effectiveness of a text message intervention promoting seat belt use among young adults: a randomized clinical trial. *JAMA Netw Open.* 2022;5(9):e2231616. https://doi.org/10.1001/jamanetworkopen.2022.31616
23. Lourens A, Sinclair M, Willems B, Young T. Education, incentive, and engineering-based interventions to promote the use of seat belts. *Cochrane Libr.* 2024;1(1):CD011218. https://doi.org/10.1002/14651858.CD011218.pub2
24. Sheveland AC, Luchman JN, Mendelson J, et al. Psychological constructs related to seat belt use: a nationally representative survey study. *Accid Anal Prev.* 2020;148:105715. https://doi.org/10.1016/j.aap.2020.105715
25. Ebert J, Xiong A, Halpern S, et al. *Summary Report: Comparative Effectiveness of Alternative Smartphone-Based Nudges to Reduce Cellphone Use While Driving: Final Report.* FHWA-HRT-22-057. Washington, DC: Federal Highway Administration; 2022.
26. Wang GX, Wang Y, Gai XS. A meta-analysis of the effects of mental contrasting with implementation intentions on goal attainment. *Front Psychol.* 2021;12:565202. https://doi.org/10.3389/fpsyg.2021.565202
27. Oettingen G. *Rethinking Positive Thinking: Inside the New Science of Motivation.* New York, NY: Current; 2015.
28. Weathers D, Poehlman TA. Defining, and understanding commitment to, activity streaks. *J Acad Mark Sci.* 2024;52(2):531–553. https://doi.org/10.1007/s11747-023-00944-4
29. DeFulio A, Rzeszutek MJ, Furgeson J, Ryan S, Rezania S. A smartphone-smartcard platform for contingency management in an inner-city substance use disorder outpatient program. *J Subst Abuse Treat.* 2021;120:108188. https://doi.org/10.1016/j.jsat.2020.108188
30. Muhlner K, DeFlavio J, Ang A, Zito M, McLellan AT, Perrochet B. Demonstration of an app-delivered digital therapeutic program for methamphetamine use disorder. *Front Psychiatry.* 2023;14:1176641. https://doi.org/10.3389/fpsyt.2023.1176641
31. Gallagher KM, Updegraff JA. Health message framing effects on attitudes, intentions, and behavior: a meta-analytic review. *Ann Behav Med.* 2012;43(1):101–116. https://doi.org/10.1007/s12160-011-9308-7
32. Zhang N, Drake SA, Ding K. Message appeals on an Instagram account promoting seat belt use that attract adolescents and young adults: elaboration-likelihood perspective study. *JMIR Form Res.* 2020;4(9):e16800. https://doi.org/10.2196/16800
33. Rothman AJ, Bartels RD, Wlaschin J, Salovey P. The strategic use of gain- and loss-framed messages to promote healthy behavior: how theory can inform practice. *J Commun.* 2006;56(suppl 1):S202–S220. https://doi.org/10.1111/j.1460-2466.2006.00290.x
34. Volpp KG, John LK, Troxel AB, Norton L, Fassbender J, Loewenstein G. Financial incentive–based approaches for weight loss. *JAMA.* 2008;300(22):2631–2637. https://doi.org/10.1001/jama.2008.804
35. Kimmel SE, Troxel AB, Loewenstein G, et al. Randomized trial of lottery-based incentives to improve warfarin adherence. *Am Heart J.* 2012;164(2):268–274. https://doi.org/10.1016/j.ahj.2012.05.005
36. Patel MS, Asch DA, Rosin R, et al. Individual versus team-based financial incentives to increase physical activity: a randomized, controlled trial. *J Gen Intern Med.* 2016;31(7):746–754. https://doi.org/10.1007/s11606-016-3627-0
37. Milkman KL, Gandhi L, Ellis SF, et al. A citywide experiment testing the impact of geographically targeted, high-pay-off vaccine lotteries. *Nat Hum Behav.* 2022;6(11):1515–1524. https://doi.org/10.1038/s41562-022-01437-0
38. Schultz W. Behavioral theories and the neurophysiology of reward. *Annu Rev Psychol.* 2006;57(1):87–115. https://doi.org/10.1146/annurev.psych.56.091103.070229
39. Wood W. *Good Habits, Bad Habits: The Science of Making Positive Changes That Stick.* 1st ed. New York, NY: Farrar, Straus and Giroux; 2019.
40. Cialdini RB. *Influence, New and Expanded: The Psychology of Persuasion.* New and Expanded ed. New York, NY: Harper Business; 2021.
41. Ebert JP, Xiong RA, Patel A, Abdel-Rahman D, McDonald CC, Delgado MK. Validation of a smartphone telematics algorithm for classifying driver trips. *Transp Res Interdiscip Perspect.* 2024;25:101109. https://doi.org/10.1016/j.trip.2024.101109
42. Hayes AF, Cai L. Using heteroskedasticity-consistent standard error estimators in OLS regression: an introduction and software implementation. *Behav Res Methods.* 2007;39(4):709–722. https://doi.org/10.3758/BF03192961

43. Blakesley RE, Mazumdar S, Dew MA, et al. Comparisons of methods for multiple hypothesis testing in neuropsychological research. *Neuropsychology*. 2009;23(2):255–264. https://doi.org/10.1037/a0012850
44. Paykin S, Menghaney M, Lin Q, Kolak M. Rural, suburban, urban classification for small area analysis. Chicago, IL: Healthy Regions & Policies Lab, Center for Spatial Data Science at the University of Chicago; 2021.
45. Governors Highway Safety Association. Seat belts. Available at: https://www.ghsa.org/state-laws/issues/seat%20belts. Accessed June 6, 2024.
46. National Center for Statistics and Analysis. Seat belt use in 2022 – use rates in states and territories. *Traffic Safety Facts*. National Highway Traffic Safety Administration. July 2023. Available at: https://crashstats.nhtsa.dot.gov/Api/Public/Publication/813487. Accessed February 27, 2025.
47. Chokshi NP, Adusumalli S, Small DS, et al. Loss-framed financial incentives and personalized goal-setting to increase physical activity among ischemic heart disease patients using wearable devices: the ACTIVE REWARD Randomized Trial. *J Am Heart Assoc*. 2018;7(12):e009173. https://doi.org/10.1161/JAHA.118.009173
48. Bonezzi A, Brendl CM, De Angelis M. Stuck in the middle: the psychophysics of goal pursuit. *Psychol Sci*. 2011;22(5):607–612. https://doi.org/10.1177/0956797611404899
49. National Safety Council. Injury Facts. Guide to calculating costs. Available at: https://injuryfacts.nsc.org/all-injuries/costs/guide-to-calculating-costs/data-details. Accessed November 7, 2023.
50. Mattson K. Insurers continue to prioritize usage-based insurance in 2023. Digital Insurance. November 13, 2023. Available at: https://www.dig-in.com/list/state-farm-progressive-geico-allstate-ubi-telematics-2023. Accessed June 11, 2024.
51. National Association of Insurance Commissioners. NAIC releases 2023 market share data. March 4, 2024. Available at: https://content.naic.org/article/naic-releases-2023-market-share-data. Accessed June 11, 2024.
52. AAA. What is usage-based insurance & is it right for you? September 29, 2021. Available at: https://www.ace.aaa.com/insurance/advocacy/what-is-usage-based-insurance.html. Accessed June 11, 2024.
53. Ben-Shahar O. Privacy protection, at what cost? Exploring the regulatory resistance to data technology in auto insurance. *J Legal Anal*. 2023;15(1):129–157. https://doi.org/10.1093/jla/laad008

How and Why Does Redlining Matter for Present-Day Health? Critical Perspectives on Causality, Cartography, and Capitalism

Carolyn Swope, MPH, Scott Markley, PhD, MS, Shannon Whittaker, PhD, MPH, and Amy Hillier, PhD, MSW

See also Winling, p. 649.

Recent years have seen an explosion of public health research on associations between historical redlining maps created by a US government agency, the Home Owners' Loan Corporation (HOLC), and present-day outcomes. Yet precisely how and why HOLC's surveys help us understand the underpinnings of present-day racial inequities remains unclear.

We apply an interdisciplinary perspective to assess the contributions and limitations of this literature, particularly with regard to causal mechanisms and theoretical explanations. While research often frames HOLC redlining as a measure of structural racism that directly shapes present-day outcomes, we look instead to racial capitalism to understand how and why racialized housing policies are implemented.

We argue that the HOLC maps represent symptoms, not causes, of systematic disinvestment in Black communities, that redlining was not produced by the federal government in isolation but was shaped by public–private collaboration and infused with capitalist logics, and that redlining interacted with many other forms of racialized housing dispossession to shape present-day riskscapes. We conclude by offering conceptual and methodological recommendations for public health researchers, including suggestions for data sources other than HOLC maps. (*Am J Public Health*. 2025;115(5):769–779. https://doi.org/10.2105/AJPH.2024.308000)

AJPH May 2025, Vol. 115, No. 5

Recent years have seen a surge of interest in historical mortgage redlining, particularly as a tangible indicator of structural racism and its effects in the United States. "Redlining" describes deeming particular neighborhoods to be risky, often based on racialized status, and implementing discriminatory lending practices accordingly. While a range of public and private entities have engaged in redlining, attention has especially focused on the Home Owners' Loan Corporation (HOLC)—a government agency formed in the 1930s to help stabilize the housing market through mortgage refinancing assistance, which conducted nationwide residential "security" surveys assessing neighborhood riskiness. Neighborhoods were assigned grades from A (best) to D ("hazardous" and colored red on accompanying maps). The increase in academic scholarship about redlining has been dramatic, facilitated by the Mapping Inequality Web site's digitization of HOLC residential security maps and area descriptions in 2016.[1] This trend is particularly marked in public health, which represents the overwhelming majority of studies on redlining (Figure 1). The turn toward recognizing and attempting to measure racism as an upstream determinant of health represents important progress. Yet how and why, precisely, HOLC's surveys help us understand the underpinnings of present-day racial inequities remains unclear.

Historian Kenneth Jackson discovered the original HOLC maps in the late 1970s and described them in his widely read 1985 book *Crabgrass Frontier*.[3] Despite his careful explanation that HOLC did not issue mortgage assistance according to its grades and argument that its maps institutionalized rather than initiated redlining, the next

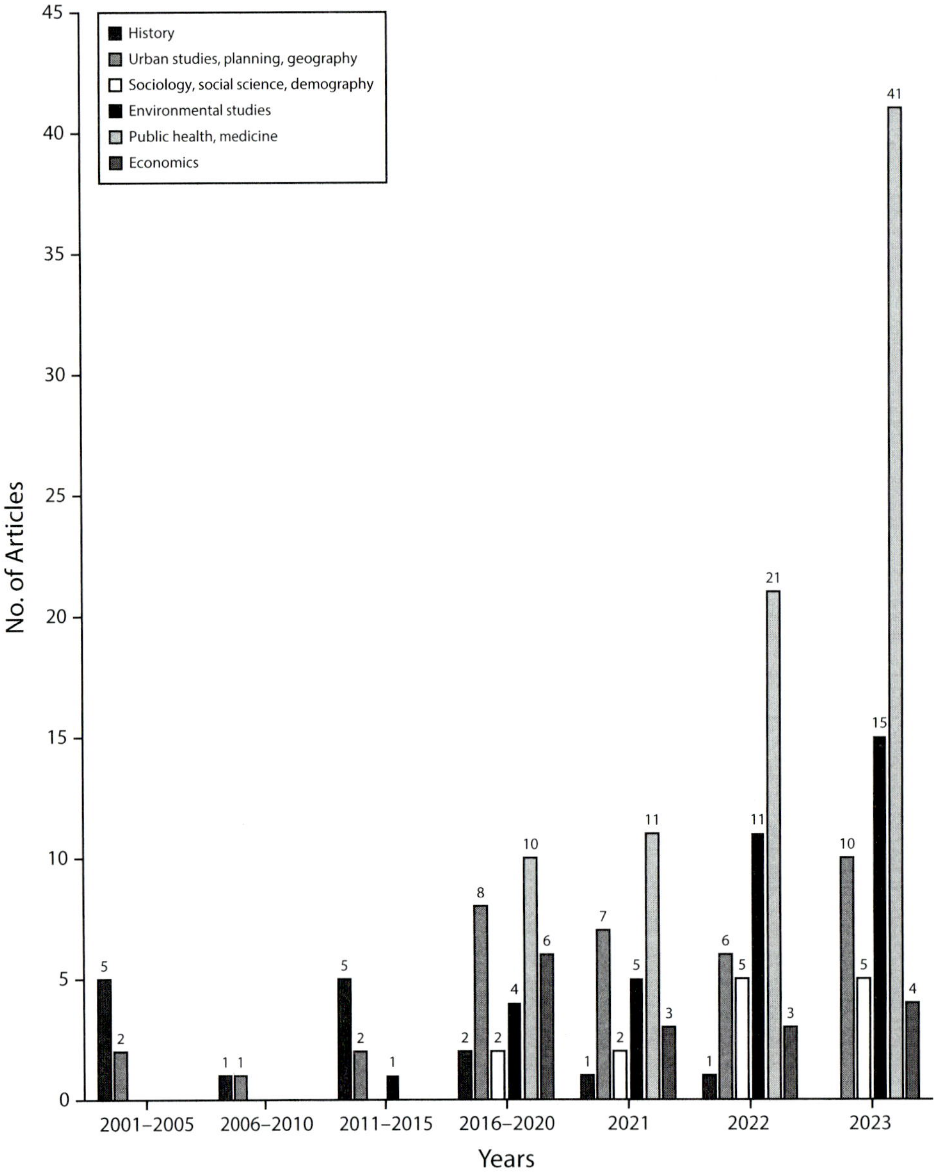

FIGURE 1— Articles About Redlining by the Home Owners' Loan Corporation (HOLC), by Discipline: United States, 2001–2023

Note. An inventory of articles published in academic journals or as academic working papers between 2001 and 2023 was created using the search terms "HOLC" and "redlining" in Google Scholar. This list was cross-referenced with a scoping review in Swope et al.[2] Academic discipline was determined primarily by the journal title and secondarily by the abstract.

2 decades of scholarship made HOLC synonymous with redlining. Subsequent scholarship from the early 2000s to the 2020s challenged this uncritical narrative and offered a more nuanced interpretation of HOLC's role in redlining, putting more attention on the Federal Housing Administration and private-sector map-making and lending practices.[4–9] But much academic scholarship, including recent public health research, overlooks this newer literature to embrace the simpler, older narrative that HOLC maps caused redlining—continuing to frame present-day health inequities as a direct outcome of HOLC grades despite the overwhelming empirical historical evidence that these maps did not inform lending decisions. Each publication seems to inspire more research—sometimes more methodologically sophisticated, sometimes focusing on a different health outcome—with no end

in sight. If HOLC redlining can be linked to heart disease and food access, why not urban tree canopy and older adult walking behavior?

In this article, we draw on our experience as scholars of geography, city planning, public health, and urban history and engage with the extensive literature about redlining across a wide range of disciplines. We assess the contributions and limitations of the literature linking HOLC redlining to the health of individuals and communities, giving special attention to the causal mechanisms and theoretical explanations offered by scholars for these relationships. While scholars often frame HOLC redlining as a measure of structural racism directly shaping present-day outcomes, we look to racial capitalism as an alternative and more useful framework. We argue that the HOLC maps represent symptoms, not causes, of systematic disinvestment in Black communities. We also argue that redlining was only one of many forms of racialized housing dispossession, one ultimately given disproportionate attention facilitated by the relative availability of digitized HOLC maps. This reframing does not mean that redlining was not racist, that the federal government was not culpable in that racism, or that the maps are not significant sources of information about discrimination and disinvestment. Rather, it draws attention to how racial differentiation and exploitation structures housing markets and policies in fundamental ways that go beyond any one process or actor, as support for capitalist profit and White supremacy shapes state policy. We conclude by offering conceptual and methodological recommendations for public health researchers, including suggestions for data sources other than HOLC maps.

TOWARD A RACIAL CAPITALISM LENS

Structural racism refers to the multitude of ways that "mutually reinforcing inequitable systems" of housing, education, health care, and criminal justice, among others, interact to exclude racialized groups from access to power, privilege, and resources—all of which are necessary to achieving optimal health.[10(p1453)] Public health scholars in recent years have begun to examine and therefore seek to quantify the impact of structurally racist policies and practices (e.g., slavery, Jim Crow laws, and mass incarceration) in persistent racialized health inequities in the United States. Prominent in this research is assessing the impact of racialized housing policies on health where studies have historically focused on the relatively downstream indicator of segregation but "overlooked the structural forces that created and reinforced segregation."[11(pS49)] HOLC redlining, as a concrete practice that is readily quantifiable, has become central to this research and accordingly has become one of the most commonly evaluated measures of structural racism in the discipline.[12]

While a structural racism perspective importantly seeks to look beyond individual-level attitudes and prejudices in explaining racism and its effects, we argue that research on structural racism has nevertheless been focused on naming racist structures and policies but with limited consideration for how and by whom they were constructed and deployed, why they were produced, and to whom the benefits accrue. Specifically, scholarship on HOLC redlining and health illustrates this limitation. For instance, studies assessing HOLC grades as a measure for structural racism rarely interrogate how and in whose interests the presence of non-White residents was linked to devaluation. Accepting appraisers' linkages of race and property value as a fait accompli obscures the underlying ideologies informing their perceptions of value and the many actors at play, framing redlining as a practice devoid from its historical context. As antiracism scholar Arun Kundnani puts it, "without an explanation of what the *structure* in structural racism is," researchers "cannot explain what sustains" ongoing bias. That is, structural forces are not simply the result of cumulative individual biases innate to White people.[13(p4)] Without such explanation, structural racism becomes a nebulous, primordial, and essentialized concept, rather than one that is intentionally constructed for specific purposes. This removal of accountability shapes structural racism as an "actorless" social determinant of health.[14] Drawing on a tradition of antiracist theory emerging from struggles over the organization of land and labor under colonialism and capitalism,[13] we instead suggest the utility of a racial capitalism lens for analyzing redlining and other processes and policies of structural racism.

A racial capitalism framework holds that the accumulation process defining the capitalist mode of production has been fundamentally shaped by White supremacy, particularly in the United States. As English and ethnic studies scholar Jodi Melamed summarizes it, for capital accumulation to occur, some people must be rendered eligible to be exploited and disposed (i.e., devalued), and "racism enshrines the[se] inequalities that capitalism requires."[15(p77)] Although some have highlighted tensions within racial capitalism scholarship[16] (e.g., whether racial division is always necessary for capitalism), we maintain that the concept appropriately identifies how aforementioned racist policies and practices in the United States perpetuate and are perpetuated by the political–economic system to produce harm for non-White groups in particular. For example, with regard to housing, the real estate industry has generated massive profits at the expense of Black and other non-White communities by valuing White presence and relationally devaluing Black presence.[17–19] In this way, a racial capitalism approach to public health allows us to see the "production and exploitation of group-differentiated premature death," as geographer Ruth Wilson Gilmore puts it[20(p28)]—not as a side-effect of racist policies and institutions whose drivers and development are unexplained, but as the direct result of capitalism's profit accumulation imperative, functioning through the (racialized) devaluation of people.

Recent interventions emphasizing racial capitalism as a key determinant of health have cogently illustrated its utility for public health researchers. Geographer Laura Pulido, for example, argues that the poisoning of Flint's water supply and resulting health problems occurred because Flint is racialized as Black and, thus, its residents were "so devalued that their lives [were] subordinated to the goals of municipal fiscal solvency."[21(p2)] Extending this thread, sociologist Whitney Laster Pirtle contends that racial capitalism should be considered a fundamental cause of the COVID-19 pandemic's racially unequal death toll. Racial capitalism has produced a situation in which Black residents are disproportionately exposed to health risk factors and isolated from protective resources, ensuring the pandemic's racially unequal outcomes through multiple pathways.[22] Philosopher Olúfẹ́mi Táíwò et al. and public health students Yesnely Flores and Harris Greenwood agree, each calling to reinterpret racial health inequities as products of racial capitalism.[23,24] Doing so, Táíwò et al. contend, adds "an explicitly political dimension" to public health scholarship[23(p21)]—in contrast to the more "actor-less" deployment of structural racism frameworks, as described previously.

Despite the nascent application of racial capitalism in public health research, work on redlining and health has yet to fully grapple with its implications. The focus has remained on the purported legacy of a past government program while downplaying or ignoring how capitalist processes both shaped it and continue to reproduce racial health inequities through other mechanisms. A racial capitalism approach shifts our attention from the physical maps to the actors and institutions that created them, and the logics that drove them. A racial capitalism approach thus places the HOLC mapping program within a political–economic context, allowing us to see it not as the archetypal case of state-sponsored discrimination but as 1 instance of what scholars of racial capitalism have called the "racist theory of value"—a definition of property value that equated Black presence with risk—being put into action.[19,25] This approach thus recognizes that persistent racial health inequities are not the outcome of 1 discriminatory program from the 1930s but are continuously being reproduced by a political–economic system that devalues Black life.

CLARIFYING THE HOME OWNERS' LOAN CORPORATION'S ROLE

We now turn to reviewing how research on redlining and health can articulate HOLC's role with greater precision to more accurately interpret associations. We discuss specific limitations in current public health redlining research, which we suggest often stem from the use of a structural racism framework without attention to the logics and actors shaping policies and to the political–economic systems in which they are embedded. And we demonstrate how a racial capitalism lens can shed light on how and why HOLC redlining matters even if we cannot attribute present-day outcomes to 1 government agency's actions in the 1930s alone.

Limited Direct Effects of Redlining Grades

Public health research on redlining has often treated HOLC grades as a way to directly quantify the enduring impact caused by an isolated historical structurally racist policy. However, in pointing to HOLC as the only culprit, this understanding overstates its direct effects, oversimplifies the complex pathways through which historical processes were developed and enacted, and misrepresents the actors and policies of true interest. Scholars across disciplines have long mistakenly assumed that HOLC used its surveys to make decisions about the agency's own investment, such that a "D" grade would result in the agency's refusal to provide financing. Furthermore, they have suggested that the maps were widely distributed, influencing private-sector lending.[5] Public health researchers have correspondingly implied or stated that HOLC grades had a direct impact on neighborhood disinvestment, which, in turn, is understood as affecting the health outcome of interest. Studies often use causal language in framing research questions and interpreting findings or seek ever more precise refinements to study design in the quest to make causal inferences. While some articles cautiously reference an "association" or "relationship," others use language like "suggest causal effect," "may be shaped," "influenced," "impacted," and "legacy," implying at least a possible causal effect. For example, the influential conceptual framing by Krieger et al.—in an article titled "Structural Racism, Historical Redlining, and Risk of Preterm Birth in New York City, 2013–2017"—concludes that "structural racism, past and present, including previous forms of racial discrimination that are now illegal, can affect current adverse health outcomes" in areas "affected by the HOLC grades."[26(p1050)]

To clarify, HOLC maps were created almost entirely after the agency had already made its loans, and the grades are not associated with the loans that it made.[5,9,27] Indeed, research has established that HOLC loaned widely in D-graded neighborhoods and, as of 1940, made loans to Black homeowners approximately proportionate to their share of the city's population.[4,28,29] This does not mean that its activities were not racist. Indeed, explicitly racist comments infused appraisals and internal agency correspondence. HOLC's loans and foreclosure sales reinforced already-existing patterns of segregation[28,29] and were intended to benefit White financial institutions who lent to Black homeowners.[28] And the very logics of "objective" economic value were already fundamentally racialized. What this evidence does mean is that HOLC's grades did not determine its decisions about whether to make loans. In addition, there is no existing evidence that its maps were widely disseminated, suggesting that they should not be viewed as directly shaping private lenders' practices, either.[5]

Assuming direct effects from HOLC grades diverts research away from questioning how redlining actually happened and identifying the true causal mechanisms that might shape present-day health outcomes. Indeed, if HOLC grades were limited in their direct effects, it raises the question of why we largely do see persistent associations in the present. In the next section, we argue that a racial capitalism approach can help answer this question through redirecting our attention to HOLC's political–economic context, such that its surveys are 1 manifestation reflecting a much more widely implemented ideology, and we consider what the surveys do "tell us as objects that likely were not used to do redlining."[5(p197)]

The Role of the Market

Public health research on redlining typically focuses exclusively on the federal government's role, as (ostensibly) distinguished from individual prejudice or incidental effects of economic processes. HOLC redlining grades accordingly seem to offer a clean, straightforward measure of structural racism in the form of state-sponsored policy. However, merely pointing to the government's role fails to interrogate the actors and sociopolitical context establishing ideologies driving the practice itself. A racial capitalism lens instead emphasizes how the market imperative for profit via segregation and racialized devaluation shaped HOLC grades—widening our understanding of redlining to encompass the private sector and its relationship with the state while pushing us to consider how these same logics infused the housing market in other forms.

While HOLC was, of course, a government agency, the government and market institutions were not wholly discrete actors. The making of HOLC's maps can be better understood as a public–private process, with "government as the vehicle and capitalism in the driver seat," as historian Destin Jenkins wrote.[30(p170)] Similarly, urban studies scholar David Imbroscio pointed out that the government did not create redlining from a tabula rasa out of ideologically isolated racism, but, rather, such policies were formed in collaboration with private-sector actors and reflected the dominant logic of existing economic markets.[31] Thus, rather than reflecting the spontaneous racism of the federal government, HOLC grades actually reflected and reproduced a shared racial–spatial ideology that many different actors, including the private sector, collaboratively implemented.

HOLC worked closely with local real estate and finance professionals to collect data and understand local markets.[27,32] Furthermore, the racist ideologies infusing HOLC's appraisal approach, linking race and property value, reflected widespread real estate theories developed and spread through networks spanning academia, the real estate and finance industries, and government. Given this "elaborate intertwining," historians LaDale Winling and Todd Michney argued that "government redlining *was* private redlining and vice versa."[32(p44)] Moreover, appraised neighborhoods had already been shaped by preexisting and concurrent policies and practices enacted by private-sector actors. Contrary to speculative claims that HOLC originated redlining, private lenders had already implemented spatially uneven lending practices, and its neighborhood appraisals took this existing mortgage availability into consideration.[9,33,34]

On a more fundamental level, HOLC did not create the racist theory of value but, rather, reproduced its existing market logics. Imbroscio pointed out that conventional analysis of redlining identifies its racism as unjustly framing Black residents as detrimental to property value because of their race rather than impartial economic criteria. Yet markets that determine "impartial" property values are not neutral, objective, and omniscient. Rather, markets are social constructions reflecting the values and biases of their creators and users. Racism had thus already structured the neighborhood values HOLC was attempting to assess, as "anti-Black beliefs *themselves* lower property values."[31(p32)] Accordingly, "the practitioners of redlining were not, on purely economic terms, wrong in their assessments. Instead, they were simply following the dictates of (perceived) market rationality."[31(p32)] Indeed, evidence suggests that Black residents largely did live in neighborhoods that could "objectively" be considered declining by economic indicators.[35] This does not mean that redlining was not a process of structural racism. Instead, it suggests that the "structure" in structural racism as it pertains to redlining is not the sum of individual appraisers' racial bias in unfairly downgrading neighborhoods based merely on Black occupancy. Rather the "structure" is the racist theory of value that fused racial and economic considerations in a capitalist housing market.

Relationship With Other Racialized Processes

The use of HOLC grades as a measure of structural racism, coupled with frequent mention of the relegation of neighborhoods with Black residents to D grades, may lead a reader to believe that the majority of residents of redlined neighborhoods were Black, redlined neighborhoods continue to have Black populations today, and most low-income Black people still live in redlined neighborhoods. However, these assumptions are not always correct, requiring greater precision and nuance in study design and interpretation for effective use of redlining as a measure of structural racism.

While redlining has become nearly synonymous with housing discrimination in public health research,[36] and indeed synonymous with racist housing policy more generally, it is only 1 form. Other racialized processes of displacement, exclusion, extraction, and disinvestment preceded, accompanied, and followed it (see Table 1 for some examples)—working together to shape and reshape neighborhoods to generate profit following the racist theory of value. For example, practices such as racial zoning and restrictive covenants shaped which neighborhoods Black residents lived in before HOLC appraisers' arrival and thus facilitated preexisting disinvestment in those neighborhoods. Nor were neighborhoods frozen at their level of investment after redlining. Policies promoting urban renewal and gentrification reversed in some neighborhoods the disinvestment and concomitant conditions that followed redlining. Indeed, redlined neighborhoods may be particularly likely to have seen such transformation, as these processes often targeted "blight" common to disinvested neighborhoods or took advantage of low property values to easily profit from revalorization. By focusing narrowly on the associations between redlining and the present day, research risks obscuring the impacts of such additional processes, absolving them—and the actors who perpetuated and profited off them—from responsibility in shaping today's conditions. Robert Gioielli identifies a tendency in research to do exactly that, terming the use of HOLC grades to singularly explain all manner of neighborhood outcomes today the "redlining vampire" and noting how it draws our attention away from the agents and policies that create new and reinforce existing forms of discrimination.[7] Thus, some recent work has emphasized that most poor Black households today do not live in redlined areas and that associations between redlining and present-day disadvantage may be explained by other processes.[37,38]

For researchers interested in structural racism, these shifting geographies of racialized disinvestment raise the question of how to account for differences in the racial composition of D-graded areas. Although Black households were almost completely concentrated in D-graded areas, not all D-graded areas were home to Black residents, and most residents of D-graded areas were not Black.[39,40] It is possible, even likely, that redlined neighborhoods with Black populations had divergent trajectories from redlined neighborhoods that did not. Thus, it is problematic to use redlining as a measure of structural racism without recognizing and exploring precisely how racialized neighborhoods were redlined. In fact, treating all D-graded areas as a single undifferentiated category could obscure a stronger association between the outcome of interest today and D-graded areas that were home to Black residents. Furthermore, the United States' demographic

TABLE 1— Select Other Racialized Processes Affecting Neighborhoods Redlined by the Home Owners' Loan Corporation: United States

Process	Description	Data Availability Examples
Restrictive racial covenants	Deed restrictions that prohibited non-White occupancy, legally enforceable until 1948.	City-level projects—such as ones run by Mapping Prejudice in Minneapolis, Mapping Segregation in DC, Chicago Covenants, and the Federal Reserve Bank of Philadelphia, among others—have begun collecting data from property deeds and publicly mapping them.
Racial zoning	Explicit legal designations that restricted occupancy in a given area of the city to a specified racial group, banned in 1917.	Racial zoning maps can be difficult to come by, but some, like Atlanta's 1922 map, survive in local archives and have been digitized.
Exclusionary zoning	Restrictive land use requirements such as large lot sizes that make it difficult to build more affordable housing types. Often accompanied by concentrating industrial uses in lower-income neighborhoods.	The National Zoning Atlas centralizes and standardizes zoning data from across the United States in a publicly accessible map.
Blockbusting and White flight	Rapid shift in neighborhood population from White to non-White—often attributable to real estate agents convincing White homeowners to sell from fear of Black residents entering the neighborhood, then reselling at a higher rate.	Historical Census data from the National Historical Geographic Information System (NHGIS), Longitudinal Tract Database (LTDB), and the S4 Lab at Brown University allow historical analyses of neighborhood-level racial change and segregation.
Predatory extraction	Charging non-White renters or homebuyers more for poorer-quality housing.	Data from the NHGIS, IPUMS USA, American Community Survey (ACS; also available through the NHGIS interface), Public Use Microdata Sample (PUMS), LTDB, and Home Mortgage Disclosure Act (HMDA) can assist analyses of predatory extraction by showing, for example, how rents or mortgage rates have varied by neighborhood racial composition.
Urban renewal	Razing areas deemed to be "blighted" or "slums," often replacing them with uses catering to higher-income people, from the 1940s to 1970s.	American Panorama has digitized project footprints and collected data on family displacement by race. The Historical Housing Unit and Urbanization Database provides historical housing unit counts in standardized neighborhood geometries. And Segregation by Design offers historical aerial imagery showing the impact of highway construction.
Housing discrimination	Denying access to housing based on personal characteristics, such as race.	HMDA data allow assessments of home lending discrimination by census tract and by individual borrowers after 1980. Data to investigate other forms of housing discrimination directly are more difficult to come by.
Present-day lending discrimination	Disproportionately denying mortgages, or making them available on differential terms, along lines of race or other characteristics.	HMDA data allow assessments of post-1980 home lending discrimination.
Discriminatory appraisals	Appraising properties in neighborhoods with many Black residents or properties occupied by Black residents lower than comparable properties in Whiter neighborhoods or properties occupied by White residents.	Federal Housing Finance Agency Home Price Index data provide single-family home values at the census-tract level for more than 400 cities. Some of these data go back to the 1970s. Though imperfect, these data could be combined with census data to assess home value differences in neighborhoods by racial composition. For more granular assessments of individual property appraisals, researchers can use local property records.
Eviction	Forcing a tenant to move out of a property.	Eviction Lab offers county-level eviction data nationwide via their online platform. However, local experts have sometimes found their data to be incomplete and their practices questionable. The Anti-Eviction Mapping Project also displays evictions for multiple cities in a series of interactive maps and other formats. Local courts track information on filed and completed eviction, although not as conveniently digitized. Note that eviction data typically only include formal legally filed evictions.

Continued

TABLE 1— Continued

Process	Description	Data Availability Examples
Foreclosure	Losing possession of a home one owns because of missed payments.	Local government sources such as courts and treasurers track data on foreclosure filings and sales, although not as conveniently digitized. While foreclosure data are also available through purchase from a number of private firms, their practices may be ethically questionable.
Disinvestment	Withdrawing or reducing capital investment in a neighborhood.	Data from HMDA, NHGIS, and the LTDB can assist analyses investigating disinvestment by showing which places are not receiving their expected share of mortgage loans or are experiencing relative income, rent, or home value decline.
Gentrification	An influx of capital investment in a neighborhood, often accompanied by a transition to residents with higher class status and racial change, typically (although not always) in recent decades.	A number of gentrification measures have been developed and tested, which can often be deployed using Census or ACS data.

composition has changed significantly since the 1930s, so redlining may have little explanatory power for the subsequent experiences of groups racialized as non-White who now make up a much larger share of the population, such as Latinx and Asian residents—at least, without careful unpacking of where these residents moved and why. This failure to account for potential differentiation in other racialized groups' experiences reflects a gap in structural racism research more broadly.[12]

Another concern is that the real relationships between redlining and present-day outcomes may be clouded if we fail to consider other processes. For example, a previously redlined neighborhood that is now gentrified might have excellent health outcomes, as environmental hazards have been remediated and residents whose health was affected by redlining have been displaced. In fact, several studies have found that HOLC grades are not associated with a present-day outcome, which authors attribute to shifting spatial patterns of spatial inequality.[41] Relatedly, focusing only on residents currently living in a neighborhood may fail to account for individual-level pathways, as affected individuals from neighborhoods that subsequently transformed may live elsewhere now (e.g., displaced by gentrification) but still bear the burden of redlining's health impacts.

Redlining is 1 snapshot in time of the widespread implementation and enforcement of the racist theory of value, but is not solely determinative of how such logics subsequently shaped redlined neighborhoods. Some neighborhoods with the same grade surely went down different trajectories because of their different populations at the time of redlining or because of the historically specific subsequent restructurings of racialized space in their city. By viewing racial capitalism as dynamically reshaping racialized geographies, researchers can more accurately explore how historical processes inform present-day environments and embodied impacts.

RECOMMENDATIONS FOR FUTURE RESEARCH

We next offer recommendations for each of the 3 areas discussed previously to advance our understanding of how historical racialized policies and processes connect to present-day health (Table 2). We do not offer methodological suggestions to improve ability to make causal inferences in research using HOLC grades. Rather, we focus on how researchers can align conceptual frameworks, research questions, and study design, including use of alternative data sources beyond those grades.

Furthermore, we urge greater investment in data infrastructure around both other forms of redlining as well as other racialized policies and processes—from zoning to foreclosures to evictions to property sales to rents to home demolitions. As Table 1 indicates, there are many other such policies and processes that still lack the type of accessible and readily usable data made available for redlining by Mapping Inequality. These processes have not necessarily been less important or consequential than redlining; rather, the lack of comparable scholarly attention likely results, at least in part, from the greater difficulty of studying them.

AJPH May 2025, Vol. 115, No. 5

TABLE 2— Methodological Suggestions and Directions for Future Research on Redlining, the Home Owners' Loan Corporation (HOLC), and Health

Opportunity to Clarify HOLC's Role	Limitations of Current Structural Racism Approach	Suggestions for Research
Limited direct effects of HOLC grades	HOLC grades were made post facto and do not reflect HOLC's actual lending patterns. Research therefore often lacks conceptual clarity on how and why historical structural racism persists into the present.	Public health researchers should align their potential construct of interest with appropriate exposure variable(s) and interpretation. Researchers should not depend on a direct impact of lending and disinvestment in their theoretical justification for the importance of studying HOLC grades and potential pathways to the outcome of interest. • Frame HOLC grades as offering a proxy for areas deemed to be "risky" by other 1930s public and private actors, if researchers are interested in the general practice of redlining by public and private actors in aggregate. HOLC's approach to assessing value likely encompassed the same factors, and indeed took into account other lenders' lending practices. However, researchers should be careful to note that they do not hypothesize direct effects stemming from loan denial, and their grades may not necessarily be an exact proxy. For example, research has found that there are meaningful differences between HOLC grades and Federal Housing Administration grades,[6] unsurprisingly given the 2 agencies had different functions. • As research relies to a greater extent on the precise borders of HOLC-graded areas (e.g., when using a boundary design or difference-in-difference approach), it also increasingly depends on the similarity between HOLC-graded areas and graded areas of redlining as actually practiced. Scholars should thus even more carefully consider their theoretical justification, and the extent to which HOLC grades are indeed an appropriate proxy for their construct of interest. • Consider whether the true interest is in historical redlining or whether present-day lending discrimination is instead more relevant (see Table 1). • Consider whether the true interest is simply the relationship between race and devaluation, rather than redlining more specifically—in which case the variable Black population share would more directly assess this question.
The role of the market	An exclusive focus on the state misattributes the form of racialized spatial devaluation, the actors involved, and the causal pathways through which it might lead to durable impacts.	Research should explore capitalism, and its exploitation of racialized hierarchies of place and personhood for profit, as itself a fundamental cause of health—interfacing with state power to shape multiple downstream mechanisms such as redlining. • Draw on frameworks such as racial capitalism and other social theory to unpack the drivers behind structurally racist policies and practices. These frameworks, through shedding light on motivations and implementation, can help identify pathways and accountable actors with more precision. • Utilize redlining maps made by private institutions, or data (e.g., from the 1940 Census) on mortgages made by private lenders. • Rather than assuming effects on grading solely attributable to racial bias, also consider how the racist theory of value infused ostensibly objective economic criteria.
Relationship with other racialized processes	Without distinguishing the racial composition of redlined neighborhoods, the framing of HOLC grades as a measure of structural racism is vague and imprecise. Furthermore, because neighborhoods have experienced shifting patterns of racialized displacement and disinvestment since the 1930s, analyses assessing structural racism in the present day must account for intervening processes.	Researchers interested in structural racism should consider differences in racial composition across redlined neighborhoods, during all time periods. • At a minimum, consider stratifying graded areas based on whether they included Black residents (or another group of interest). More research comparing trajectories of D-graded areas with Black populations versus other racialized groups is also necessary.[39,40] • Do not control for the racial composition in 1940 as a confounder. This approach situates race as exogenous to the exposure-outcome relationship. Because the racist theory of value suffused grading decisions, there is not a reliable way to isolate the effect of race and appropriately compare neighborhoods without its influence. • Account not only for Black population at the time of HOLC's surveys but also in subsequent decades. For example, some cities had very small Black populations in the 1930s, but neighborhoods with any Black residents at that time quickly became majority-Black. Future research might compare present-day health outcomes in neighborhoods that today are all predominantly Black but that at the time of redlining had no versus small versus large Black populations. • While very little research has examined the relationship between redlining and racialized groups beyond the Black-White binary, future research could consider the relationship between redlining grades and other racialized populations (e.g., Latinx, Asian), both at the time of redlining and in subsequent decades as these populations grew. Researchers should also recognize the dynamic nature of racialized spatial inequality across time. • Consider additionally accounting for the impacts of racialized processes such as urban renewal or gentrification, which occurred between redlining and the present, utilizing some of the data sources suggested in Table 1. • Conceptually, rather than framing HOLC redlining as the origin of segregation, recognize how it built on preexisting segregation shaped by additional processes.

CONCLUSION

To understand the true effects of structurally racist policies like redlining and to grasp how neighborhoods became racialized and thereby redlined, researchers must more fully unpack the actual practice of redlining and employ appropriate theoretical frameworks. Without this intentional engagement, HOLC redlining will remain an imprecise measurement of oppression for racialized communities in the United States. Instead, centering racial capitalism as a fundamental cause of health inequity helps illuminate how and why redlining matters for present-day health.

Moving forward, stronger collaboration between public health scholars and urban historians and other disciplines can offer important context to inform these conceptual frameworks in examining the historical roots of present-day health injustice. Funders should support and incentivize innovative work in this area, adopting an interdisciplinary and theoretically engaged approach. Journal editors can further promote this more productive line of scholarship by setting expectations that submissions on redlining should adequately engage with historical and theoretical considerations. Such work can aid policymakers and practitioners in understanding agents and drivers perpetuating historically rooted health inequity and in developing appropriate strategies for identifying neighborhoods that most need support in the present, as targeting HOLC-redlined neighborhoods (the subject of numerous policy proposals) may be inaccurate and inefficient. Indeed, as recent public health scholarship has begun to urge,[42] further research on redlining must not come at the cost of awareness of and action on current drivers of racialized riskscapes and concomitant health inequities. More broadly, we urge public health scholarship to embrace politicized analyses of the drivers of health injustice, attentive to the political–economic drivers that inform the policies and practices that shape our everyday lives. AJPH

ABOUT THE AUTHORS

Carolyn Swope is with the Urban Planning Program, Graduate School of Architecture, Planning and Preservation, Columbia University, New York, NY. Scott Markley is with the National Zoning Atlas. Shannon Whittaker is with the Center for Innovation in Social Science, Boston University, Boston, MA. Amy Hillier is with the University of Pennsylvania School of Social Policy and Practice, Philadelphia.

CORRESPONDENCE

Correspondence should be sent to Carolyn Swope, MPH, Schermerhorn Extension 659, 1200 Amsterdam Ave, New York, NY 10027 (e-mail: cbs2164@columbia.edu). Reprints can be ordered at https://www.ajph.org by clicking the "Reprints" link.

PUBLICATION INFORMATION

Full Citation: Swope C, Markley S, Whittaker S, Hillier A. How and why does redlining matter for present-day health? Critical perspectives on causality, cartography, and capitalism. *Am J Public Health*. 2025;115(5):769–779.

Acceptance Date: December 18, 2024.

DOI: https://doi.org/10.2105/AJPH.2024.308000

ORCID iDs:

Carolyn Swope https://orcid.org/0000-0002-5982-5950

Shannon Whittaker https://orcid.org/0000-0003-2890-5314

CONTRIBUTORS

C. Swope conceptualized the commentary and led the project. A. Hillier served as senior author. All authors contributed to drafting, critically reviewing, and revising the article.

CONFLICTS OF INTEREST

S. Markley reports employment at the National Zoning Atlas, a data set mentioned in the article.

HUMAN PARTICIPANT PROTECTION

This study did not involve human participants.

REFERENCES

1. Digital Scholarship Lab. Mapping Inequality. Available at: https://dsl.richmond.edu/panorama/redlining. Accessed July 12, 2018.
2. Swope CB, Hernández D, Cushing LJ. The relationship of historical redlining with present-day neighborhood environmental and health outcomes: a scoping review and conceptual model. *J Urban Health*. 2022;99(6):959–983. https://doi.org/10.1007/s11524-022-00665-z
3. Jackson KT. *Crabgrass Frontier: The Suburbanization of the United States*. New York, NY: Oxford University Press; 1985.
4. Fishback P, Rose J, Snowden KA, Storrs T. New evidence on redlining by federal housing programs in the 1930s. *J Urban Econ*. 2024;141. https://doi.org/10.1016/j.jue.2022.103462
5. Markley S. Federal 'redlining' maps: a critical reappraisal. *Urban Stud*. 2023;61(2):195–213. https://doi.org/10.1177/00420980231182336
6. Xu W. Legacies of institutionalized redlining: a comparison between speculative and implemented mortgage risk maps in Chicago, Illinois. *Hous Policy Debate*. 2022;32(2):249–274. https://doi.org/10.1080/10511482.2020.1858924
7. Gioielli R. The Tyranny of the Map: Rethinking Redlining. *The Metropole*. November 3, 2022. Available at: https://themetropole.blog/2022/11/03/the-tyranny-of-the-map-rethinking-redlining. Accessed November 4, 2022.
8. Crossney KB, Bartelt DW. The legacy of the Home Owners' Loan Corporation. *Hous Policy Debate*. 2005;16(3-4):547–574. https://doi.org/10.1080/10511482.2005.9521555
9. Hillier AE. Redlining and the Home Owners' Loan Corporation. *J Urban Hist*. 2003;29(4):394–420. https://doi.org/10.1177/0096144203029004002
10. Bailey ZD, Krieger N, Agénor M, Graves J, Linos N, Bassett MT. Structural racism and health inequities in the USA: evidence and interventions. *Lancet*. 2017;389(10077):1453–1463. https://doi.org/10.1016/S0140-6736(17)30569-X
11. Mehdipanah R, McVay KR, Schulz AJ. Historic redlining practices and contemporary determinants of health in the Detroit metropolitan area. *Am J Public Health*. 2023;113(suppl 1):S49–S57. https://doi.org/10.2105/AJPH.2022.307162
12. Hing AK, Chantarat T, Fashaw-Walters S, Hunt SL, Hardeman RR. Instruments for racial health equity: a scoping review of structural racism measurement, 2019–2021. *Epidemiol Rev*. 2024;46(1):1–26. https://doi.org/10.1093/epirev/mxae002
13. Kundnani A. *What Is Antiracism?: And Why It Means Anticapitalism*. Brooklyn, NY: Verso Books; 2023.
14. Wien S, Miller AL, Kramer MR. Structural racism theory, measurement, and methods: a scoping review. *Front Public Health*. 2023;11:1069476. https://doi.org/10.3389/fpubh.2023.1069476.
15. Melamed J. Racial capitalism. *Critical Ethnic Studies*. 2015;1(1):76–85. https://doi.org/10.5749/jcritethnstud.1.1.0076
16. Paret M, Levenson Z. Two racial capitalisms: Marxism, domination, and resistance in Cedric Robinson and Stuart Hall. *Antipode*. 2024;56(5):1802–1829. https://doi.org/10.1111/anti.13054
17. Taylor KY. *Race for Profit: How Banks and the Real Estate Industry Undermined Black Homeownership*. Chapel Hill, NC: The University of North Carolina Press; 2019.

18. Markley SN, Hafley TJ, Allums CA, Holloway SR, Chung HC. The limits of homeownership: racial capitalism, Black wealth, and the appreciation gap in Atlanta. *Int J Urban Reg Res.* 2020;44(2):310–328. https://doi.org/10.1111/1468-2427.12873
19. Abrams C. *Forbidden Neighbors: A Study of Prejudice in Housing.* New York, NY: Harper; 1955.
20. Gilmore RW. *Golden Gulag: Prisons, Surplus, Crisis, and Opposition in Globalizing California.* Oakland, CA: University of California Press; 2007.
21. Pulido L. Flint, environmental racism, and racial capitalism. *Capitalism Nat Socialism.* 2016;27(3):1–16. https://doi.org/10.1080/10455752.2016.1213013
22. Laster Pirtle WN. Racial capitalism: a fundamental cause of novel coronavirus (COVID-19) pandemic inequities in the United States. *Health Educ Behav.* 2020;47(4):504–508. https://doi.org/10.1177/1090198120922942
23. Táíwò OO, Fehrenbacher AE, Cooke A. Material insecurity, racial capitalism, and public health. *Hastings Cent Rep.* 2021;51(6):17–22. https://doi.org/10.1002/hast.1293
24. Flores YA, Greenwood HM. The future of public health must be radical: incorporating racial capitalism. *Health Educ Behav.* 2023;50(4):473–476. https://doi.org/10.1177/10901981231166572
25. Markley SN. Planning spatial obsolescence: residential segregation and the racist theory of (anti-)value. *Environ Plan D.* 2024;42(5-6):758–775. https://doi.org/10.1177/02637758241261218
26. Krieger N, Van Wye G, Huynh M, et al. Structural racism, historical redlining, and risk of preterm birth in New York City, 2013–2017. *Am J Public Health.* 2020;110(7):1046–1053. https://doi.org/10.2105/AJPH.2020.305656
27. Michney TM. How the City Survey's redlining maps were made: a closer look at HOLC's Mortgage Rehabilitation division. *J Plann Hist.* 2022;21(4):316–344. https://doi.org/10.1177/15385132211013361
28. Michney TM, Winling L. New perspectives on New Deal housing policy: explicating and mapping HOLC loans to African Americans. *J Urban Hist.* 2020;46(1):150–180. https://doi.org/10.1177/0096144218819429
29. Hillier AE. Who received loans? Home Owners' Loan Corporation lending and discrimination in Philadelphia in the 1930s. *J Plann Hist.* 2003;2(1):3–24. https://doi.org/10.1177/1538513202239694
30. Jenkins D. Who segregated America? In: Marcus S, Zaloom C, eds. *Think in Public.* New York, NY: Columbia University Press; 2019:169–178. https://doi.org/10.7312/marc19008-015
31. Imbroscio D. Race matters (even more than you already think): racism, housing, and the limits of the color of law. *J Race Ethn City.* 2020;2(1):29–53. https://doi.org/10.1080/26884674.2020.1825023
32. Winling LC, Michney TM. The roots of redlining: academic, governmental, and professional networks in the making of the New Deal lending regime. *J Am Hist.* 2021;108(1):42–69. https://doi.org/10.1093/jahist/jaab066
33. Markley S. Tabulating Home Owners' Loan Corporation area description sheet data. *Environ Plan B Urban Anal City Sci.* 2022;50(1):268–280. https://doi.org/10.1177/23998083221133112
34. Greer J. The Home Owners' Loan Corporation and the development of the residential security maps. *J Urban Hist.* 2013;39(2):275–296. https://doi.org/10.1177/0096144212436724
35. Fishback PV, LaVoice J, Shertzer A, Walsh RP. The HOLC maps: how race and poverty influenced real estate professionals' evaluation of lending risk in the 1930s. *J Econ Hist.* 2023;83(4):1019–1056. https://doi.org/10.1017/S0022050723000475
36. Cross RI, Huỳnyh J, Bradford NJ, Francis B. Racialized housing discrimination and population health: a scoping review and research agenda. *J Urban Health.* 2023;100(2):355–388. https://doi.org/10.1007/s11524-023-00725-y
37. Mallach A. Shifting the redlining paradigm: the Home Owners' Loan Corporation maps and the construction of urban racial inequality. *Hous Policy Debate.* 2024;34(6):891–917. https://doi.org/10.1080/10511482.2024.2321226
38. Graetz N, Esposito M. Historical redlining and contemporary racial disparities in neighborhood life expectancy. *Soc Forces.* 2022;102(1):1–22. https://doi.org/10.1093/sf/soac114
39. Markley SN, Holloway SR. Underestimating racism? Decoupling race and redlining. *Ann Assoc Am Geogr.* 2024;114(7):1464–1482. https://doi.org/10.1080/24694452.2024.2350993
40. Smith RB, Painter G. People and place: does the reason for redlining impact the long-term trajectory of neighborhoods. *J Urban Aff.* 2023:1–19. https://doi.org/10.1080/07352166.2023.2288593
41. Lynch EE, Malcoe LH, Laurent SE, Richardson J, Mitchell BC, Meier HCS. The legacy of structural racism: associations between historic redlining, current mortgage lending, and health. *SSM Popul Health.* 2021;14:100793. https://doi.org/10.1016/j.ssmph.2021.100793
42. Jacoby SF. Home Owners' Loan Corporation maps and place-based injury risks: a complex history. *Am J Public Health.* 2023;113(4):356–358. https://doi.org/10.2105/AJPH.2023.307242

Housing Quality Metric (HQM): Neighborhood-Level Data, Housing Quality, and Population Health

Veronica Garrison, DrPH, MPH, Peter J. Ashley, DrPH, MPH, Alyssa J. Moran, ScD, MPH, RD, Thomas K. M. Cudjoe, MD, MPH, MA, Eliana M. Perrin, MD, MPH, and Craig Evan Pollack, MD, MHS

See also Fenelon, p. 637, and Routhier, p. 640.

Objectives. To develop a national, tract-level measure of neighborhood housing quality and test its validity by examining associations with population health metrics.

Methods. Using microdata from the 2021 American Housing Survey postfit to the 2018–2022 American Community Survey, we developed the Housing Quality Metric (HQM), which predicts the likelihood that a US census tract contains a large share of poor-quality housing units across 3 domains: physical inadequacy, housing cost burden, and poor neighborhood perception. We then used regression models to assess the ecological association between HQM and area-level measures of adult population health (fair or poor general health, poor mental health, and poor physical health) from the PLACES data set.

Results. Census tract HQM score was significantly associated with a higher predicted proportion of adults self-reporting all 3 examined negative health status outcomes in both unadjusted and adjusted models.

Conclusions. HQM presents the first national, tract-level measure of poor housing quality that has significant associations with adult population health status.

Public Health Implications. HQM can be used to target resources and interventions in ways that may better capture the complex relationship between housing quality and population health than existing measures of housing quality. (*Am J Public Health*. 2025;115(5):780–788. https://doi.org/10.2105/AJPH.2024.307962)

AJPH May 2025, Vol. 115, No. 5

The rise of tenements in the 19th century brought a public health focus on housing quality. Overcrowded, poorly ventilated apartment buildings were viewed as places where diseases could easily spread and fire was hard to contain. More recently, practitioners and policymakers have returned to this history by reexamining the ways that housing conditions can affect health and well-being across the life span. Healthy People 2030 identifies the importance of "housing and homes," and the US Department of Housing and Urban Development's (HUD) strategic plan included an objective to "advance policies that recognize housing's role as essential to health."[1,2]

Traditionally, housing quality has been defined by federal agencies as the physical conditions within a housing unit, often focusing on factors associated with lead poisonings, falls, and chronic respiratory illnesses (e.g., mold, presence of pests).[3–6] HUD's physical inadequacy metric suggests that fewer than 2% of occupied units meet the criteria for the most serious physical problems,[7] whereas authors from the Centers for Disease Control and Prevention (CDC) used a more expansive definition and found that more than one fifth (21.3%) of 2007 and 2009 occupied housing units were designated as "unhealthy."[8] Nonfederal researchers have also sought to quantify housing adequacy.[9–12]

Although current estimates provide national rates of physical inadequacy, there are no estimates available for small geographic areas across the nation. Physical housing conditions are likely to vary across the United States because of housing being constructed at different time points and a range of other factors. Local estimates of poor housing quality are critical to understanding the drivers of poor health before resources and interventions can be deployed.

Moreover, physical housing quality is 1 of multiple aspects of housing quality shown to affect health. Swope and Hernández suggest that, in addition to physical adequacy, housing affects health via cost, stability, and neighborhood context.[13] Together with the model by Leifheit et al., these conceptual frameworks situate housing within structural factors that reinforce health disparities.[14] This broader view of housing aligns with empirical evidence; 8.53 million US households have worst-case housing needs, a measure commonly used to define poor affordability.[15] Being housing cost burdened has been correlated with numerous adverse health outcomes, such as physical health, mental health status, and adverse childhood experiences.[16–21] Neighborhood disadvantage has been linked to a wide variety of health behaviors, health status, and health care utilization.[22–25] Indices of housing cost burden and neighborhood context, when used in isolation, do not capture tradeoffs made across housing quality dimensions.

To standardize quality designations that include multiple domains of housing quality affecting health, we developed the Housing Quality Metric (HQM) data set. The HQM identifies US census tracts with large shares of housing units with poor housing quality across 3 domains: physical inadequacy, housing cost burden, and poor neighborhood perception. We then tested the validity of these measures by assessing their association with adult population health.

METHODS

We used 2 data sets with complementary strengths to generate the HQM. The American Housing Survey (AHS) provides detailed information on housing quality. The AHS is nationally representative but lacks adequate sample size to estimate housing quality at small geographic levels. By contrast, the American Community Survey (ACS) has detailed sociodemographic characteristics by census tract but lacks specific information on housing quality. Therefore, we used the AHS to build models on the observed likelihood of a household reporting poor-quality housing based on a wide range of covariates. We then applied the coefficients from these models (postfit) to covariates from ACS data to generate a predicted probability of a household facing each domain of poor housing quality.

We aggregated predictions by census tract to estimate the likelihood that the jurisdiction contained a large share of poor-quality occupied housing units. We linked the HQM with tract-level health data (PLACES) to explore the relationship between neighborhood-level poor housing quality and population health status.

Data Sources

2021 American Housing Survey. The AHS is the nation's most comprehensive nationally representative housing survey, providing data on housing and neighborhood quality, housing costs, and recent moves for a wide range of housing types. For this study, we excluded vacant units from analyses as well as housing units with missing responses for outcome variables. The final 2021 AHS sample consisted of approximately 56 000 (unweighted) occupied housing units.

American Community Survey, 2018 to 2022. Sent to approximately 3.5 million people annually, the ACS gathers key demographic information on individuals and households. We used 2018–2022 5-year ACS estimates to ensure sufficient sample size when summarizing by tract.

PLACES data. Released by the CDC, PLACES: Local Data for Better Health data use small-area estimations to calculate the prevalence of health outcomes at the census tract level from a range of data sources, including the Behavioral Risk Factor Surveillance System and Census Bureau data.[26] We excluded census tracts with a population of fewer than 50 people. Because of data collection issues, estimates for Florida are not available in the 2023 data release.[27]

Measures

2021 Housing Quality Metric (HQM). We employed several steps to develop the HQM (Appendix A, available as a supplement to the online version of this article at http://www.ajph.org), using an approach to small-area estimation that has been employed previously.[28–30]

Step 1: Selection of housing outcomes. We used 2021 AHS data to identify 3 domains of poor housing quality that align with existing conceptual models: physical inadequacy, housing cost burden, and poor neighborhood perception. We required outcomes derived from variables likely to be included in future AHS data collection to allow for an eventual change over time analyses. We further required that the variables had adequate sample size and a low level of missingness. We did not include housing stability, which is a fourth indicator of housing quality, because of the lack of available AHS data; however, there are efforts under way to develop a housing insecurity index that can be incorporated into future HQM data sets.[31]

Housing units were defined as "physically inadequate" if any of the following 6 conditions were reported:

i. exposure to mold or moisture (e.g., large area of mold or leaks),
ii. exposure to pest allergens (e.g., cockroaches and rodents),
iii. poor interior conditions (e.g., holes in the floor, ceiling, or walls),
iv. heating and cooling issues (e.g., unsafe heating methods or lack of equipment),
v. plumbing issues (e.g., frequent breakdowns, lack of connection to a sewage system), or
vi. electrical problems (e.g., exposed electrical wire, incorrect usage of extension cords).

We selected items on the basis of availability within the full AHS sample (e.g., not included in the healthy homes module, an infrequent module), not having high levels of missingness (e.g., vacant units), sufficient sample size (e.g., indoor stair issues was excluded), variables reported for all housing units (e.g., multifamily building residents did not receive external conditions questions), and expert consensus. "Housing cost burdened" was defined as a household paying more than 30% of their income on combined housing and utility costs.[15] We used 7 questions to define "poor neighborhood perception," including the reported presence of poor-quality schools, presence of petty crime, presence of serious crime, high risk for disasters, proximity to buildings with barred windows, proximity to abandoned or vandalized buildings, and presence of trash or litter within ½ block of the housing unit. The outcome of poor neighborhood perception was defined as a dichotomous outcome (0–1 poor neighborhood conditions reported, ≥ 2 poor neighborhood conditions reported) based on sample distribution. Online Appendix B outlines AHS variables and questions used to define each housing quality domain; online Appendix C shows the national prevalence of each domain, including subfactors used to define each.

Step 2: Data standardization. Since B coefficients from the AHS model were to be postfitted to ACS data, we standardized covariates in the AHS and the ACS to facilitate data integration (online Appendix D).[32] This required that AHS and ACS ask about the same construct and that the responses be used in the same way across data sets (e.g., same categories). We compared distributions of selected variables between data sets and found them to be similar (online Appendix E). Neither data set captures information for persons living in group quarters.

Step 3: Model development. We modeled household exposure to poor housing quality using AHS as a function of person-level, household-level, housing, and geographic characteristics. We selected covariates on the basis of availability within both data sets, inclusion in prior relevant studies, and consultation with experts. We used sampling weights to account for complex survey design. We examined physical inadequacy and poor neighborhood perception using an ordinal dependent variable and ordered logistic regression models, but results were similar to binary outcome models. To ensure consistency across each of the 3 housing quality domain, the binary logistic regression model was selected for modeling purposes for all three. Full model results are available in online Appendix F. Pearson goodness-of-fit statistics showed that for all 3 models, the χ^2 values were low relative to the degrees of freedom and the *P* values were high, indicating appropriate model fit. Additionally, multicollinearity was not a concern for selected covariates (online Appendix G).

Step 4: Postfit data. We used AHS model results to predict housing quality for each ACS housing unit. The AHS and ACS models used the same covariates as standardized in step 2, with logistic regression B coefficients from each AHS model applied (postfit) to the ACS household-level responses. For each of the 3 AHS quality domains, ACS households received a score of less than 1, indicating how likely the household was to experience each respective outcome (higher score = higher probability). To ensure proper fit, predicted ACS probability scores among households were compared alongside AHS household-level observed outcome prevalence rates by model attribute (online Appendix H). During data standardization processes described in step 2, we excluded observations with high levels of missingness (n < 100) prior to postfit, resulting in limited missingness during the postfit process. When we examined the percentage difference between observed rates in the AHS and predicted rates in the ACS, estimates were, on average, different by less than 1 percentage point for all domains.

Step 5: Summarization by geography. Predicted probabilities for individual ACS households were then summarized by census tract. We calculated both the predicted mean and median; we selected the mean metric for final estimates because of closer agreement with observed AHS rates. The final metric for each housing quality domain is the predicted percentage of occupied households in each census tract likely to experience poor-quality housing. This metric is a continuous variable ranging from 0.0 to 1.0. For this study, we used national quartile thresholds to define "high-risk" areas, but researchers can independently define thresholds when using raw HQM data. We used suppression processes for geographies with insufficient data or unstable estimates. The 2021 HQM provided data for 83 353 census tracts using 2020 boundaries; some tracts have null estimates to protect confidentiality. We also developed, tested, and validated county-level and state-level estimates, which are publicly available for download at housinghealth.org and in the article's online data appendix at http://www.ajph.org.

Lastly, we assigned census tracts an HQM score of 0 to 3. For every instance of a census tract scoring in the top national quartile for any of the 3 separate housing quality issues, we added 1 point; census tracts that scored in no top quartiles scored 0, whereas census tracts that scored in all 3 top quartiles scored 3. We tested alternative thresholds (online Appendix I), and researchers may apply alternative cutpoints or use continuous domain variables.

Population health status. We used 3 health status variables from 2023 PLACES data to quantify the percentage of adults aged 18 years and older in a census tract reporting (1) fair or poor general health; (2) poor mental health, defined as mental health not good for 14 or more days; and (3) poor physical health, defined as physical health not good for 14 days or more. PLACES estimates are based on 2021 Behavioral Risk Factor Surveillance System data.

Statistical Analysis

We mapped ordinal HQM scores for census tracts and linked them with population health data using 11-digit census tract codes. At the census tract level, we first tested the association between HQM scores and each health outcome using χ^2 tests. We used regression models to associate each continuous health status variable with the HQM ordinal score as the main predictor, unadjusted and adjusted for neighborhood-level characteristics (e.g., poverty rate and the prevalence of certain household types). In secondary analyses, separate regression models examined each domain of housing quality separately with each health status measure. We conducted analyses using SAS Enterprise Guide 8.3 (SAS Institute Inc, Cary, NC) and ArcGIS Pro 3.0 (ESRI, Redlands, CA).

RESULTS

Approximately 63.3% (SE = 0.27) of occupied housing units, or approximately 81 million occupied households, experienced at least 1 of 3 domains of poor housing quality. Nearly one third (32.4%; SE = 0.28) reported at least 1 major physical inadequacy in the home, 34.3% (SE = 0.27) were housing cost burdened, and approximately one quarter (22.1%; SE = 0.27) reported poor neighborhood perception.

One fifth (19.3%) of census tracts had a high prevalence of only 1 isolated housing quality issue (HQM score = 1), 12.6% of census tracts had a large share of poor housing quality issues across only 2 domains (HQM score = 2), and approximately 10.2% of census tracts had a high concentration of all 3 poor housing quality issues (HQM score = 3; Figure 1). Notably, there was wide distribution across the United States for the highest-risk tracts (HQM score = 3), with 44 states including at least 1 of these highest-risk tracts. Table 1 shows the characteristics of all census tracts overall and by the number of concentrated housing quality issues. Census tracts with higher cumulative HQM scores had lower average household incomes, lower levels of college education, fewer owner-occupied homes, and more Black residents.

Examining each HQM domain separately reveals significant national variability. The highest-risk tracts for physical inadequacy were clustered in the West Coast and the Southwest (online Appendix K). Consistent with prior research on housing cost burden, most top-quartile tracts for the housing cost burdened domain were clustered in the Northeast and West Coast (online Appendix L). A large share of units that self-reported poor neighborhood perception were in the South (online Appendix M).

Predicted Prevalence of Adverse Adult Health Status

Figure 2 displays the unadjusted, linear relationship between the mean

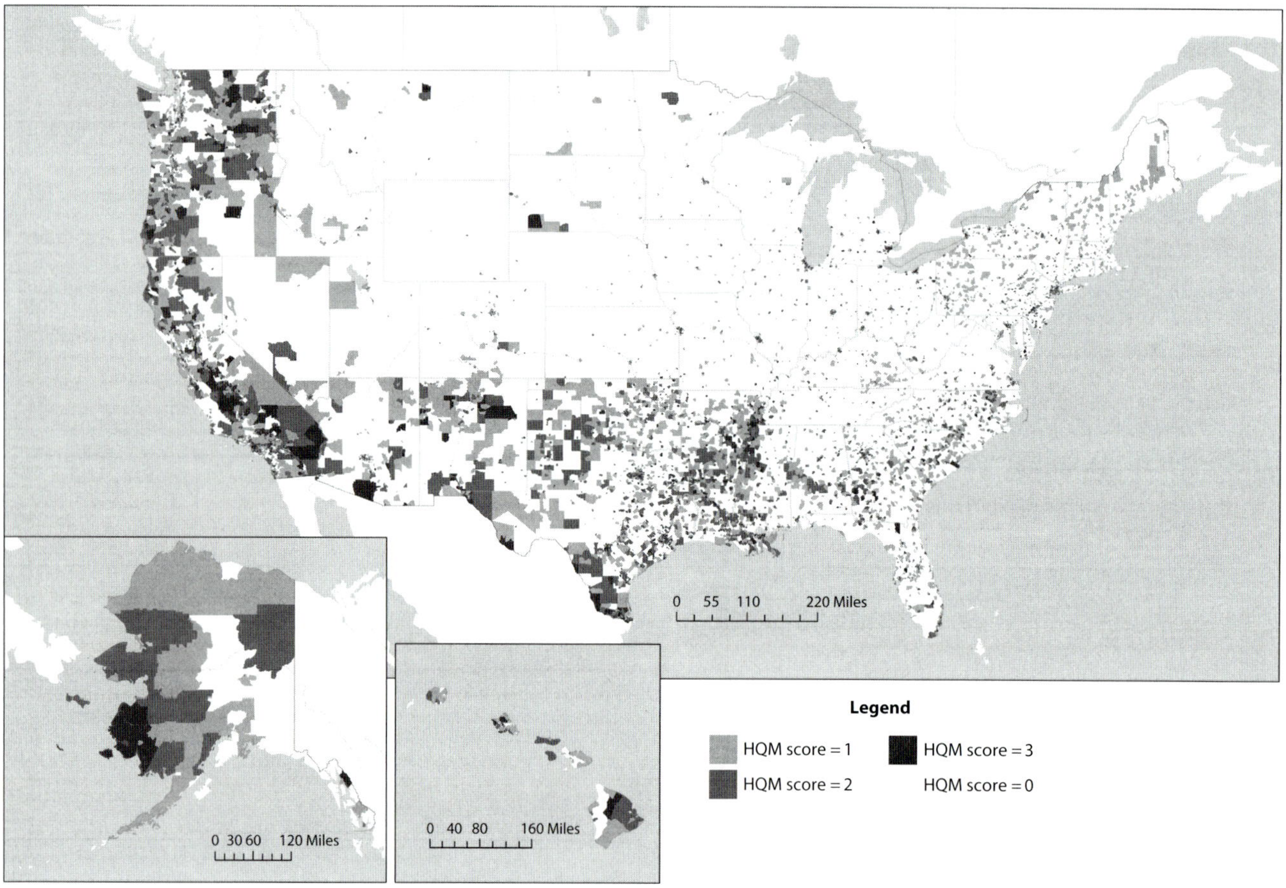

FIGURE 1— Housing Quality Metric (HQM) Score (0–3) Based on the Concentrated Presence of Poor Housing Quality Among US Census Tracts: 2021 HQM Data Set

Note. Data source is the 2021 HQM data set. Census tract HQM score ranges from 0 to 3, depending on how many dimensions of poor housing quality are identified within the respective jurisdiction. The 3 poor housing quality domains are (a) physically inadequate, (b) housing cost burdened, and (c) poor neighborhood perception. National quartile cutpoints represent the top national quartile for each domain. To score 1 point for the physically inadequate domain, the predicted percentage of occupied units within the census tract was 35.42% or higher. To score 1 point for the housing cost burdened domain, the predicted percentage of occupied units within the census tract was 42.38% or higher. To score 1 point for the poor neighborhood perception domain, the predicted percentage of occupied units within the census tract was 17.02% or higher. All domains scores were summed to develop final HQM score, ranging from 0 to 3.

predicted prevalence of adverse health status outcomes and the HQM cumulative count of neighborhood-level poor housing quality issues. Approximately 14.8% of adults were estimated to be in fair or poor self-rated health in census tracts with a HQM score of zero, increasing in a stepwise fashion to a point where 26.5% of adults lived in tracts with an HQM score of 3. Poor physical health was estimated to be 10.9% in tracts with a HQM score of zero and 15.1% in tracts with a score of 3. There was a 5.2 percentage-point lower prevalence of poor mental health reported in tracts with HQM scores of zero versus 3. Results were attenuated but remained statistically significant in models that adjusted for census tract sociodemographic characteristics, with a higher prevalence of poor health found in census tracts with higher HQM scores (Table 2).

In secondary analyses, we examined the association between each separate domain of poor housing quality with each population health metric (online Appendix J). Results showed a significant association between each domain of poor housing quality and each neighborhood health metric in both unadjusted and adjusted relationships.

DISCUSSION

The HQM data set predicts the proportion of occupied households within a census tract that have poor-quality housing based on a household's physical condition, housing cost burden, and perceived neighborhood quality. We found

TABLE 1— Mean of US Census Tract Characteristics by Housing Quality Metric (HQM) Score (0–3) Based on the Presence of Poor Housing Quality: United States, 2021 HQM Data Set Linked With the 2018–2022 American Community Survey

Characteristic	HQM Score (0–3)				
	All (0–3)	0	1	2	3
% households living below poverty level	13.9	9.1	14.7	19.5	27.5
% adults aged ≥ 25 y with college degree	19.6	22.1	20.2	16.4	12.1
% 1-person households	31.3	33.6	30.6	28.2	25.7
% households with children (aged < 18 y)	30.0	29.4	28.6	30.3	33.5
% households with older adults (aged ≥ 60 y)	41.7	44.4	40.5	38.2	35.6
% owner-occupied households	5.1	5.9	5.3	4.2	2.9
% persons who identify as only White	65.7	78.6	60.7	44.3	35.7
% persons who identify as only Black	13.5	6.7	13.2	25.2	30.1
% persons who identify as only Asian	5.2	4.4	7.5	6.0	5.1

Note. Census tract HQM score ranges from 0 to 3, depending on how many domains of poor housing quality are identified within the respective jurisdiction. The 3 poor housing quality domains are (a) physically inadequate, (b) housing cost burdened, and (c) poor neighborhood perception. National quartile cutpoints represent the top national quartile for each dimension. To score 1 point for the physically inadequate domain, the predicted percentage of occupied units within the census tract was 35.42% or higher. To score 1 point for the housing cost burdened domain, the predicted percentage of occupied units within the census tract was 42.38% or higher. To score 1 point for the poor neighborhood perception domain, the predicted percentage of occupied units within the census tract was 17.02% or higher. All domain scores were summed to develop final HQM score ranging from 0 to 3.

that over 40% of US census tracts were categorized as having high prevalence of at least 1 aspect of poor-quality housing, whereas 10% (approximately 8000 census tracts) had a high concentration of all 3 housing quality issues. Findings underscore an abundance of unmet housing quality needs within the US occupied housing stock.

When we merged housing quality data with population health data, we found that census tracts with poor housing quality had higher prevalence of poor general health, mental health,

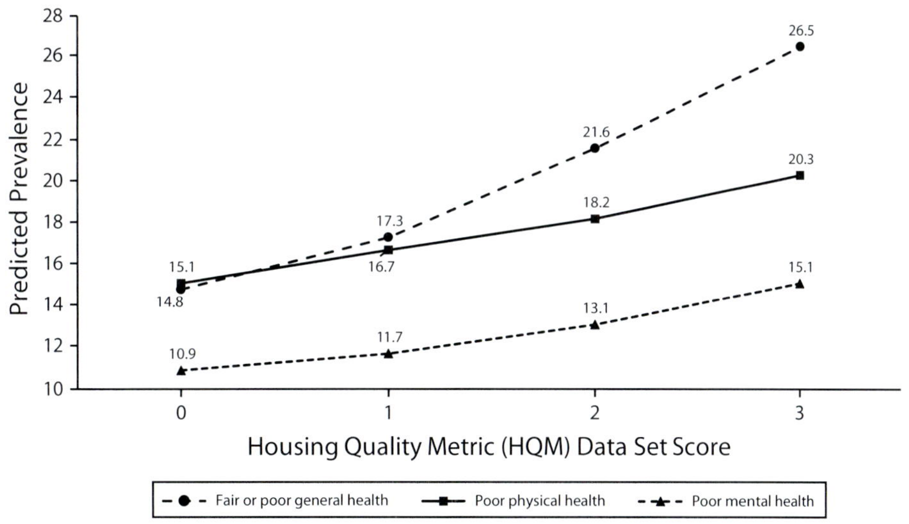

FIGURE 2— Predicted Prevalence of Self-Reported Negative Health Status Among Adults by Housing Quality Metric (HQM) Score (0–3) Based on the Presence of Poor Housing Quality: United States, 2021 HQM Data Set Linked With 2023 PLACES: Local Data for Better Health

Note. For all 3 health status outcomes, generalized linear model procedures revealed a significant relationship ($P < .001$) between HQM score and the health outcome. R-square values were 0.225 for poor physical health, 0.317 for mental health, and 0.384 for fair or poor general health.

TABLE 2— Linear Regression Results for Population Health Estimates by Housing Quality Metric (HQM) Score, Unadjusted and Adjusted for Neighborhood-Level Variables: United States, 2021 Housing Quality Metric Data Set Linked With the 2018–2022 American Community Survey and the 2023 PLACES: Local Data for Better Health

	Predicted Prevalence of Adults Self-Reporting Fair or Poor General Health, B (SE)		Predicted Prevalence of Adults Self-Reporting Poor Physical Health, B (SE)		Predicted Prevalence of Adults Self-Reporting Poor Mental Health, B (SE)	
	Unadjusted	Adjusted[a]	Unadjusted	Adjusted[a]	Unadjusted	Adjusted[a]
HQM Score						
0 (Ref)	1	1	1	1	1	1
1	2.50 (0.07)	1.00 (0.04)	0.79 (0.04)	0.11 (0.02)	1.65 (0.04)	0.40 (0.02)
2	6.81 (0.07)	3.27 (0.05)	2.23 (0.04)	0.61 (0.02)	3.14 (0.04)	0.61 (0.03)
3	11.69 (0.07)	5.19 (0.05)	4.25 (0.03)	1.29 (0.03)	5.22 (0.03)	0.94 (0.03)
Constant	14.8 (0.03)	13.9 (0.11)	10.9 (0.02)	10.8 (0.05)	15.08 (0.02)	20.2 (0.06)
R^2	0.38	0.77	0.22	0.74	0.31	0.72

Note. All $P < .001$.
[a]Adjusted for tract-level continuous variables including percentage of households living below the poverty rate, percentage of households where the education status of the head of household is college degree or higher, percentage of 1-person households, percentage of households with children, percentage of households with older adults, and percentage of owner-occupied households.

and physical health among adults, even after adjustment for neighborhood-level characteristics. This finding lends validity to results and underscores the importance of the HQM as a novel approach to investigating housing quality as an important social determinant of health, especially for administrators and policymakers that can combine HQM estimates with local knowledge and expertise.

Generally, neighborhoods with a lower number of owners, more households below the poverty level, and more households with children had higher rates of poor housing quality. Neighborhoods with poor housing quality were also more likely to have a higher proportion of Black residents; which is reflective of historical and contemporary practices and policies.[33] The result is increased exposure to poor housing quality in ways that may systematically exacerbate health disparities.

The HQM is composed of 3 housing quality domains that overlap and diverge in ways that have not been well understood in prior research. Each housing quality domain represents distinct issues, a finding consistent with prior research on tradeoffs that households make when deciding where to live. Physical housing quality is often the most important attribute in residential choice, and "intent to move" studies show an increased preference for neighborhood-level factors such as localized amenities and safety.[34–38]

The association between HQM and neighborhood health adds to the robust evidence based on neighborhood determinants of health. The stepwise gradient is especially notable, which, together with the sensitivity analyses, suggests that each dimension of poor housing quality is associated with worse neighborhood health outcomes. This is consistent with a growing body of evidence examining the relationship between various aspects of housing quality and health status. For example, HIV researchers have linked viral suppression with housing quality status and examined geographic trends.[39,40] Another recent study using state Medicaid data found that health data are associated with housing quality, and vice versa.[41]

Limitations

This study has several limitations. First, study covariates used for predictive modeling estimates were limited to variables available in both surveys and focused on head-of-household characteristics rather than member-level characteristics. One notable shortcoming is that White heads of households were overrepresented in AHS compared with ACS data. Second, both AHS and ACS responses are self-reported, meaning that self-report bias could affect estimates. However, when constructs such as poor neighborhood perception are examined, self-reported observations about neighborhood quality are often accurate metrics, especially compared with more objective measures.[42,43] Third, housing quality indicators were limited to metrics available in the full AHS data set. Several markers, such as indoor air quality (e.g., secondhand smoke exposure), safety measures for young children, water quality, and external issues such as roof and foundation problems, were asked to only a part of the sample and therefore not included. Self-reported extreme cold as an indicator of housing quality was also excluded because of the potential for natural disasters like the 2021 Texas power crisis to affect results. Additional analyses including this measure did not change the associations between HQM and health (data not shown).

Fourth, there are approximately 16 million vacant homes in the United States. Vacant units were excluded from HQM analyses because of a lack of information about property quality. This exclusion might affect estimates, especially in states with high shares of unoccupied housing units. Fifth, the association with health outcomes represents an ecological, cross-sectional analysis and thus is not causal in nature. Sixth, PLACES data are based on self-reported responses, a type of information bias that is likely nondifferential. Lastly, the surveys used for underlying data are primarily conducted in English and Spanish, therefore reducing the generalizability of the HQM for households where English and Spanish are not the primary household language (~7% of households).

Implications

The HQM represents a novel effort to measure multiple domains of poor housing quality. The resulting measure can be used by a wide range of stakeholders to examine neighborhood-level quality, affordability, and perception within and across census tracts and to make data-informed decisions. HQM is designed to be flexible: policymakers may decide to use national cutpoints consistent with the current study or define areas of need with reference to specific jurisdictions. HQM data may be combined with information from local data sources—including, for example, funding allocations—to better understand a community's unique housing, social, and public health needs. Future research could leverage HQM estimates to investigate the association between HQM and individual-level outcomes. It will also be important to examine the correlation between the HQM and other national data sets of neighborhood quality and opportunity—including, for example, the Opportunity Atlas,[44] the Area Deprivation Index,[45] and the Child Opportunity Index.[46]

Conclusions

This study provides the first national, neighborhood-level estimates of poor housing quality domains among the US occupied housing stock and demonstrates an association with neighborhood health status. The development of estimates for poor housing quality allows researchers, administrators, and policymakers to quantify housing quality within jurisdictions. AJPH

ABOUT THE AUTHORS

Veronica Garrison is with the Office of Policy Development and Research, US Department of Housing and Urban Development, Washington, DC. At the time of this study, Peter J. Ashley was with the Office of Lead Hazard Control and Healthy Homes, US Department of Housing and Urban Development, Washington, DC, and Alyssa J. Moran was with the Johns Hopkins Bloomberg School of Public Health, Baltimore, MD. Thomas K. M. Cudjoe is with the Division of Geriatric Medicine and Gerontology, Johns Hopkins School of Medicine, Baltimore. Eliana M. Perrin is with the Department of Pediatrics, Johns Hopkins School of Medicine and Johns Hopkins School of Nursing, Baltimore. Craig E. Pollack is with the Department of Health Policy and Management, Johns Hopkins Bloomberg School of Public Health and Johns Hopkins School of Nursing, Baltimore.

CORRESPONDENCE

Correspondence should be sent to Craig E. Pollack, MD, MHS, Johns Hopkins University, 601 N Caroline St, 7th Floor, Baltimore, MD 21287 (e-mail: Cpollac2@jhmi.edu). Reprints can be ordered at https://www.ajph.org by clicking the "Reprints" link.

PUBLICATION INFORMATION

Full Citation: Garrison V, Ashley PJ, Moran AJ, Cudjoe TKM, Perrin EM, Pollack CE. Housing Quality Metric (HQM): neighborhood-level data, housing quality, and population health. *Am J Public Health*. 2025;115(5):780–788.

Acceptance Date: November 25, 2024.

DOI: https://doi.org/10.2105/AJPH.2024.307962

ORCID iD:

Thomas K. M. Cudjoe https://orcid.org/0000-0002-2590-209X

CONTRIBUTORS

V. Garrison had full access to all of the data in the study and takes responsibility for the integrity of the data and the accuracy of the data analysis. V. Garrison, P. J. Ashley, A. Moran, T. K. M. Cudjoe, E. M. Perrin, and C. E. Pollack conceptualized and designed the study. V. Garrison and C. E. Pollack acquired, analyzed, and interpreted data. V. Garrison drafted the manuscript and performed statistical analysis. P. J. Ashley, A. Moran, T. K. M. Cudjoe, E. M. Perrin, and C. E. Pollack critically revised the manuscript for important intellectual content. C. E. Pollack supervised the study.

ACKNOWLEDGMENTS

T. K. M. Cudjoe was supported by a National Institutes of Health (award K23AG075191).

Note. The findings and conclusions in this report are those of the authors and do not necessarily represent those of the US Department of Housing and Urban Development.

CONFLICTS OF INTEREST

T. K. M. Cudjoe receives consulting fees outside the submitted work from Papa, Inc and Edenbridge Healthcare. From September 2019 to July 2022, Johns Hopkins entered into a contract with the US Department of Housing and Urban Development for C. E. Pollack to work part time on a temporary assignment assisting the agency on housing and health issues. C. E. Pollack reports stock ownership in Gilead Pharmaceuticals and is on the board of the American Association of Service Coordinators.

HUMAN PARTICIPANT PROTECTION

This research was declared "Non-Human Subjects" by the Johns Hopkins Bloomberg School of Public Health institutional review board.

REFERENCES

1. US Dept of Health and Human Services. Healthy People 2030 Objectives and Measures. Available at: https://health.gov/healthypeople/objectives-and-data/about-objectives/healthy-people-2030-objectives-and-measures. Accessed January 1, 2022.

2. US Department of Housing and Urban Development. FY 2022-2026 HUD Strategic Plan. Available at: https://www.hud.gov/HUD-FY22-26-Strategic-Plan-Focus-Areas. Accessed March 20, 2022.
3. Shiue I, Bramley G. Environmental chemicals mediated the effect of old housing on adult health problems: US NHANES, 2009–2010. *Environ Sci Pollut Res Int.* 2015;22(2):1299–1308. https://doi.org/10.1007/s11356-014-3468-5
4. Kanchongkittiphon W, Mendell MJ, Gaffin JM, Wang G, Phipatanakul W. Indoor environmental exposures and exacerbation of asthma: an update to the 2000 review by the Institute of Medicine. *Environ Health Perspect.* 2015;123(1):6–20. https://doi.org/10.1289/ehp.1307922
5. Matte TD, Jacobs DE. Housing and health—current issues and implications for research and programs. *J Urban Health.* 2000;77(1):7–25. https://doi.org/10.1007/BF02350959
6. Jacobs DE, Wilson J, Dixon SL, Smith J, Evens A. The relationship of housing and population health: a 30-year retrospective analysis. *Environ Health Perspect.* 2009;117(4):597–604. https://doi.org/10.1289/ehp.0800086
7. Eggers F, Moumen F. American Housing Survey: housing adequacy and quality as measured by the AHS. 2013. https://doi.org/10.2139/ssrn.2284174
8. Raymond J, Wheeler W, Brown MJ; Centers for Disease Control and Prevention (CDC). Inadequate and unhealthy housing, 2007 and 2009. *MMWR Suppl.* 2011;60(1):21–27.
9. Routhier G. Beyond worst case needs: measuring the breadth and severity of housing insecurity among urban renters. *Hous Policy Debate.* 2018;29(2):235–249. https://doi.org/10.1080/10511482.2018.1509228
10. Mundra K, Sharma A. Housing adequacy gap for minorities and immigrants in the US: evidence from the 2009 American Housing Survey. *J Housing Research.* 2015;24(1):55–72.
11. Eggers FJ, Moumen F. *American Housing Survey: A Measure of (Poor) Housing Quality.* Washington, DC: US Dept of Housing and Urban Development; 2013.
12. Chu MT, Fenelon A, Rodriguez J, Zota AR, Adamkiewicz G. Development of a multidimensional housing and environmental quality index (HEQI): application to the American Housing Survey. *Environ Health.* 2022;21(1):56. https://doi.org/10.1186/s12940-022-00866-8
13. Swope CB, Hernández D. Housing as a determinant of health equity: a conceptual model. *Soc Sci Med.* 2019;243:112571. https://doi.org/10.1016/j.socscimed.2019.112571
14. Leifheit KM, Schwartz GL, Pollack CE, Linton SL. Building health equity through housing policies: critical reflections and future directions for research. *J Epidemiol Community Health.* 2022;76(8):759–763. https://doi.org/10.1136/jech-2021-216439
15. Alvarez TA, Steffen BL. Worst case housing needs: 2023 report to Congress. US Dept of Housing and Urban Development. May 2023. Available at: https://www.huduser.gov/portal/publications/Worst-Case-Housing-Needs-2023.html. Accessed January 28, 2025.
16. Shamsuddin S, Campbell C. Housing cost burden, material hardship, and well-being. *Hous Policy Debate.* 2022;32(3):413–432. https://doi.org/10.1080/10511482.2021.1882532
17. Acolin A, Reina V. Housing cost burden and life satisfaction. *J Hous Built Environ.* 2022;37(4):1789–1815. https://doi.org/10.1007/s10901-021-09921-1
18. Kuroki M. Housing affordability and mental health in the United States: 2013–2020. *Ment Health Prev.* 2023;29:200261. https://doi.org/10.1016/j.mhp.2023.200261
19. Nobari TZ, Whaley SE. Severe housing-cost burden and low-income young children's exposure to adverse experiences: a cross-sectional survey of WIC participants in Los Angeles County. *Matern Child Health J.* 2021;25(2):321–329. https://doi.org/10.1007/s10995-020-03032-z
20. Park GR, Seo BK. Housing cost burden and material hardship among older adults: how do they influence psychological health?. *Int J Geriatr Psychiatry.* 2022;37(8). https://doi.org/10.1002/gps.5790
21. Jenkins Morales M, Robert SA. Housing cost burden and health decline among low- and moderate-income older renters. *J Gerontol B Psychol Sci Soc Sci.* 2022;77(4):815–826. https://doi.org/10.1093/geronb/gbab184
22. Elliott DS, Wilson WJ, Huizinga D, Sampson RJ, Elliott A, Rankin B. The effects of neighborhood disadvantage on adolescent development. *J Res Crime Delinq.* 1996;33(4):389–426. https://doi.org/10.1177/0022427896033004002
23. Ross CE. Neighborhood disadvantage and adult depression. *J Health Soc Behav.* 2000;41(2):177–187. https://doi.org/10.2307/2676304
24. Durfey SNM, Kind AJH, Buckingham WR, DuGoff EH, Trivedi AN. Neighborhood disadvantage and chronic disease management. *Health Serv Res.* 2019;54(suppl 1):206–216. https://doi.org/10.1111/1475-6773.13092
25. Pollack CE, Blackford AL, Du S, Deluca S, Thornton RLJ, Herring B. Association of receipt of a housing voucher with subsequent hospital utilization and spending. *JAMA.* 2019;322(21):2115–2124. https://doi.org/10.1001/jama.2019.17432
26. Centers for Disease Control and Prevention. PLACES. Available at: https://www.cdc.gov/places. Accessed March 2023.
27. Centers for Disease Control and Prevention. PLACES. Current Release Notes. Available at: https://www.cdc.gov/places/help/data-notes/index.html. Accessed July 2023.
28. El Emam K, Brown A, AbdelMalik P, et al. A method for managing re-identification risk from small geographic areas in Canada. *BMC Med Inform Decis Mak.* 2010;10(1):18. https://doi.org/10.1186/1472-6947-10-18
29. Muller CJ, MacLehose RF. Estimating predicted probabilities from logistic regression: different methods correspond to different target populations. *Int J Epidemiol.* 2014;43(3):962–970. https://doi.org/10.1093/ije/dyu029
30. Garrison VEH, Ashley PJ. Identifying jurisdictions at risk of containing housing units with deteriorated paint: results and targeting implications for the US Department of Housing and Urban Development. *J Public Health Manag Pract.* 2021;27(6):546–557. https://doi.org/10.1097/PHH.0000000000001191
31. Murdoch J, Brahmachari M, Okyere D, Moumen F. *Measuring Housing Insecurity: Index Development Using American Housing Survey Data.* Washington, DC: US Dept of Housing and Urban Development; June 2023.
32. Eggers FJ, US Dept of Housing and Urban Development. Comparison of housing information from the American Housing Survey and the American Community Survey. Contract No. C-CHI-00839. September 2007. Available at: https://www.census.gov/content/dam/Census/programs-surveys/ahs/working-papers/comparison_hsg.pdf. Accessed September 1, 2022.
33. Rothstein R. *The Color of Law: A Forgotten History of How Our Government Segregated America.* New York, NY: Liveright Publishing; 2017.
34. Louviere J, Timmermans H. Hierarchical information integration applied to residential choice behavior. *Geogr Anal.* 1990;22(2):127–144. https://doi.org/10.1111/j.1538-4632.1990.tb00200.x
35. Abraham JE, Hunt JD. Specification and estimation of nested logit model of home, workplaces, and commuter mode choices by multiple-worker households. *Transp Res Rec.* 1997;1606(1):17–24. https://doi.org/10.3141/1606-03
36. Molin E, Oppewal H, Timmermans H. Group-based versus individual-based conjoint preference models of residential preferences: a comparative test. *Environ Plan A.* 1999;31(11):1935–1947. https://doi.org/10.1068/a311935
37. Srour IM, Kockelman KM, Dunn TP. Accessibility indices: connection to residential land prices and location choices. *Transp Res Rec.* 2002;1805(1):25–34. https://doi.org/10.3141/1805-04
38. Kim JH, Pagliara F, Preston J. The intention to move and residential location choice behaviour. *Urban Stud.* 2005;42(9):1621–1636. https://doi.org/10.1080/00420980500185611
39. Clemenzi-Allen A, Geng E, Christopoulos K, et al. Degree of housing instability shows independent "dose-response" with virologic suppression rates among people living with human immunodeficiency virus. *Open Forum Infect Dis.* 2018;5(3):ofy035. https://doi.org/10.1093/ofid/ofy035
40. Aidala AA, Wilson MG, Shubert V, et al. Housing status, medical care, and health outcomes among people living with HIV/AIDS: a systematic review. *Am J Public Health.* 2016;106(1):e1–e23. https://doi.org/10.2105/AJPH.2015.302905
41. Chakraborty O, Dragan KL, Ellen IG, et al. Housing-sensitive health conditions can predict poor-quality housing. *Health Aff (Millwood).* 2024;43(2):297–304. https://doi.org/10.1377/hlthaff.2023.01008
42. Hale L, Hill TD, Friedman E, et al. Perceived neighborhood quality, sleep quality, and health status: evidence from the Survey of the Health of Wisconsin. *Soc Sci Med.* 2013;79:16–22. https://doi.org/10.1016/j.socscimed.2012.07.021
43. Ross CE, Mirowsky J. Disorder and decay: the concept and measurement of perceived neighborhood disorder. *Urban Aff Rev.* 1999;34(3):412–432. https://doi.org/10.1177/107808749903400304
44. Chetty R, Friedman JN, Hendren N, Jones MR, Porter SR. *The Opportunity Atlas: Mapping the Childhood Roots of Social Mobility.* Cambridge, MA: National Bureau of Economic Research; 2018. NBER Working Paper 25147.
45. Kind AJH, Buckingham W. Making neighborhood disadvantage metrics accessible: The Neighborhood Atlas. *N Engl J Med.* 2018;378(26):2456–2458. https://doi.org/10.1056/NEJMp1802313
46. Noelke C, McArdle N, DeVoe B, et al. Child Opportunity Index 3.0: technical documentation. 2024. Available at: https://www.diversitydatakids.org/sites/default/files/file/COI30_TechDoc_20241004.pdf. Accessed January 28, 2025.

COVID-19 Policies and Sexually Transmitted Infections in 22 US States, January 2020–December 2021

Catherine C. Pollack, PhD, Georgia H. Redd, MSE, MPH, Collin M. Timm, PhD, and Yukari C. Manabe, MD

See also Fitzpatrick and Tucker, p. 628, and Pinto et al., p. 631.

Objectives. To quantify the effects of 5 jurisdiction-level COVID-19 policies on chlamydia, gonorrhea, and syphilis rates in 22 US jurisdictions between January 2020 and December 2021.

Methods. We applied a mixed-effects, negative binomial, interrupted time series model to estimate the impact that each policy of interest had on reported cases.

Results. Mandatory stay-at-home periods were associated with a decrease in reported chlamydia (incident rate ratio [IRR] = 0.75; 95% confidence interval [CI] = 0.71, 0.80) and gonorrhea (IRR = 0.85; 95% CI = 0.78, 0.94) cases. We also observed decreased chlamydia case reporting when gatherings were restricted to 10 people (IRR = 0.88; 95% CI = 0.85, 0.92), masking was recommended (IRR = 0.90; 95% CI = 0.85, 0.97), or polymerase chain reaction testing was limited to symptomatic individuals (IRR = 0.72; 95% CI = 0.67, 0.77). Universal vaccine access corresponded to decreases in reported gonorrhea (IRR = 0.83; 95% CI = 0.75, 0.92) but increases in syphilis (IRR = 1.33; 95% CI = 1.04, 1.70) cases. We also observed effects by sex, race, and ethnicity.

Conclusions. COVID-19 policies had disparate effects on sexually transmitted infection rates that varied across demographic groups. Overall results were attenuated after the first lockdown period (March–May 2020), but demographic variations persisted. (*Am J Public Health*. 2025;115(5):789–798. https://doi.org/10.2105/AJPH.2024.307957)

AJPH May 2025, Vol. 115, No. 5

COVID-19 pandemic policies had profound effects on the broader disease landscape. Global decreases in respiratory diseases were observed during their typical seasons in 2020 and 2021, potentially attributable to restrictions alleviating COVID-19 spread.[1] Simultaneously, stay-at-home orders restricted health care access.[2] Sexually transmitted infection (STI) rates were especially affected by the COVID-19 pandemic. Drastic decreases in US rates of chlamydia, gonorrhea, and syphilis were observed in March and April 2020, corresponding with stringent stay-at-home restrictions and STI clinic staff reassignments.[3,4]

The driving factors behind these decreases and the subsequent resurgence of gonorrhea and syphilis are unclear but may relate to changes in sexual behaviors or decreases in testing and screening access.[5,6] One study among men who have sex with men noted that 25% experienced difficulties accessing STI testing services, and a majority reported decreases in sexual behavior in early 2020 that increased after stay-at-home requirements were lifted.[7] A separate study found increases in sexual partnership during the initial lockdown and subsequent period.[8] Another study found higher rates of chlamydia and gonorrhea in US counties with high COVID-19 case counts, suggesting that COVID-19 policy adherence affected STI rates; however, that study looked only at aggregate 2020 rates and did not directly examine policies.[9]

Literature on the impacts of COVID-19 on STI rates in the United States has focused on the initial shutdown period, limiting understanding on how policies may have affected later shifts in STI rates. Longer longitudinal studies also provide more opportunities to explore the effects of other COVID-19 policies, such as masking requirements, vaccination, and testing access. Furthermore, the majority of studies present nationwide results, which preclude examination of jurisdiction-specific policies. Understanding the implications of specific infectious disease policies can help inform decision-making in future disease outbreaks. We evaluated the impact of 5 COVID-19 policies (i.e., stay-at-home requirements, gathering restrictions, masking requirements, testing access, and vaccination access) on the rates of chlamydia, gonorrhea, and syphilis in the United States between January 2020 and December 2021.

METHODS

We compiled external data on 5 distinct COVID-19 policies and monthly counts of chlamydia, gonorrhea, and syphilis across multiple US jurisdictions. Details on data collection and the corresponding statistical analyses are enumerated.

Data Collection

We sent requests for monthly aggregated count data between 2019 and 2022 for chlamydia, gonorrhea, and syphilis to 59 US jurisdictions with their own public health department. We also requested counts by sex, race, and ethnicity. We adjusted all received data per 100 000 population using the US Census Bureau's American Community Survey 5-year data for the corresponding jurisdiction and demographic group.[10]

We extracted COVID-19 policies from the Oxford COVID-19 Government Response Tracker, which contains 24 distinct COVID-19 policies.[11] We limited our analysis to 5 policies that we hypothesized would affect STI rates (Table 1). We considered restrictions on gatherings and stay-at-home requirements "community health practices." We considered masking requirements, testing access, and vaccination access "individual health practices." We rounded the policy implementation date to the start of the month to align with monthly STI data. We hypothesized that stricter community health practices and masking requirements would be associated with fewer reported STI cases, as these policies may reduce high-risk sexual behavior frequency and clinic access. We hypothesized that increased testing and vaccination access would be associated with increased reported STI rates, given that infection status awareness and increased protection may result in a reversal of protective behaviors and increased clinic access.

TABLE 1— COVID-19 Policies Included in the Analysis: 22 US States, January 2020–December 2021

Policy	Levels	Category
Gathering restrictions	No restriction (Ref) Restrictions on gatherings of > 1000 individuals Restrictions on gatherings of 101–1000 individuals Restrictions on gatherings of 11–100 individuals Restrictions on gatherings of ≤ 10 individuals	Community
Stay-at-home requirements	No restriction (Ref) Recommended Required with exceptions Required without exceptions	Community
Masking requirements	No restriction (Ref) Recommended Required in some shared spaces Required in occupied shared spaces Required in occupied or unoccupied shared spaces	Individual
PCR testing access	No policy (Ref) Access for specific[a] symptomatic individuals Access for any symptomatic individual Access for anyone via drive-through tests	Individual
Vaccine access	No vaccination (Ref) Available for 1 key group[b] Available for 2 key groups Available for all key groups Available for all key groups plus select individuals Universal availability	Individual

Note. PCR = polymerase chain reaction.
[a]Specific groups included essential workers, close contacts of individuals with confirmed COVID-19, and individuals who had recently traveled internationally.
[b]We defined key groups as essential workers, immunocompromised individuals, and those aged 65 years and older.

Statistical Analysis

We constructed mixed-effects negative binomial interrupted time series models for each policy exposure and STI outcome combination. Interrupted time series models are used in health services research to model immediate and long-term effects of policies relative to a prepolicy period.[12] We chose a negative binomial model to account for the strictly positive nature of the outcome. We chose a mixed-effects model with a random effect for jurisdiction to account for repeated measures in a jurisdiction over time. Therefore, all models had the following structure:

$$\hat{y}_{s,d,i} = \beta_0 + \beta_1 X_1 + \beta_2 I_{2,s} + \beta_3 X_{3,s} + [\beta_4 I_{4,s} + \ldots + \beta_n I_{n,s}] + u_s, \quad (1)$$

where $\hat{y}_{s,d,i}$ represents the estimated population-adjusted case counts for disease d in jurisdiction s for month i;

β_0 represents a fixed-effects intercept; $\beta_1 X_{i,1}$ represents the number of months since January 1, 2020 (the study origin); $\beta_2 I_{2,S}$ represents whether the month was before or after policy implementation (with β_2 interpreted as the immediate effect during the month when the policy was enacted); $\beta_3 X_{3,S}$ represents the number of months after policy enactment (with β_3 interpreted as the long-term policy impact); $\beta_4 I_4$ through $\beta_n I_{n,s}$ represent policy stringency as determined by the Oxford COVID-19 Government Response Tracker compared with a reference of no policy; and u_S represents a random intercept per jurisdiction.[11] We ran separate models for each policy–disease combination, resulting in 15 models (3 diseases and 5 policies) for the main analysis.

Given that behaviors may have differed from March through May 2020 because of the overarching national lockdowns, we conducted a sensitivity analysis with June 2020 as the origin for 4 of the 5 policies. We excluded vaccination access from this sensitivity analysis, because vaccines were unavailable during the excluded period. For all analyses, we considered a *P* value less than .05 statistically significant. We performed all analyses in R version 4.3.0 using RStudio version 2023.06.0 + 421 (RStudio, Boston, MA).

RESULTS

Of 59 contacted jurisdictions, 50 (84.7%) replied to initial contact. Of respondents, 22 (44%) provided monthly aggregated count data. Jurisdictional representation was geographically diverse, with 7 from the South (32%), 6 from the Midwest (27%), 5 from the West (23%), and 4 from the Northeast (18%). Additional data on sex, race, and ethnicity were provided for 19 of 22 (86.4%) jurisdictions (Figure 1). We evaluated sex for men and women, as most jurisdictions provided binary data for this demographic. We evaluated race (i.e., White, Black/African American, Asian, American Indian/Alaska Native [AIAN], Native Hawaiian/Pacific Islander) and ethnicity (i.e., non-Hispanic/non-Latino, Hispanic/Latino) for the most consistent categories reported across jurisdiction.

We removed counts for additional race/ethnicity categories not listed

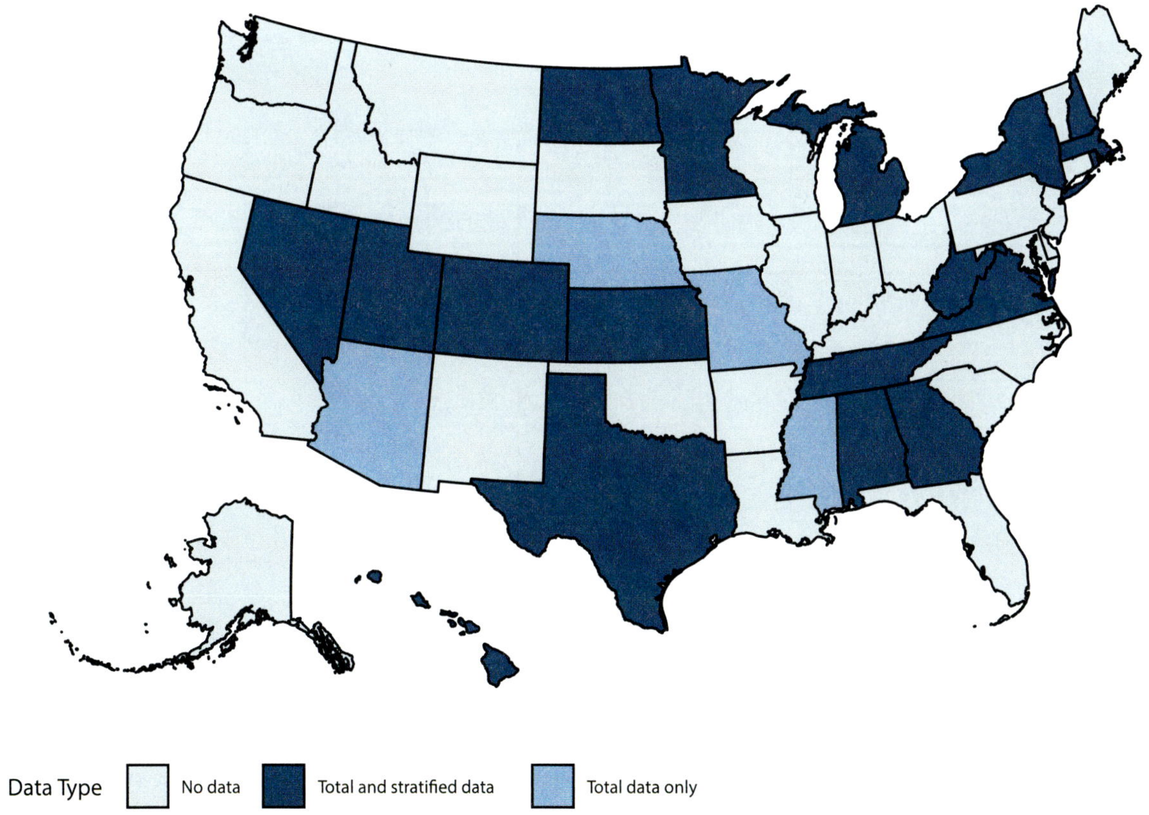

FIGURE 1— Jurisdictions Providing Data for the Study: 22 US States, January 2020–December 2021

Note. All jurisdictions shown in light blue provided monthly, aggregated data. Jurisdictions shown in dark blue provided additional monthly aggregated data by sex, race, and ethnicity.

(including "other") to avoid comparing groups that were inconsistent between jurisdictions. We excluded jurisdictions without demographic data for a category from that subanalysis. We aggregated data by the jurisdictions according to their established policies and procedures. Appendix A (available as a supplement to the online version of this article at http://www.ajph.org) provides jurisdiction data notes.

COVID-19 Community Health Policy Impact

For chlamydia and gonorrhea, mandatory stay-at-home periods were associated with decreases in average disease rates (Figure 2). There were 25% fewer reported chlamydia cases (incident rate ratio [IRR] = 0.75; 95% confidence interval [CI] = 0.71, 0.80; $P < .001$) and 15% fewer gonorrhea cases (IRR = 0.85; 95% CI = 0.78, 0.94; $P = .001$) on average compared with periods without restrictions. This was consistent in the majority of demographic subgroups to varying degrees (Appendix B, available as a supplement to the online version of this article at http://www.ajph.org). Hispanic individuals had the greatest average decrease for both chlamydia (IRR = 0.61; 95% CI = 0.55, 0.69; $P < .001$) and gonorrhea (IRR = 0.71; 95% CI = 0.61, 0.81; $P < .001$). Mandatory stay-at-home periods were not associated with syphilis rates.

Recommended stay-at-home periods had an effect on gonorrhea but not chlamydia. There were 15% more gonorrhea cases on average (IRR = 1.15; 95% CI = 1.09, 1.21; $P < .001$) during recommended stay-at-home periods than during no policy periods, with the largest increase among women (IRR = 1.24; 95% CI = 1.16, 1.32; $P < .001$). Recommended stay-at-home periods had no statistical effect on overall syphilis rates. There were changes among demographic groups, with Asians experiencing the greatest average decrease (IRR = 0.53; 95% CI = 0.28, 0.98; $P = .043$).

Gathering size restrictions had varying impacts (Appendix C, available as a supplement to the online version of this article at http://www.ajph.org). When gatherings were restricted to 10 people, chlamydia decreased by 12% on average (IRR = 0.88; 95% CI = 0.85, 0.92; $P < .001$) compared with no policy periods, with Hispanic individuals experiencing the greatest decrease (IRR = 0.85; 95% CI = 0.79, 0.92; $P < .001$). When gatherings were restricted to 1000 people, men (IRR = 0.86; 95% CI = 0.75, 0.98; $P = .025$) and Hispanic individuals

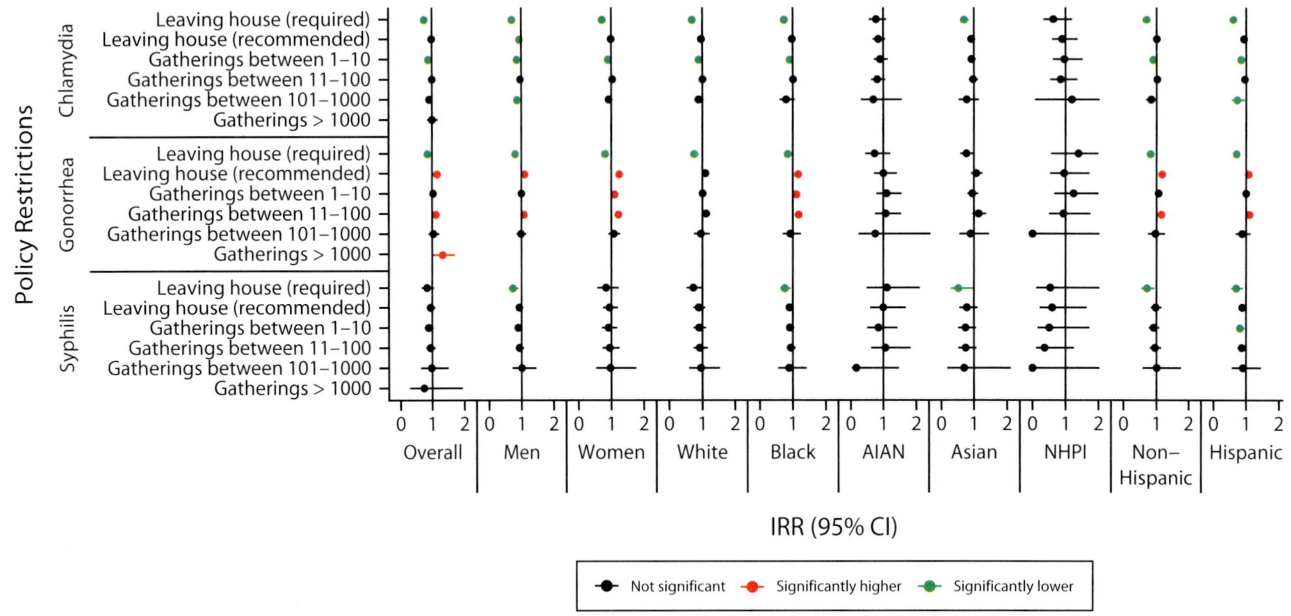

FIGURE 2— Estimated Effects of COVID-19 Community Health Policies on Chlamydia, Gonorrhea, and Syphilis Rates per 100 000 Persons: 22 US States, January 2020–December 2021

Note. AIAN = American Indian/Alaska Native; CI = confidence interval; IRR = incident rate ratio; NHPI = Native Hawaiian/Pacific Islander. Red points with IRR > 1 indicate a significantly increased rate of the sexually transmitted infection of interest during the month of policy enactment compared with a period of no policy restrictions, and green points with IRR < 1 indicate a significantly decreased rate. Black points indicate no significant difference. Missing points indicate that not enough jurisdictions provided data for that category to create a model, and missing CIs denote especially tight bands that were not present given the figure scale.

(IRR = 0.73; 95% CI = 0.56, 0.96; *P* = .024) experienced case decreases.

Although gonorrhea cases overall were not significantly affected during these periods, Black individuals (IRR = 1.11; 95% CI = 1.01, 1.21; *P* = .025) and women (IRR = 1.10; 95% CI = 1.02, 1.18; *P* = .016) had significantly more average cases than in periods without restrictions. This effect persisted when gathering sizes were relaxed, with additional demographic groups (i.e., men, non-Hispanic, Hispanic) experiencing a significant increase in cases. Syphilis rates were not significantly affected by gathering restrictions.

COVID-19 Individual Health Policy Impact

When masking was recommended, there were 10% fewer average chlamydia cases (IRR = 0.90; 95% CI = 0.85, 0.97; *P* = .003) than in periods without masking policies (Figure 3). This trend was consistent across demographic groups, with the largest effect among AIAN individuals (IRR = 0.54; 95% CI = 0.35, 0.83; *P* = .005). When masking was always required in shared spaces, chlamydia cases were higher among women (IRR = 1.07; 95% CI = 1.01, 1.14; *P* = .024) and non-Hispanic individuals (IRR = 1.12; 95% CI = 1.04, 1.21; *P* = .003) than in no policy periods (Appendix D, available as a supplement to the online version of this article at http://www.ajph.org). Overall gonorrhea cases increased by 32% on average (IRR = 1.32; 95% CI = 1.23, 1.43; *P* < .001) during these periods, an effect shared by many demographic groups. We observed no significant effect for syphilis.

The impact of COVID-19 polymerase chain reaction (PCR) testing access on STI rates was consistent (Appendix E, available as a supplement to the online version of this article at http://www.ajph.org). Observed STI rates decreased as PCR testing was restricted to symptomatic individuals in limited populations (e.g., those who had recently traveled internationally, essential workers). There were 20% fewer gonorrhea cases (IRR = 0.80; 95% CI = 0.72, 0.90; *P* < .001), 28% fewer chlamydia cases (IRR = 0.72; 95% CI = 0.67, 0.78; *P* < .001), and 29% fewer syphilis cases (IRR = 0.71; 95% CI = 0.55, 0.91; *P* = .006) on average compared with periods when PCR testing access was not measured, an effect paralleled across most demographic subgroups. When PCR tests were readily available to any individual, effects diverged.

We found fewer average chlamydia cases (IRR = 0.87; 95% CI = 0.80, 0.95; *P* = .002), more average gonorrhea

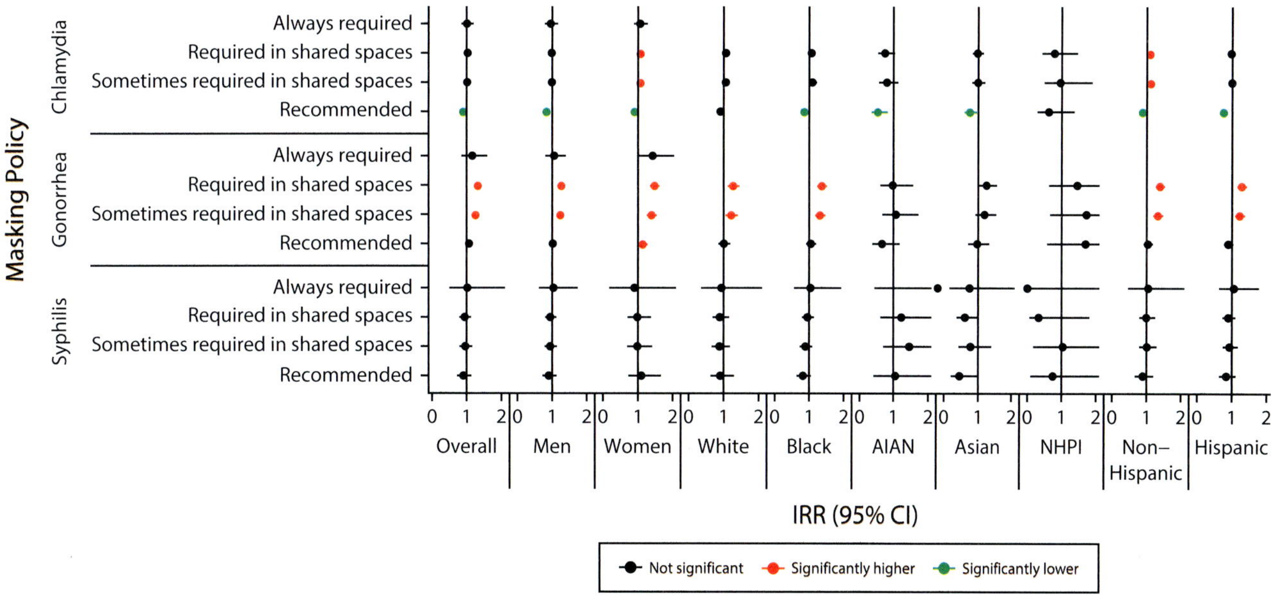

FIGURE 3— Estimated Effects of COVID-19 Masking Policies on Chlamydia, Gonorrhea, and Syphilis Rates per 100 000 Persons: 22 US states, January 2020–December 2021

Note. AIAN = American Indian/Alaska Native; CI = confidence interval; IRR = incident rate ratio; NHPI = Native Hawaiian/Pacific Islander. Red points with IRR > 1 indicate a significantly increased rate of the sexually transmitted infection of interest during the month of policy enactment compared with a period of no policy restrictions, and green points with IRR < 1 indicate a significantly decreased rate. Black points indicate no significant difference. Missing points indicate that not enough jurisdictions provided data for that category to create a model, and missing CIs denote especially tight bands that are not present given the figure scale.

cases (IRR = 1.19; 95% CI = 1.04, 1.37; $P = .011$), and no significant change in syphilis cases (IRR = 0.83; 95% CI = 0.63, 1.09; $P = .182$). Women (IRR = 1.25; 95% CI = 1.07, 1.46; $P = .006$) and Hispanic individuals (IRR = 1.33; 95% CI = 1.09, 1.62; $P = .006$) had a significant increase in gonorrhea cases when testing was more readily available than in no policy periods.

Vaccination access had a contradictory impact relative to other policies (Appendix F, available as a supplement to the online version of this article at http://www.ajph.org). Although vaccine access did not have an overall effect on chlamydia cases, men (IRR = 1.17; 95% CI – 10.6, 1.28; P – .001), White individuals (IRR = 1.21; 95% CI = 1.08, 1.36; $P = .001$), non-Hispanic individuals (IRR = 1.20; 95% CI = 1.09, 1.32; $P < .001$), and Hispanic individuals (IRR = 1.28; 95% CI = 1.10, 1.48; $P = .001$) experienced increases when vaccines became universally available. There were 33% more syphilis cases on average (IRR = 1.33; 95% CI = 1.04, 1.70; $P = .022$) than in periods when COVID-19 vaccines were unavailable. There were 13% fewer gonorrhea cases on average (IRR = 0.83; 95% CI = 0.75, 0.92; $P = .001$) when vaccines were universally available, with women experiencing a significant decrease (IRR = 0.83; 95% CI = 0.73, 0.93; $P = .002$).

Sensitivity Analysis

When we excluded March to May 2020 from the analysis, the overall impact of each policy on STI rates was no longer statistically significant. Substantial differences remained for select demographic groups. There were 16% fewer average chlamydia cases in men (IRR = 0.84; 95% CI = 0.74, 0.97; $P = .017$) and 24% fewer in Hispanic individuals (IRR = 0.76; 95% CI = 0.59, 0.98; $P = .037$) when gatherings were restricted to 1000 persons or fewer than in periods without restrictions. No significant associations were found for other demographic subgroups or STIs.

There were 13% fewer chlamydia cases in women (IRR = 0.87; 95% CI = 0.77, 0.98), 22% fewer in Hispanic individuals (IRR = 0.79; 95% CI = 0.62, 0.99; $P = .043$), and 32% fewer in Asian individuals (IRR = 0.68; 95% CI = 0.47, 1.00; $P = .048$) on average when stay-at-home requirements were mandatory than in periods without stay-at-home policies. There were 24% fewer gonorrhea cases in men (IRR = 0.76; 95% CI = 0.62, 0.93; $P = .006$), 35% fewer in Hispanic individuals (IRR = 0.65; 95% CI = 0.49, 0.86; $P = .003$), 34% fewer in White individuals (IRR = 0.66; 95% CI = 0.48, 0.92; $P = .013$), and 23% fewer in Black individuals (IRR = 0.77; 95% CI = 0.59, 1.00; $P = .048$) on average when stay-at-home requirements were mandatory. All other stay-at-home associations were not statistically significant.

On average, chlamydia cases among Hispanic individuals were 48% lower (IRR = 0.52; 95% CI = 0.31, 0.88; $P = .015$) during periods when masking was recommended than during periods without masking requirements. There were 30% more chlamydia cases in Asian individuals (IRR = 1.30; 95% CI = 1.08, 1.58; $P = .006$) on average when masking was sometimes required in shared public spaces. There were 37% fewer gonorrhea cases in men (IRR = 0.63; 95% CI = 0.47, 0.84; $P = .002$), 34% fewer in women (IRR = 0.66; 95% CI = 0.56, 0.95; $P = .025$), 43% fewer in non-Hispanic individuals (IRR = 0.57; 95% CI = 0.40, 0.82; $P = .002$), 59% fewer in Hispanic individuals (IRR = 0.41; 95% CI = 0.28, 0.61; $P < .001$), 35% fewer in White individuals (IRR = 0.65; 95% CI = 0.46, 0.92; $P = .016$), 57% fewer in Black individuals (IRR = 0.43; 95% CI = 0.22, 0.83; $P = .012$), and 96% fewer in AIAN individuals (IRR = 0.06; 95% CI = 0.01, 0.71; $P = .025$) on average when masks were recommended. During these same periods, there were 73% more cases of syphilis in White individuals (IRR = 1.73; 95% CI = 1.03, 2.92; $P = .040$) on average. All other masking associations were not statistically significant.

There were 33% fewer gonorrhea cases in Hispanic individuals (IRR = 0.67; 95% CI = 0.48, 0.92; $P = .015$) and 74% fewer in Asian individuals (IRR = 0.26; 95% CI = 0.08, 0.89; $P = .032$) on average when PCR testing was only available to symptomatic persons than in periods without PCR testing access policies. All other PCR testing associations were not statistically significant.

DISCUSSION

To our knowledge, this study is the first to quantify the consequences of 5 COVID-19 policies (i.e., stay-at-home requirements, gathering restrictions, masking requirements, testing access, and vaccination access) on chlamydia, gonorrhea, and syphilis rates across the United States. In 22 geographically diverse jurisdictions, chlamydia decreased when stay-at-home requirements were mandatory, gathering restrictions were most restrictive, masking was recommended, and PCR tests were universally available. Gonorrhea cases decreased when stay-at-home requirements were mandatory and vaccines were more available, and they rose when gathering restrictions were loosened and testing access increased. Syphilis was largely unaffected by community health policies, whereas universal vaccination access corresponded with case increases. The magnitude and significance of these effects varied across demographics and period. Although the overall association between COVID-19 policies and STI rates were attenuated after the first US lockdown, relationships in select demographic groups persisted. These heterogeneous results suggest the complex impact diverse public health policies can have on STI rates across demographic groups.

We selected the 5 evaluated COVID-19 policies to capture various facets of health behavior. Stay-at-home requirements and gathering restrictions were contagion mitigation policies that, although effective, were highly divisive.[13,14] Thus, these policies are likely to be reserved for crises and may demonstrate how the most stringent emergency policies for 1 disease affect another. However, masking policies are less burdensome and may offer a middle ground for contagion mitigation that balances easy implementation with effectiveness. Yet the political partisanship of masking may inhibit their utility in future infectious disease outbreaks. The restrictive nature of these policies led to our hypothesis that increases in their stringency would be associated with a decrease in STI rates.

In addition, testing and vaccine policies may influence human behavior. Previous work has shown that patients diagnosed with influenza traveled less frequently during their illness than during illness-free periods, suggesting that knowledge of disease state may influence behaviors.[15] Thus, we hypothesized that widespread knowledge of COVID-19 status (as measured through testing access) would similarly affect sexual behaviors and thus STI rates. We hypothesized that vaccination availability would have a similar effect, as patients vaccinated against COVID-19 may be more likely to reengage in sexual behaviors after lockdown. Alternatively, taking a COVID-19 test and receiving a vaccination are health-seeking behaviors that decrease transmission, and individuals exhibiting these behaviors may also be less likely to engage in high-risk behaviors that could increase their STI risk.[16]

Researchers have speculated that the STI decrease during the US national lockdown was attributable to reduced access to sexual health services.[3–5,7,17,18] Others have argued that it may be owing to sexual behavior changes.[1,19,20] Our results support the clinic access hypothesis, as we observed significantly fewer chlamydia and gonorrhea cases when stay-at-home orders were mandated and when gatherings were limited to 10 or fewer people (chlamydia only). This effect disappeared when we excluded March to May 2020, even though similar lockdown policies were reintroduced in select jurisdictions afterward. This supports the idea that closing clinics and reducing testing services—not the lockdowns—contributed to the decreases in testing. However, the policies affected almost every demographic group individually after this period. These results align with the hypothesis that increased stringency in stay-at-home orders and gathering restrictions would be associated with lower STI rates. Future work should examine each group individually to identify unique determinants that affected these results and have long-term influences on sexual health service access.

Periods with the most stringent masking policies were not significantly associated with STI rates. However, this shifted as masking policies loosened. Whereas gonorrhea cases increased when masks were sometimes required, chlamydia cases decreased when masking was recommended. This effect differed among women and non-Hispanic individuals, who experienced significant increases in cases when masking was sometimes required. These increases may also be connected to clinic reopenings and resumption of regular testing, and chlamydia increases among women and non-Hispanic individuals may suggest that they resumed normal visits earlier than did others. These findings were partially aligned with our hypothesis, and variations may be attributable to adherence, which we did not measure in this study.

Similarly, although COVID-19 vaccine access was not associated overall with chlamydia, we observed an increase uniquely among men, Hispanic individuals, and White individuals when the vaccine became universally available. This may suggest that these individuals were last to return to regular clinic visits, especially because universal COVID-19 vaccine access was not granted until spring 2021. It could also indicate a resurgence in sexual behavior among these groups, an effect observed directly after national lockdowns both in and outside the United States.[5,21,22] However, testing and vaccination access are critical components of policy adherence that we did not measure, which could explain the lack of an overall relationship between COVID-19 vaccine access and STI rates.

There is limited earlier work measuring associations between COVID-19 policies and STI rates. One study among men who have sex with men in the Netherlands found a decrease in STIs during the nationwide lockdown that was not significant during subsequent policy shifts.[21] There were fewer chlamydia and gonorrhea cases among men in this study when stay-at-home and gathering restrictions were implemented after the main lockdown period. Because earlier work evaluated only men who have sex with men, future work should stratify analyses by sexual behavior to determine what role this may play. Another study found no association between adherence to nonpharmaceutical COVID-19 policies and a history of STI among adolescent and young adult Black men, although temporality of the STI relative to policy enactment was not evaluated.[23] By contrast, we found a marked association between policy implementation and STI rates among both Black/African American individuals and men.

We hypothesize that our results demonstrate challenges in testing access that differentially affected demographic groups. The decrease in STI rates during the complete shutdown period correlates with data in other work that showed that STI testing decreased during the same period.[6] The dramatic increase in congenital syphilis shown in other work suggests that sexual behaviors and STI transmission still occurred during this time window.[24] Given this pattern, we expected that syphilis rates in our study would also change dramatically; however, syphilis rates did not fluctuate widely. We hypothesize that this discrepancy is attributable to testing and treatment changes that remained after lockdown orders were rescinded. The racial and ethnic differences in STI rates after lockdown suggest that there may have been additional inequitable access to testing and STI services in particular groups. Thus, our results emphasize the crucial need to identify areas for technical and process innovations that can enhance equitable access to testing.

Limitations

Several study limitations are of note. First, the ecological nature of this study precluded our ability to establish causality and may have obfuscated individual trends. Future work could directly evaluate COVID-19 policy adherence and STI rates over time, especially beyond the initial lockdown. This could also confirm the precise temporality of cases relative to policy implication, as we assumed policy implementation on the first of every month.

Second, data were not available for certain demographic groups, and future work could repeat this analysis for those groups, including men who have sex with men. Similarly, although the public health jurisdictions that provided data were geographically diverse, they were not comprehensive. We hypothesize that this did not affect results, assuming jurisdictions are missing at random.

Third, given the heterogeneity in individual jurisdictions, we did not adjust models for jurisdiction-level variables, thereby potentially exaggerating the observed effects. Similarly, we did not incorporate substate policies specific to a certain county or city into our analysis, as data were not available at a lower level of geography. We assumed that state policies superseded local policies, but future work could examine the effect of more localized policies on STI rates (especially for jurisdictions where the city and state policies differed).

Finally, our chosen model, although straightforward in interpretation, assumed a linear relationship and serial correlation that did not diminish over time. Future work could explore alternative model structures (e.g., an autoregressive integrated moving average) to assess the relationship between COVID-19 policy stringency and STI rates.

Conclusions

COVID-19 stay-at-home orders, gathering restrictions, masking requirements, PCR testing access, and vaccine access had differential effects across demographic groups and STI rates. Chlamydia decreased with more stringent community health policies, whereas gonorrhea decreased for more stringent policies before increasing when policies were loosened. Syphilis was unaffected except when vaccines became universally available, which corresponded to case increases. Aggregated impacts became statistically insignificant when policy effects were limited to June 2020 onward but persisted among demographic groups. Taken together, these results suggest that more stringent community health COVID-19 policies had a greater influence on STI rates than did less stringent individual health policies. These relationships could be mediated by policy adherence or testing access, which we did not capture and which should be examined in future work. Before enacting new policies for a disease, policymakers and health experts should consider how they may fit into the broader disease landscape, including both overall and group-specific consequences. AJPH

ABOUT THE AUTHORS

Catherine C. Pollack is with the Decision Systems Group, Johns Hopkins University Applied Physics Laboratory, Laurel, MD. Georgia H. Redd and Collin M. Timm are with the Applied Biological Sciences Group, Johns Hopkins University Applied Physics Laboratory. Yukari C. Manabe is with the Division of Infectious Diseases, Johns Hopkins University School of Medicine, Baltimore, MD.

CORRESPONDENCE

Correspondence should be sent to Catherine C. Pollack, 7707 Montpelier Rd, MPE3-E165, Laurel, MD 20273 (e-mail: catherine.pollack@jhuapl.edu).

PUBLICATION INFORMATION

Full Citation: Pollack CC, Redd GH, Timm CM, Manabe YC. COVID-19 policies and sexually transmitted infections in 22 US states, January 2020–December 2021. *Am J Public Health*. 2025;115(5):789–798.

Acceptance Date: November 20, 2024.

DOI: https://doi.org/10.2105/AJPH.2024.307957

ORCID iDs:
Catherine C. Pollack https://orcid.org/0000-0002-7434-5306

Georgia H. Redd https://orcid.org/0009-0005-6860-3638

Collin M. Timm https://orcid.org/0000-0002-7804-5044

Yukari C. Manabe https://orcid.org/0000-0001-8619-5598

CONTRIBUTORS

C. C. Pollack and G. H. Redd analyzed the data. C. C. Pollack and C. M. Timm collected the data and drafted the initial version of the article. C. C. Pollack, C. M. Timm, and Y. C. Manabe formulated the research question, designed the analysis, and revised and approved the final version of the article.

ACKNOWLEDGMENTS

Research reported in this article was supported by the National Institute of Biomedical Imaging and Bioengineering of the National Institutes of Health, National Institutes of Health (NIH; award U54EB007958).

We would like to acknowledge Kaitlin Lovett, Damon Duquaine, and the following jurisdictional public health departments: the Alabama Department of Public Health; the Colorado Department of Public Health & Environment, Office of STI/HIV/VH; the Georgia Department of Public Health, STD Program; the State of Hawaii Department of Health, Harm Reduction Services Branch, Clinic and Field Services Section; the Kansas Department of Health & Environment, Section on Disease Intervention; the Massachusetts Department of Public Health, Bureau of Infectious Disease and Laboratory Sciences, Office of Integrated Surveillance and Information Services; the Michigan Department of Health and Human Services, Bureau of HIV and STI Programs; the Minnesota Department of Health, HIV, STD, TB Section; the Missouri Department of Health and Senior Services, Division of Community and Public Health; the Nebraska Department of Health and Human Services; the Nevada Department of Health and Human Services, Office of Analytics; the New Hampshire Department of Health and Human Services; the New York State Department of Health, Bureau of HIV and STI Field Services; the New York City Department of Health and Mental Hygiene, Division of Disease Control, Bureau of Hepatitis, HIV, and Sexually Transmitted Infections; the North Dakota Department of Health and Human Services, Public Health Division, Sexually Transmitted and Bloodborne Diseases Unit; the Rhode Island Department of Health, Division of Emergency Preparedness and Infectious Disease, Center for HIV, Viral Hepatitis, STD, and TB Epidemiology; the Tennessee Department of Health, HIV/STD/Viral Hepatitis Program; the Texas Department of State Health Services, HIV/STD Prevention and Care Unit; the Utah Department of Health & Human Services, HEART (HIV/STD Elimination, Analysis, Response & Treatment) Program; the Virginia Department of Health, Office of Epidemiology; the West Virginia Department of Health & Human Resources, Division of STD, HIV, Hepatitis and Tuberculosis, Office of Epidemiology and Prevention Services; and states that made their data publicly available.

Note. The content of this article is solely the responsibility of the authors and does not necessarily represent the official views of the NIH.

CONFLICTS OF INTEREST

The authors have no potential or actual conflicts of interest from funding or affiliation-related activities.

HUMAN PARTICIPANT PROTECTION

This study was exempt from institutional review board approval because all data were provided at an aggregated level.

REFERENCES

1. Chow EJ, Uyeki TM, Chu HY. The effects of the COVID-19 pandemic on community respiratory virus activity. *Nat Rev Microbiol*. 2023;21(3): 195–210. https://doi.org/10.1038/s41579-022-00807-9
2. Gertz AH, Pollack CC, Schultheiss MD, Brownstein JS. Delayed medical care and underlying health in the United States during the COVID-19 pandemic: a cross-sectional study. *Prev Med Rep*. 2022;28:101882. https://doi.org/10.1016/j.pmedr.2022.101882
3. Pagaoa M, Grey J, Torrone E, Kreisel K, Stenger M, Weinstock H. Trends in nationally notifiable sexually transmitted disease case reports during the US COVID-19 pandemic, January to December 2020. *Sex Transm Dis*. 2021;48(10):798–804. https://doi.org/10.1097/OLQ.0000000000001506
4. Wright SS, Kreisel KM, Hitt JC, Pagaoa MA, Weinstock HS, Thorpe PG. Impact of the COVID-19 pandemic on Centers for Disease Control and Prevention–funded sexually transmitted disease programs. *Sex Transm Dis*. 2022;49(4):e61–e63. https://doi.org/10.1097/OLQ.0000000000001566
5. Berzkalns A, Thibault CS, Barbee LA, Golden MR, Khosropour C, Kerani RP. Decreases in reported sexually transmitted infections during the time of COVID-19 in King County, WA: decreased transmission or screening? *Sex Transm Dis*. 2021; 48(8 suppl):S44–S49. https://doi.org/10.1097/OLQ.0000000000001463
6. Pinto CN, Niles JK, Kaufman HW, et al. Impact of the COVID-19 pandemic on chlamydia and gonorrhea screening in the US. *Am J Prev Med*. 2021;61(3):386–393. https://doi.org/10.1016/j.amepre.2021.03.009
7. Pampati S, Emrick K, Siegler AJ, Jones J. Changes in sexual behavior, PrEP adherence, and access to sexual health services because of the COVID-19 pandemic among a cohort of PrEP-using MSM in the South. *J Acquir Immune Defic Syndr*. 2021;87(1): 639–643. https://doi.org/10.1097/QAI.0000000000002640
8. Hamill MM, Yu T, Armington GS, Hsieh YH, Manabe YC, Melendez JH. Factors associated with new sexual partnerships during the COVID-19 pandemic: a survey of online sexually transmitted infection testing platform users. *Sex Transm Dis*. 2022;49(10):695–699. https://doi.org/10.1097/OLQ.0000000000001675
9. Pollack CC, Bradburne J, Lee NK, et al. A national, county-level evaluation of the association between COVID-19 and sexually transmitted infections within the United States in 2020. *Sex Transm Dis*. 2023;50(8):536–542. https://doi.org/10.1097/OLQ.0000000000001818
10. US Census Bureau. American Community Survey 5-year data (2009–2021). December 12, 2024. Available at: https://www.census.gov/data/developers/data-sets/acs-5year.html. Accessed February 2, 2025.
11. Hale T, Angrist N, Goldszmidt R, et al. A global panel database of pandemic policies (Oxford COVID-19 Government Response Tracker). *Nat Hum Behav*. 2021;5(4):529–538. https://doi.org/10.1038/s41562-021-01079-8
12. Ewusie JE, Soobiah C, Blondal E, Beyene J, Thabane L, Hamid JS. Methods, applications and challenges in the analysis of interrupted time series data: a scoping review. *J Multidiscip Healthc*. 2020;13: 411–423. https://doi.org/10.2147/JMDH.S241085
13. Fowler JH, Hill SJ, Levin R, Obradovich N. Stay-at-home orders associate with subsequent decreases in COVID-19 cases and fatalities in the United States. *PLoS One*. 2021;16(6):e0248849. https://doi.org/10.1371/journal.pone.0248849
14. Deane C, Parker K, Gramlich J. A year of US public opinion on the coronavirus pandemic. March 5, 2021. Available at: https://www.pewresearch.org/social-trends/2021/03/05/a-year-of-u-s-public-opinion-on-the-coronavirus-pandemic. Accessed September 30, 2024.
15. Vigfusson Y, Karlsson TA, Onken D, et al. Cell-phone traces reveal infection-associated behavioral change. *Proc Natl Acad Sci U S A*. 2021;118(6): e2005241118. https://doi.org/10.1073/pnas.2005241118
16. Shank F, Korovich M, Nicoletti A, Angelone DJ, Jones MC. The influence of health-related behavior profiles on college students' perceptions of COVID-19 safety measures. *J Community Health*. 2024;49(4):1–9. https://doi.org/10.1007/s10900-024-01342-9
17. Tao J, Napoleon SC, Maynard MA, et al. Impact of the COVID-19 pandemic on sexually transmitted infection clinic visits. *Sex Transm Dis*. 2021;48(1): e5–e7. https://doi.org/10.1097/OLQ.0000000000001306
18. Nagendra G, Carnevale C, Neu N, Cohall A, Zucker J. The potential impact and availability of sexual health services during the COVID-19 pandemic. *Sex Transm Dis*. 2020;47(7):434–436. https://doi.org/10.1097/OLQ.0000000000001198
19. Holt M, Chan C, Broady TR, et al. Adjusting behavioural surveillance and assessing disparities in the impact of COVID-19 on gay and bisexual

men's HIV-related behaviour in Australia. *AIDS Behav*. 2023;27(2):518–534. https://doi.org/10.1007/s10461-022-03788-1

20. Hammoud MA, Maher L, Holt M, et al. Physical distancing due to COVID-19 disrupts sexual behaviors among gay and bisexual men in Australia: implications for trends in HIV and other sexually transmissible infections. *J Acquir Immune Defic Syndr*. 2020;85(3):309–315. https://doi.org/10.1097/QAI.0000000000002462
21. de la Court F, Boyd A, Coyer L, et al. The impact of COVID-19-related restrictions in 2020 on sexual healthcare use, pre-exposure prophylaxis use, and sexually transmitted infection incidence among men who have sex with men in Amsterdam, the Netherlands. *HIV Med*. 2023;24(2):212–223. https://doi.org/10.1111/hiv.13374
22. Storer D, Prestage G, McManus H, et al. Relationship between sexual behaviors with non-committed relationship partners and COVID-19 restrictions and notification rates: results from a longitudinal study of gay and bisexual men in Australia. *Sex Res Social Policy*. 2023;20(2):825–836. https://doi.org/10.1007/s13178-022-00733-8
23. Ratnayake A, Campbell MB, Gomes G, Kissinger PJ. Are prior sexual risk behaviors associated with adherence to COVID-19 preventative behaviors among young Black men? *Sex Transm Dis*. 2023;50(10):687–691. https://doi.org/10.1097/OLQ.0000000000001851
24. Gregory ECW, Ely DM. Trends and characteristics in maternal syphilis rates during pregnancy: United States, 2016–2022. NCHS Data Brief. 2024;(496):1–8. Available at: https://www.cdc.gov/nchs/data/databriefs/db496.pdf. Accessed February 18, 2025.

Sexually Transmitted Infection Disparities and Social Determinants of Health in California, 2013–2021

Esther E. Gotlieb, MPH, Nicole O. Burghardt, MPH, Jiawen Hu, PhD, Kathleen Jacobson, MD, and Robert E. Snyder, PhD, MPH

Objectives. To characterize the intersection of social determinants of health, measured as the availability of community opportunities for healthy living, and sexually transmitted infections (STIs) in California.

Methods. Geocoded 2013–2021 California bacterial STI cases were aggregated into Healthy Places Index (HPI) quartiles. Communities in the lowest scoring HPI quartile have the fewest opportunities for healthy living, while communities in the highest scoring quartile have the most opportunities.

Results. As community opportunities became more available, bacterial STI risk decreased. Asian people had the lowest bacterial STI rates, while Black/African American people had the highest. As community opportunities increased, White people had the largest overall STI risk reduction, Native Hawaiian and other Pacific Islander people had the smallest reduction, Hispanic/Latino people had equivalent gonorrhea and early syphilis risk, and American Indian/Alaska Native people had equivalent chlamydia risk.

Conclusions. Although STI incidence decreased as community opportunities increased, people of different racial and ethnic identities were differentially affected. Because the availability of community opportunities is not enough to mitigate racial health disparities, more work is needed to ensure community-level STI prevention efforts are accessible and inclusive. (*Am J Public Health.* 2025;115(5):799–807. https://doi.org/10.2105/AJPH.2024.307963)

AJPH May 2025, Vol. 115, No. 5

In California from 2013 to 2022, cases of chlamydia increased by 15%, gonorrhea by 106%, early syphilis by 159%, and syphilis of late or unknown duration by 340%. While the majority of bacterial sexually transmitted infection (STI) cases were among Hispanic/Latino people, Black/African American people had the highest bacterial STI rates compared with all other racial and ethnic groups in the state. In 2022, when compared with Asian people, who had the lowest bacterial STI rates, Black/African American people had 7 times the risk of early syphilis, 8 times the risk of chlamydia, and more than 10 times the risk of gonorrhea. Although bacterial STI rates have remained elevated among American Indian/Alaska Native (AI/AN) people, from 2020 to 2021, early syphilis rates among AI/AN people increased by 27% (69% increase among AI/AN females), the largest increase among all races or ethnicities in that time period, and remained steady into 2022. From 2021 to 2022, early syphilis rates among Native Hawaiian and other Pacific Islander (NHOPI) people increased by 15% (42% among NHOPI females), the largest increase compared with all other racial and ethnic groups over that time period. Bacterial STI rates in California are also significantly different between men and women—there have been consistently higher chlamydia rates among females, and higher gonorrhea and syphilis rates among males.[1]

Social, political, and structural contexts that contribute to differences in disease risk between populations (social determinants of health [SDoH]) are the community conditions in which individuals live, work, grow, learn, and play.[2–4] The opportunity to access neighborhood resources, such as health care, housing, employment, and transportation impact health and well-being.[3] SDoH that are important for sexual health include safe, quality, and stable housing; economic stability; and judgment-free and nondiscriminatory health care services.[4] Structural racism, an SDoH that is a root cause of racial health disparities is "the totality of ways in which societies foster [racial] discrimination, via mutually reinforcing [inequitable] systems . . . that in turn reinforce discriminatory beliefs, values, and distribution of resources."[5(p1455)] Political, economic, social, and cultural institutional decisions contributed to socially and racially segregated communities and community divestments, leading to disparate access to power, wealth, and neighborhood opportunities needed to support health and well-being.[5] The disenfranchisement, forced assimilation, and segregation experienced by Indigenous communities; slavery, violence, marginalization, and Jim Crow laws experienced by Black/African American people; and discriminatory laws and immigration policies experienced by Hispanic/Latino people are institutional practices with lasting, devastating consequences that have resulted in unequal access to community opportunities to lead healthy lives and contribute to present-day racial health disparities.[6] Exposure to adverse SDoH, such as racism, discrimination, lack of economic opportunities, inadequate health care coverage, and insufficient educational opportunities, impact individual opportunities for healthy living.[6] Characterizing neighborhood SDoH, or the availability of opportunities for healthy living in a community, may identify opportunities for interventions that would improve health outcomes among people who live in that same area.

Incorporating SDoH into routine public health surveillance enables identification and characterization of modifiable SDoH that contribute to disease disparities and subsequent identification of at-risk populations that would benefit from interventions to reduce disease burden. Nationally, the Centers for Disease Control and Prevention (CDC) began integrating SDoH into public health activities and the CDC's infrastructure through a workgroup, forums, and centralized access to SDoH resources, recognizing that incorporating SDoH into public health infrastructure improves health outcomes and reduces health disparities.[7] Improvements to SDoH impact health outcomes differentially by race and ethnicity; however, more research is needed to identify the extent to which SDoH moderate STI racial health disparities.[8,9] Using the California Healthy Places Index (HPI), we describe how SDoH, as measured by the availability of community opportunities for healthy living, impacts STI incidence, and the extent to which SDoH reduce STI risk. The HPI leverages data to identify communities with the fewest resources to equitably support community-level investments and policy decisions. The HPI has been used to identify and prioritize public health efforts, such as funding allocation, vaccine distribution, and COVID-19 testing resource allotments.[10] The findings from this analysis will help identify disproportionally affected populations and prioritize interventions for STI prevention.

METHODS

The HPI is a composite geospatial index of community conditions related to life expectancy that was designed by the Public Health Alliance of Southern California.[11] The HPI is a validated index to measure the availability of community opportunities that support healthy living and developed from community-level SDoH with actionable policy and program implications.[12] The HPI is composed of 23 community indicators aggregated into 8 domains: economic, education, social, transportation, neighborhood, housing, clean environment, and health care access. To construct the index, the Public Health Alliance of Southern California scored and divided 2010 US census tracts into quartiles. Areas in the lowest scoring quartile (HPI quartile 1) represented areas with the fewest community opportunities for healthy living, while areas in the highest scoring quartile (HPI quartile 4) represented areas with the most community opportunities for healthy living. The HPI was intentionally designed and recommended to be used as quartiles because "in the California policy environment, people living in the 25% most disadvantaged census tracts are often earmarked for increased investments."[13(p2)] Census tracts with populations of fewer than 1500 people or with more than 50% of the population living in group quarters (e.g., correctional facilities or skilled nursing facilities) were not scored and were excluded (3.31% of California census tracts; n = 267).

All cases of chlamydia, gonorrhea, early syphilis (including primary, secondary, and early nonprimary nonsecondary syphilis), and syphilis of late or unknown duration that were reported to the California Department of Public Health from 2013 to 2021 were eligible for inclusion. Individuals' home addresses were geocoded using ArcMap version 10.7.1 to 2010 US census tracts.[14] Individuals without addresses to geocode or whose home addresses geocoded to medical provider addresses, correctional facilities, or military bases were excluded. Cases among people from

Los Angeles and San Francisco Counties were excluded because their addresses during the study period were not available (Study Methods A, available as a supplement to the online version of this article at https://ajph.org).

HPI scores for each STI case were determined from the census tract where the person resided. We used the χ^2 test to compare demographic characteristics of people who lived in each HPI quartile by STI (chlamydia, gonorrhea, early syphilis, and syphilis of late or unknown duration). We used the Kruskal–Wallis test to compare median ages and the χ^2 test to compare gender, race, and ethnicity between individuals, using an α of 0.05 to determine statistical significance. We categorized gender identity as (1) male/transgender male, (2) female/transgender female, and (3) other/unknown (unknown gender identity/declined to answer/genderqueer or nonbinary/identity not listed). Race and ethnicity were available as mutually exclusive categories, following federal Office of Management and Budget standards.

We calculated incidence rates and incidence rate ratios by HPI quartile and for each STI, and by gender, race, and ethnicity. We calculated incidence by using the cumulative number of STI cases reported from 2013 to 2021, by census tract. A person was included as a case at the point in time when they were diagnosed. A person could be included multiple times if they had multiple, unique, nonrelated STI diagnoses. The years of 2013 to 2021 were selected as the analysis period to increase the depth of a similar analysis conducted during this time period, which described syphilis rates by HPI quartile.[15] The current analysis expands on the previous analysis by including additional STIs (chlamydia and gonorrhea) and by assessing findings by gender, race, and ethnicity. The 2017 American Community Survey 5-year population estimates were aggregated by HPI quartile to obtain the incidence rate per 100 000 persons.[16] We generated the data analysis for this study by using SAS software, version 9.4 (SAS Institute, Cary, NC).[17]

RESULTS

A total of 1 368 744 (80.23%) STI cases were geocoded (of 1 706 039 reported) and included in the analysis (984 812/1 221 050 total [80.65%] chlamydia cases, 295 850/372 809 total [79.36%] gonorrhea cases, 52 576/63 569 total [82.71%] early syphilis cases, and 35 506/48 611 total [73.04%] syphilis of late or unknown duration cases). Most patients reported as cases of gonorrhea (59.24%), early syphilis (80.38%), and syphilis of late or unknown duration (63.10%) were male/transgender male, while most chlamydia cases were reported in females/transgender females (67.57%; Table 1).

A total of 337 295 (19.77% of total) cases (236 238 chlamydia cases, 76 959 gonorrhea cases, 10 993 early syphilis cases, and 13 105 syphilis of late or unknown duration cases) had no address information available or did not geocode to addresses in communities assigned an HPI score. Compared with individuals in areas without an HPI score, those with chlamydia, gonorrhea, and early syphilis assigned an HPI score were significantly younger, while all individuals with bacterial STIs had significantly different distributions of gender, race, and ethnicity ($P < .001$; Table A, available as a supplement to the online version of this article at https://ajph.org).

The distribution of STI cases significantly ($P < .001$) decreased as HPI quartile scores increased for chlamydia (31.97% of individuals resided in the lowest scoring HPI quartile vs 15.38% of individuals in the highest scoring HPI quartile), gonorrhea (33.63% of individuals resided in the lowest scoring HPI quartile vs 15.18% of individuals in the highest scoring HPI quartile), early syphilis (31.93% of individuals resided in the lowest scoring HPI quartile vs 16.89% of individuals in the highest scoring HPI quartile), and syphilis of late or unknown duration (41.55% of individuals resided in the lowest scoring HPI quartile vs 11.00% of individuals in the highest scoring HPI quartile; Table 1).

STI incidence rates were highest in the lowest scoring HPI quartile and lowest in the highest scoring HPI quartile. Residents who lived in areas in the lowest scoring HPI quartile had 2.30 (95% confidence interval [CI] = 2.24, 2.36) times the risk of early syphilis, 2.53 (95% CI = 2.51, 2.54) times the risk of chlamydia, 2.69 (95% CI = 2.66, 2.72) times the risk of gonorrhea, and 4.59 (95% CI = 4.43, 4.76) times the risk of syphilis of late or unknown duration, compared with residents who lived in areas in the highest scoring HPI quartile (Table 2).

Black/African American people who lived in the lowest scoring HPI quartile had the highest bacterial STI incidence rates, while Asian people who lived in the highest scoring HPI quartile had the lowest bacterial STI incidence rates compared with people of other racial and ethnic groups in all other HPI quartiles. When comparing risk within each race and ethnicity group, Asian people who lived in areas in the lowest scoring HPI quartile had 2.36 (95% CI = 2.28, 2.44) times the risk of chlamydia compared with Asian people in the highest

TABLE 1— Demographic Characteristics of Sexually Transmitted Infections Among Geocoded Individuals Who Resided in a Census Tract With a California Healthy Places Index (HPI) Score: California, 2013–2021

Characteristic	Sexually Transmitted Infection, No. (%) or Median (IQR)			
	Chlamydia (n = 984 812)	Gonorrhea (n = 295 850)	Early Syphilis (n = 52 576)	Syphilis of Late or Unknown Duration (n = 35 506)
Age, y	23 (20–29)	27 (22–35)	33 (26–44)	33 (26–43)
Gender				
Male/transgender male	317 786 (32.27)	175 265 (59.24)	42 259 (80.38)	22 406 (63.10)
Female/transgender female	665 426 (67.57)	120 014 (40.57)	10 288 (19.57)	13 070 (36.81)
Other/unknown[a]	1 600 (0.16)	571 (0.19)	29 (0.06)	30 (0.08)
Race/ethnicity				
American Indian or Alaska Native	3 297 (0.33)	1 420 (0.48)	250 (0.48)	155 (0.44)
Asian	35 610 (3.62)	9 324 (3.15)	2 503 (4.76)	1 401 (3.95)
Black or African American	86 159 (8.75)	43 486 (14.70)	5 152 (9.80)	3 605 (10.15)
Hispanic or Latino	240 355 (24.41)	72 404 (24.47)	20 555 (39.10)	15 552 (43.80)
Native Hawaiian and other Pacific Islander	4 180 (0.42)	1 088 (0.37)	236 (0.45)	144 (0.41)
White	159 342 (16.18)	65 332 (22.08)	16 851 (32.05)	7 960 (22.42)
Multiracial	3 426 (0.35)	1 439 (0.49)	495 (0.94)	242 (0.68)
Other	63 555 (6.45)	15 887 (5.37)	1 349 (2.57)	1 104 (3.11)
Unknown	388 888 (39.49)	85 470 (28.89)	5 185 (9.86)	5 343 (15.05)
HPI quartile*				
1 (fewest community opportunities for healthy living)	314 854 (31.97)	99 506 (33.63)	16 787 (31.93)	14 753 (41.55)
2	285 181 (28.96)	84 865 (28.69)	14 879 (28.30)	10 017 (28.21)
3	233 312 (23.69)	66 558 (22.50)	12 028 (22.88)	6 831 (19.24)
4 (most community opportunities for healthy living)	151 465 (15.38)	44 921 (15.18)	8 882 (16.89)	3 905 (11.00)

Note. IQR = interquartile range.
[a]Other/unknown gender includes unknown gender identity, declined to answer, genderqueer or nonbinary, and gender identity not listed.
*$P < .001$ produced using χ^2 test of association.

scoring HPI quartile, while White people who lived in areas in the lowest scoring HPI quartile had 3.06 (95% CI = 2.93, 3.19) times the risk of early syphilis, 3.18 (95% CI = 3.11, 3.26) times the risk of gonorrhea, and 6.55 (95% CI = 6.12, 7.00) times the risk of syphilis of late or unknown duration compared with White people living in the highest scoring HPI quartile, the highest rate ratios compared with all other racial and ethnic groups with those conditions.

Conversely, NHOPI people who lived in the lowest scoring HPI quartile had 0.74 (95% CI = 0.47, 1.16) times the risk of early syphilis, 0.76 (95% CI = 0.69, 0.84) times the risk of chlamydia, 0.92 (95% CI = 0.76, 1.11) times the risk of gonorrhea, and 1.35 (95% CI = 0.79, 2.34) times the risk of syphilis of late or unknown duration compared with NHOPI people living in the highest scoring HPI quartile, the lowest rate ratios compared with all other racial and ethnic groups. AI/AN people who lived in the lowest scoring HPI quartile had nearly an equal risk of chlamydia (1.18; 95% CI = 1.05, 1.34) as AI/AN people who lived in the highest scoring HPI quartile. Hispanic/Latino people who lived in the lowest scoring HPI quartile had nearly an equal risk of early syphilis (1.07; 95% CI = 1.02, 1.12) and gonorrhea (1.22; 95% CI = 1.19, 1.26) as Hispanic/Latino people who lived in the highest scoring HPI quartile (Table 3). When describing risk within each HPI quartile, compared with Asian people (the reference population with the lowest bacterial STI rates), STI risk increased as HPI scores increased for all Black/African American, NHOPI, and Hispanic/Latino people with any bacterial STI; AI/AN people with chlamydia, gonorrhea, and early syphilis; and White people with chlamydia (Table B, available as a supplement to the online version of this article at https://ajph.org).

All bacterial STI rates were highest in the lowest scoring HPI quartile and

TABLE 2— Rates of Sexually Transmitted Infections Among Geocoded Individuals Who Resided in a Census Tract With a California Healthy Places Index (HPI) Score, by HPI Quartile: California, 2013–2021

	HPI Quartile[a]			
Sexually Transmitted Infection	**1**	**2**	**3**	**4**
Chlamydia				
Rate/100 000	5 332.01	4 074.17	3 085.59	2 110.85
RR (95% CI)	2.53 (2.51, 2.54)	1.93 (1.92, 1.94)	1.46 (1.45, 1.47)	1 (Ref)
Gonorrhea				
Rate/100 000	1 685.12	1 212.41	880.24	626.03
RR (95% CI)	2.69 (2.66, 2.72)	1.94 (1.91, 1.96)	1.41 (1.39, 1.42)	1 (Ref)
Early syphilis				
Rate/100 000	284.29	212.57	159.07	123.78
RR (95% CI)	2.30 (2.24, 2.36)	1.71 (1.67, 1.76)	1.29 (1.25, 1.32)	1 (Ref)
Syphilis of late or unknown duration				
Rate/100 000	249.84	143.11	90.34	54.42
RR (95% CI)	4.59 (4.43, 4.76)	2.63 (2.53, 2.73)	1.66 (1.60, 1.73)	1 (Ref)

Note. CI = confidence interval; RR = rate ratio.
[a]Quartiles defined as 1 = fewest community opportunities for healthy living to 4 = most community opportunities for healthy living.

lowest in the highest scoring HPI quartile among both males/transgender males and females/transgender females. Across each HPI quartile, females/transgender females consistently had higher rates of chlamydia compared with males/transgender males, while males/transgender males consistently had higher rates of gonorrhea, early syphilis, and syphilis of late or unknown duration compared with females/transgender females. Compared with female/transgender female residents in the highest scoring HPI quartile, female/transgender female residents in the lowest scoring HPI quartile had 3.20 (95% CI = 3.17, 3.22) times the risk of chlamydia, 4.71 (95% CI = 4.62, 4.80) times the risk of gonorrhea, 8.83 (95% CI = 8.15, 9.53) times the risk of early syphilis, and 9.51 (95% CI = 8.86, 10.21) times the risk of syphilis of late or unknown duration. Compared with male/transgender male residents in the highest scoring HPI quartile, male/transgender male residents in the lowest scoring HPI quartile had 1.63 (95% CI = 1.61, 1.65) times the risk of chlamydia, 1.69 (95% CI = 1.65, 1.74) times the risk of early syphilis, 1.89 (95% CI = 1.86, 1.92) times the risk of gonorrhea, and 3.13 (95% CI = 3.00, 3.26) times the risk of syphilis of late or unknown duration (Table 4).

DISCUSSION

From 2013 to 2021, the cumulative STI incidence in California was lowest in communities where residents had the most community opportunities to lead healthy lives. However, the impact of community opportunities on STI outcomes varied by subpopulation. Not only did changes in the availability of community opportunities differentially impact each racial and ethnic group, but racial and ethnic health disparities, as measured by STI rate ratios between a given racial or ethnic group and the racial or ethnic group with the lowest STI rates (Asian), also were worse as community opportunities became more available among AI/AN, Black/African American, Hispanic/Latino, and NHOPI people (Table B, available as a supplement to the online version of this article at https://ajph.org). This suggests that the presence of community opportunities, as measured by HPI or other social indices, does not benefit all racial and ethnic groups equally, and living in communities with more opportunities to be healthy may not be enough alone to mitigate racial health disparities. Black and Brown populations had the smallest in magnitude reductions in STI risk as community opportunities became more available. This could be a function of the multigenerational effects of structural racism and other programs, practices, and policies that are neither inclusive nor relevant to these communities.

Both males/transgender males and females/transgender females had reduced STI risk as community opportunities were more available; however, females/transgender females had a larger decrease in STI risk as

TABLE 3— Rates of Sexually Transmitted Infections Between Communities With the Most Opportunities for Healthy Living and Fewest Opportunities for Healthy Living Among Geocoded Individuals Who Resided in a Census Tract With a California Healthy Places Index (HPI) Score, by HPI Quartile and Race/Ethnicity: California, 2013–2021

	HPI Quartile,[a] Rate/100 000 or RR (95% CI)				
Sexually Transmitted Infection	**1**	**2**	**3**	**4**	**HPI Quartile 1: HPI Quartile 4**
Chlamydia					
American Indian or Alaska Native	2 873.53	2 932.16	3 322.93	2 429.49	1.18 (1.05, 1.34)
Asian	1 654.51	1 187.11	997.01	701.67	2.36 (2.28, 2.44)
Black or African American	8 626.90	6 701.21	5 858.24	4 773.23	1.81 (1.77, 1.85)
Hispanic or Latino	2 762.57	2 405.90	2 086.58	1 869.56	1.48 (1.46, 1.50)
Native Hawaiian and other Pacific Islander	3 381.67	3 590.89	3 976.42	4 450.20	0.76 (0.69, 0.84)
White	2 213.59	1 613.93	1 333.67	988.66	2.24 (2.21, 2.27)
Gonorrhea					
American Indian or Alaska Native	1 555.53	1 139.97	1 152.93	1 117.01	1.39 (1.17, 1.67)
Asian	410.03	335.07	246.30	188.37	2.18 (2.04, 2.32)
Black or African American	4 773.82	3 274.27	2 654.02	2 336.53	2.04 (1.98, 2.11)
Hispanic or Latino	812.26	707.79	638.88	664.60	1.22 (1.19, 1.26)
Native Hawaiian and other Pacific Islander	997.15	932.37	1 009.62	1 088.57	0.92 (0.76, 1.11)
White	1 159.79	686.66	482.04	364.34	3.18 (3.11, 3.26)
Early syphilis					
American Indian or Alaska Native	249.12	264.79	165.23	167.55	1.49 (0.94, 2.45)
Asian	106.40	103.06	66.52	44.83	2.37 (2.08, 2.70)
Black or African American	559.72	371.47	305.97	338.61	1.65 (1.51, 1.81)
Hispanic or Latino	223.70	199.51	185.13	209.83	1.07 (1.02, 1.12)
Native Hawaiian and other Pacific Islander	173.42	179.54	265.09	234.98	0.74 (0.47, 1.16)
White	299.39	175.31	120.95	97.93	3.06 (2.93, 3.19)
Syphilis of late or unknown duration					
American Indian or Alaska Native	205.67	158.87	73.43	48.87	4.21 (1.94, 10.85)
Asian	77.60	53.49	36.82	23.29	3.33 (2.83, 3.92)
Black or African American	444.60	256.52	199.66	163.32	2.72 (2.41, 3.09)
Hispanic or Latino	207.06	143.95	113.23	101.48	2.04 (1.91, 2.18)
Native Hawaiian and other Pacific Islander	168.60	141.75	107.17	124.68	1.35 (0.79, 2.34)
White	202.21	85.64	50.01	30.89	6.55 (6.12, 7.00)

Note. CI = confidence interval; RR = rate ratio.
[a]Quartiles defined as 1 = fewest community opportunities for healthy living to 4 = most community opportunities for healthy living.

community opportunities became more available compared with males/transgender males. This difference is perhaps reflective of gender differences in health care–seeking behaviors; regular engagement in prenatal care (and subsequent STI screening), especially among those who live in areas with more community opportunities for healthy living; and higher STI rates among different demographics of males/transgender males living in both high and low scoring HPI quartiles, such as men who have sexual contact with other men.

Findings from this work are consistent with similar studies that described the effects of SDoH on syphilis risk. Though overall rate ratios were similar between this work and previous work that used the HPI to characterize syphilis morbidity, we highlight large risk differences between people of different genders, races, and ethnicities.[15] Our findings that SDoH differentially impact people of different racial and ethnic identities were consistent with

TABLE 4— Rates of Sexually Transmitted Infections Between Communities With the Most Opportunities for Healthy Living and Fewest Opportunities for Healthy Living Among Geocoded Individuals Who Resided in a Census Tract With a California Healthy Places Index (HPI) Score, by HPI Quartile and Gender: California, 2013–2021

	HPI Quartile,[a] Rate/100 000 or RR (95% CI)				
Sexually Transmitted Infection	**1**	**2**	**3**	**4**	**HPI Quartile 1: HPI Quartile 4**
Chlamydia					
Male/transgender male	2878.33	2556.37	2183.00	1765.01	1.63 (1.61, 1.65)
Female/transgender female	7797.89	5552.15	3953.76	2438.68	3.20 (3.17, 3.22)
Gonorrhea					
Male/transgender male	1719.52	1436.85	1134.03	909.57	1.89 (1.86, 1.92)
Female/transgender female	1644.32	987.50	630.10	349.18	4.71 (4.62, 4.80)
Early syphilis					
Male/transgender male	391.35	348.32	279.07	231.10	1.69 (1.65, 1.74)
Female/transgender female	175.71	79.08	42.05	19.94	8.83 (8.15, 9.53)
Syphilis of late or unknown duration					
Male/transgender male	267.16	188.38	132.10	85.38	3.13 (3.00, 3.26)
Female/transgender female	232.06	98.34	49.51	24.41	9.51 (8.86, 10.21)

Note. CI = confidence interval; RR = rate ratio.
[a]Quartiles defined as 1 = fewest community opportunities for healthy living to 4 = most community opportunities for healthy living.

findings from a scoping review focused on adolescents, which described how SDoH, such as economic stability, social contexts, and the built environment, had differential impacts on health and education outcomes by race, ethnicity, and gender.[8] Other work described how SDoH differentially impacted mental health outcomes of Black and White populations and other health outcomes between people of different gender identities and sexual orientations.[18] While limited studies exist on how SDoH have differentially impacted sexual health outcomes in different populations, sexual health efforts in California routinely utilize SDoH to inform prevention efforts, respond to STI disparities, and reduce discrimination and stigmatization.

The use of public health surveillance data to understand the effects of SDoH on STI incidence can identify populations with high STI morbidity and limited access to community resources, and support systemic changes that identify and eliminate structural drivers of racism. Furthermore, by incorporating race and ethnicity into routine analyses, opportunities for racial health equity are more directly centered in public health activities and enable interventions to reduce and prevent racial health disparities. In California, structured public health interventions, policy updates, syndemic approaches to sexual health, and systemic prevention efforts have directly resulted from the identification of structural drivers of population-specific health disparities. Expanded syphilis screening recommendations in California include all sexually active persons aged 15 to 44 years, regardless of gender identity or sexual orientation, a structural-level intervention that can reduce disparities and stigmatization.[19] Routine STI screening guidelines among people living with HIV or using doxycycline postexposure prophylaxis (doxyPEP) for STI prevention or preexposure prophylaxis for HIV prevention were also developed (in part) in response to inequities in STI and HIV burden among men who have sex with men.[20] Expanded emergency department syphilis screening guidelines were designed to reach underserved populations and respond to the growing congenital syphilis crisis.[21] Policy reformations through the 340B Drug Discount Program expanded access to Bicillin (penicillin G benzathine injectable suspension), enabling treatment to many underserved populations.[22] The California Department of Public Health's statewide strategic plan to address HIV, hepatitis C virus, and STIs intentionally centered equity and racial justice to mitigate and prevent racial health disparities.[23] Future work can more directly explore how equity-focused interventions that extend beyond the community mitigate health disparities and quantify the impacts of interventions on STI burden using causal inference methodology. Incorporating SDoH into public health prevention activities enables improvements to the communities in which people live and ultimately yield more equitable health outcomes.

Limitations

There were several limitations to this study. First, around 19.8% of STI cases had missing addresses; were geocoded to a provider, military, or correctional facility; or were geocoded to census tracts not assigned an HPI score (Table C, available as a supplement to the online version of this article at https://ajph.org). These excluded cases were significantly different than cases that did geocode to tracts with an HPI score. Among people with chlamydia, gonorrhea, and early syphilis, the excluded population was significantly older, and there were significantly different distributions of gender and race and ethnicity between excluded and included persons ($P < .001$; Table A). However, given that the population without a geocoded residential address may reflect more adverse conditions (e.g., unstable or temporary housing, intermittent and variable access to medical care, incarceration), and we would expect this population to have a higher STI risk, this would be a conservative bias and underestimate the magnitude of disparities. This, however, assumes that all of these excluded people would have ended up residing in lower HPI census tracts, which is not assured, so the true impact of this exclusion bias cannot be assessed (Table A).

Second, neighborhood composition and boundaries were defined using census tracts. While neighborhood-based work presumes tracts as distinguishable areas, actual neighborhoods may encompass several census tracts.[24] Artificial geographic boundaries can change and therefore are subject to providing inaccurate findings, further subject to the modifiable areal unit problem.[25] Third, place-based research is subject to the ecological fallacy such that inferences could be made about an individual based on their respective HPI quartile of residence.[26,27] Fourth, limiting cases to those with a single home address does not account for mobile populations and may not include the full extent of a person's daily activities or account for time spent in other communities.[28,29]

Finally, to capture the extent to which racial health disparities exist, it is imperative to accurately capture an individual's racial and ethnic identity. California STI surveillance bases its reporting of race and ethnicity on guidelines from the federal Office of Management and Budget (i.e., as singular, mutually exclusive groups). These guidelines result in racial misclassification and chronic underreporting of disease burden in different racial and ethnic groups as people who identify as more than 1 race or ethnicity are often not included in surveillance reporting, thus potentially undercounting the magnitude in which racial and ethnic disparities exist.[30] Future work addressing racial health disparities could consider the effect of mutually exclusive race and ethnicity reporting categories on underreporting, and incorporate non–mutually exclusive race and ethnicity groups into the analysis.

Public Health Implications

This research adds to the growing body of STI racial and health equity literature by describing how people of different racial and ethnic groups are differentially impacted by the community conditions in which they live. In California, policy changes designed with equity in mind have enabled greater access to STI medication, development of screening guidelines to prevent health disparities and adverse health outcomes, opt-out emergency department testing and empiric treatment, early recommendations for doxyPEP, and utilization of evidence-based models to address SDoH critical for optimal sexual health.[20–23,31] Findings from this work can be used to prioritize STI prevention efforts among populations at greater risk for STIs, help to understand barriers and solutions within communities, and strategize additional ways of reducing health disparities among populations with a disproportionate STI burden. AJPH

ABOUT THE AUTHORS

Esther E. Gotlieb, Nicole O. Burghardt, Jiawen Hu, Kathleen Jacobson, and Robert E. Snyder are with the Sexually Transmitted Diseases Control Branch, Division of Communicable Disease Control, Center for Infectious Diseases, California Department of Public Health, Richmond and Sacramento, CA.

Note. The findings and conclusions in this article are those of the authors and do not necessarily represent the views or opinions of the California Department of Public Health or the California Health and Human Services Agency.

CORRESPONDENCE

Correspondence should be sent to Esther E. Gotlieb, 850 Marina Bay Parkway, Building P, 2nd Floor, Richmond, CA 94804-6403 (e-mail: esther.gotlieb@cdph.ca.gov). Reprints can be ordered at https://www.ajph.org by clicking the "Reprints" link.

PUBLICATION INFORMATION

Full Citation: Gotlieb EE, Burghardt NO, Hu J, et al. Sexually transmitted infection disparities and social determinants of health in California, 2013–2021. *Am J Public Health*. 2025;115(5): 799–807.

Acceptance Date: November 27, 2024.

DOI: https://doi.org/10.2105/AJPH.2024.307963

ORCID iDs:
Esther E. Gotlieb https://orcid.org/0009-0002-3458-0456

Nicole O. Burghardt https://orcid.org/0000-0002-4278-0821

Kathleen Jacobson https://orcid.org/0000-0002-4988-2329

Robert E. Snyder https://orcid.org/0000-0001-9743-0872

CONTRIBUTORS

E. E. Gotlieb wrote the article with support from N. O. Burghardt, J. Hu, K. Jacobson, and R. E. Snyder. E. E. Gotlieb performed the analysis. J. Hu prepared the data. R. E. Snyder conceptualized and designed the analysis. N. O. Burghardt and R. E. Snyder supervised this work.

CONFLICTS OF INTEREST

The authors have no conflicts of interest to disclose.

HUMAN PARTICIPANT PROTECTION

Analysis of public health surveillance data is a routine public health activity. This project (2024-097) was reviewed by the California Health and Human Services Committee for the Protection of Human Subjects and was considered "Not Research or Exempt."

REFERENCES

1. California Department of Public Health. Sexually Transmitted Diseases Control Branch Data. 2023. Available at: https://www.cdph.ca.gov/Programs/CID/DCDC/Pages/STD-Data.aspx. Accessed April 3, 2023.
2. Centers for Disease Control and Prevention. Social Determinants of Health (SDOH). 2024. Available at: https://www.cdc.gov/about/priorities/why-is-addressing-sdoh-important.html?CDC_AAref_Val=https://www.cdc.gov/about/sdoh/index.html. Accessed February 19, 2025.
3. Swope CB, Hernández D. Housing as a determinant of health equity: a conceptual model. *Soc Sci Med.* 2019;243:112571. https://doi.org/10.1016/j.socscimed.2019.112571
4. Hogben M, Leichliter JS. Social determinants and sexually transmitted disease disparities. *Sex Transm Dis.* 2008;35(12):S13–S18. https://doi.org/10.1097/OLQ.0b013e31818d3cad
5. Bailey ZD, Krieger N, Agénor M, Graves J, Linos N, Bassett MT. Structural racism and health inequities in the USA: evidence and interventions. *Lancet.* 2017;389(10077):1453–1463. https://doi.org/10.1016/S0140-6736(17)30569-X
6. Egede LE, Walker RJ, Williams JS. Addressing structural inequalities, structural racism, and social determinants of health: a vision for the future. *J Gen Intern Med.* 2024;39(3):487–491. https://doi.org/10.1007/s11606-023-08426-7
7. Lipshutz JA, Hall JE, Penman-Aguilar A, Skillen E, Naoom S, Irune I. Leveraging social and structural determinants of health at the Centers for Disease Control and Prevention: a systems-level opportunity to improve public health. *J Public Health Manag Pract.* 2022;28(2):E380–E389. https://doi.org/10.1097/PHH.0000000000001363
8. Monroe P, Campbell JA, Harris M, Egede LE. Racial/ethnic differences in social determinants of health and health outcomes among adolescents and youth ages 10–24 years old: a scoping review. *BMC Public Health.* 2023;23(1):410. https://doi.org/10.1186/s12889-023-15274-x
9. Johnson Lyons S, Gant Z, Jin C, Dailey A, Nwangwu-Ike N, Satcher Johnson A. A census tract-level examination of differences in social determinants of health among people with HIV, by race/ethnicity and geography, United States and Puerto Rico, 2017. *Public Health Rep.* 2022;137(2):278–290. https://doi.org/10.1177/0033354921990373
10. Public Health Alliance of Southern California. HPI Into Action. 2022. Available at: https://www.healthyplacesindex.org/hpi-into-action. Accessed June 12, 2024.
11. Public Health Alliance of Southern California. California Healthy Places Index 3.0. 2022. Available at: https://healthyplacesindex.org. Accessed March 9, 2023.
12. Maizlish N, Delaney T, Dowling H, et al. California Healthy Places Index: frames matter. *Public Health Rep.* 2019;134(4):354–362. https://doi.org/10.1177/0033354919849882
13. Public Health Alliance of Southern California. Healthy Places Index Guidance. 2023. Available at: https://phasocal.org/wp-content/uploads/2023/06/PHA_HPI_Guidance_Report523_4.pdf. Accessed September 30, 2024.
14. ArcGIS Mapping Software, version 10.7.1. Redlands, CA: Environmental Systems Research Institute; 2019.
15. Johnson KA, Snyder RE, Tang EC, et al. Geospatial social determinants of health correlate with disparities in syphilis and congenital syphilis cases in California. *Pathogens.* 2022;11(5):547. https://doi.org/10.3390/pathogens11050547
16. US Census Bureau. Selected characteristics, 2013–2017 American Community Survey 5-year estimates. 2018. Available at: https://data.census.gov. Accessed October 3, 2024.
17. SAS version 9.4. Cary, NC: SAS Institute Inc; 2016.
18. Kammer-Kerwick M, Cox K, Purohit I, Watkins SC. The role of social determinants of health and social position in mental health: an examination of the moderating effects of race, ethnicity, and gender on depression through the All of Us dataset. Preprint. Posted online November 16, 2023. medRxiv. 23298593. https://doi.org/10.1101/2023.11.16.23298593
19. California Department of Public Health. California Department of Public Health (CDPH) updates syphilis screening recommendations. 2024. Available at: https://www.cdph.ca.gov/Programs/OPA/Pages/CAHAN/CDPH-Updates-Syphilis-Screening-Recommendations.aspx. Accessed October 15, 2024.
20. California Department of Public Health. California sexually transmitted infections (STI) screening recommendations. 2022. Available at: https://www.cdph.ca.gov/Programs/CID/DCDC/Pages/California-STI-Screening-Recommendations.aspx. Accessed October 15, 2024.
21. California Department of Public Health. Implementation guide: Screening for HIV, hepatitis C, and syphilis in emergency departments. 2025. Available at: https://www.cdph.ca.gov/Programs/CID/DCDC/Pages/STI/Implementation-Guides/Emergency-Departments.aspx. Accessed February 20, 2025.
22. Department of Health and Human Services. 340B Drug Pricing Program; Administrative Dispute Resolution. RIN 0906–AB28. 2022;(73516):11. Available at: https://www.govinfo.gov/content/pkg/FR-2022-11-30/pdf/2022-25752.pdf. Accessed September 3, 2024.
23. Office of AIDS and STD Control Branch. Ending the epidemics: addressing human immunodeficiency virus (HIV), hepatitis C virus (HCV), and sexually transmitted infections (STIs) in California. *Integrated Statewide Strategic Plan Overview 2022–2026.* 2021:12. Available at: https://www.cdph.ca.gov/programs/cid/doa/cdph%20document%20library/cdph_stratplan2021_final_ada.pdf. Accessed September 3, 2024.
24. Logan JR. Relying on the census in urban social science. *City Community.* 2018;17(3):540–549. https://doi.org/10.1111/cico.12331
25. Delmelle EM, Desjardins MR, Jung P, et al. Uncertainty in geospatial health: challenges and opportunities ahead. *Ann Epidemiol.* 2022;65:15–30. https://doi.org/10.1016/j.annepidem.2021.10.002
26. Gottlieb LM, Francis DE, Beck AF. Uses and misuses of patient- and neighborhood-level social determinants of health data. *Perm J.* 2018;22(4 suppl):18-078. https://doi.org/10.7812/TPP/18-078
27. Shih YT, Bradley C, Yabroff KR. Ecological and individualistic fallacies in health disparities research. *J Natl Cancer Inst.* 2023;115(5):488–491. https://doi.org/10.1093/jnci/djad047
28. Sheehan CM, Gotlieb EE, Ayers SL, et al. Neighborhood conditions and type 2 diabetes risk among Latino adolescents with obesity in Phoenix. *Int J Environ Res Public Health.* 2022;19(13):7920. https://doi.org/10.3390/ijerph19137920
29. Kwan M-P. From place-based to people-based exposure measures. *Soc Sci Med.* 2009;69(9):1311–1313. https://doi.org/10.1016/j.socscimed.2009.07.013
30. Agency for Healthcare Research and Quality. 3. Defining categorization needs for race and ethnicity data. In: *Race, Ethnicity, and Language Data: Standardization for Health Care Quality Improvement.* 2018. Available at: https://www.ahrq.gov/research/findings/final-reports/iomracereport/reldata3.html. Accessed August 21, 2024.
31. California Department of Public Health. Doxycycline post-exposure prophylaxis (doxy-PEP) for the prevention of bacterial sexually transmitted infections (STIs). 2023. Available at: https://www.cdph.ca.gov/Programs/CID/DCDC/CDPH%20Document%20Library/CDPH-Doxy-PEP-Recommendations-for-Prevention-of-STIs.pdf. Accessed August 29, 2024.